CONTEMPORARY HEMATOLOGY

Judith E. Karp, M.D., Series Editor

For further volumes:
http://www.springer.com/series/7681

Elihu H. Estey · Frederick R. Appelbaum
Editors

Leukemia and Related Disorders

Integrated Treatment Approaches

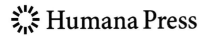 Humana Press

Editors

Elihu H. Estey, M.D.
Professor of Medicine
Division of Hematology
University of Washington
School of Medicine
Member, Fred Hutchinson Cancer Research Center
Attending Physician, Seattle Cancer Care Alliance
Seattle, WA USA

Frederick R. Appelbaum, M.D.
Professor of Medicine
Head, Division of Oncology
Director, Clinical Research Division Fred Hutchinson Cancer Research Center
Executive Director, Seattle Cancer Care Alliance
University of Washington
School of Medicine
Seattle, WA USA

ISBN 978-1-60761-564-4   e-ISBN 978-1-60761-565-1
DOI 10.1007/978-1-60761-565-1
Springer New York Dordrecht Heidelberg London

Library of Congress Control Number: 2011944980

Printed on acid-free paper

Humana Press is part of Springer Science+Business Media (www.springer.com)

Preface

There is no shortage of multiauthored books describing management of acute and chronic leukemias and myelodysplastic syndromes. However, we believe that this book has several distinctive features. All the authors are members of a single academic center. While the authors' views on treatment approaches necessarily differ, the book's single-center nature will hopefully provide the reader with a relatively unified approach to management. This theme is furthered by the inclusion of three chapters on the role of allogeneic transplant, befitting the Fred Hutchinson Cancer Research Center's long history of leadership in this discipline. There are both chapters on supportive care and on long-term complications of successful treatment, another long-standing interest of the center. The authors' expertise has prompted the editors to give them wide latitude in writing the chapters. In general, the chapters combine a thorough review of the literature and their own perspectives. The editors are confident that the chapters are uniformly excellent and informative.

The focus of this book is clinical. The intended audience is thus all physicians treating patients with acute or chronic leukemias or myelodysplasia. The many questions the authors receive from community oncologists suggest that this audience is large.

Seattle, WA, USA   Elihu H. Estey
Seattle, WA, USA   Frederick R. Appelbaum

Acknowledgment

The editors appreciate the authors' expertise and hard work, which made this book possible.

Contents

Contributors

K. Scott Baker, M.D., M.S. Department of Pediatrics, University of Washington School of Medicine, Seattle, WA, USA

Clinical Research Division, Fred Hutchinson Cancer Research Center, Seattle, WA, USA

Michael Boeckh, M.D. Vaccine and Infectious Diseases and Clinical Research Divisions, Fred Hutchinson Cancer Research Center, Seattle, WA, USA

Allergy and Infectious Diseases Division, University of Washington School of Medicine, Seattle, WA, USA

Andrew Coveler, M.D. Division of Medical Oncology, Department of Medicine, University of Washington School of Medicine, Seattle, WA, USA

Clinical Research Division, Fred Hutchinson Cancer Research Center, Seattle, WA, USA

Colleen Delaney, M.D., M.Sc. Department of Pediatrics, University of Washington School of Medicine, Seattle, WA, USA

Clinical Research Division, Fred Hutchinson Cancer Research Center, Seattle, WA, USA

Meghan Delaney, DO, PMH Department of Laboratory Medicine, Assistant Medical Director, Puget Sound Blood Center, Seattle, WA, USA

Elihu H. Estey, M.D. Division of Hematology, University of Washington School of Medicine, Seattle, WA, USA

Member, Fred Hutchinson Cancer Research Center, Seattle, WA, USA

Attending Physician, Seattle Cancer Care Alliance, Seattle, WA, USA

Terry B. Gernsheimer, M.D. Division of Hematology, Department of Medicine, University of Washington School of Medicine, Seattle, WA, USA

Transfusion Services, Seattle Cancer Care Alliance, Seattle, WA, USA

Puget Sound Blood Center, Seattle, WA, USA

Jonathan A. Gutman, M.D. Department of Medical Oncology, University of Colorado School of Medicine, Aurora, CO, USA

Paul J. Martin, M.D. Clinical Research Division, Fred Hutchinson Cancer Research Center, Seattle, WA, USA

Debra K. Mattson, PA-C Vaccine and Infectious Diseases and Clinical Research Divisions, Fred Hutchinson Cancer Research Center, Seattle, WA, USA

Laura F. Newell, M.D. Division of Hematology, Department of Medicine, University of Washington School of Medicine, Seattle, WA, USA

Vivian G. Oehler, M.D. Clinical Research Division, Fred Hutchinson Cancer Research Center, Seattle, WA, USA

Division of Hematology, Department of Medicine, University of Washington School of Medicine, Seattle, WA, USA

John M. Pagel, M.D., Ph.D. Associate Professor, Department of Medicine, University of Washington School of Medicine, Seattle, WA, USA

Associate Fred Hutchinson Cancer Research Center, Seattle, WA, USA

Steven A. Pergam, M.D., MPH Vaccine and Infectious Diseases and Clinical Research Divisions, Fred Hutchinson Cancer Research Center, Seattle, WA, USA

Allergy and Infectious Diseases Division, University of Washington School of Medicine, Seattle, WA, USA

Jerald P. Radich, M.D. Clinical Research Division, Fred Hutchinson Cancer Research Center, Seattle, WA, USA

Department of Clinical Research and Oncology, University of Washington School of Medicine, Seattle, WA, USA

Gunnar Bjarni Ragnarsson, M.Sc., M.D. Department of Clinical Research, University of Washington Medical Center, Seattle, WA, USA

Clinical Research Division, Fred Hutchinson Cancer Research Center, Seattle, WA, USA

Emily Jo Rajotte, M.S., M.P.H. Survivorship, Program Manager, Clinical Research Division, Fred Hutchinson Cancer Research Center, Seattle, WA, USA

Aravind Ramakrishnan, M.D. Department of Medicine, University of Washington School of Medicine, Seattle, WA, USA

Clinical Research Division, Fred Hutchinson Cancer Research Center, Seattle, WA, USA

Brenda M. Sandmaier, M.D. Department of Medicine, University of Washington School of Medicine, Seattle, WA, USA

Clinical Research Division, Fred Hutchinson Cancer Research Center, Seattle, WA, USA

Bart Lee Scott, M.D. Clinical Research Division, Fred Hutchinson Cancer Research Center, Seattle, WA, USA

Department of Medicine, University of Washington Medical Center, Seattle, WA, USA

Andrei R. Shustov, M.D. Division of Hematology, University of Washington School of Medicine, Seattle, WA, USA

Kelly M. Smith, M.D. Divisions of Hematology and Oncology, University of Washington School of Medicine, Seattle, WA, USA

Brent L. Wood, M.D., Ph.D. Department of Laboratory Medicine, University of Washington Medical Center, Seattle, WA, USA

Frederick R. Appelbaum, M.D. Professor of Medicine Head, Division of Oncology Director, Clinical Research Division Fred Hutchinson Cancer Research Center, Executive Director, Seattle Cancer Care Alliance, University of Washington, School of Medicine, Seattle, WA, USA

Chapter 1
Acute Myeloid Leukemia (AML)

Elihu H. Estey

Abstract The diagnosis of AML rests on demonstration that the marrow contains > 20% blasts of myeloid lineage. The overarching therapeutic decision is whether the patient should receive standard or investigational therapy. Appreciation of prognostic factors predicting response to the former is fundamental to this decision. These factors include those associated with early death (for example performance status) and with resistance (for example cytogenetics and various genetic markers). The latter is the principal cause of therapeutic failure even in fit patients in their 70s. Here we review pre- and post-treatment prognostic factors and discuss various new therapeutic options.

Keywords AML • Immature myeloid cells • Blasts • Bone marrow failure • Anemia • Neutropenia • Infection • Leukemia

Introduction

The fundamental lesion in acute myeloid leukemia (AML) is the accumulation of abnormal immature myeloid cells ("blasts") that are defective in their ability to differentiate into mature progeny. The result is bone marrow failure, although the degree of such failure does not correlate with the amount of accumulation as measured by marrow or blood blast counts. The most common symptom of marrow

E.H. Estey, M.D. (✉)
Division of Hematology, University of Washington School of Medicine,
825 Eastlake Ave E, 98109 Seattle, WA, USA

Member, Fred Hutchinson Cancer Research Center, Seattle, WA, USA

Attending Physician, Seattle Cancer Care Alliance, Seattle, WA, USA
e-mail: eestey@seattlecca.org

E.H. Estey and F.R. Appelbaum (eds.), *Leukemia and Related Disorders:*
Integrated Treatment Approaches, Contemporary Hematology,
DOI 10.1007/978-1-60761-565-1_1, © Springer Science+Business Media, LLC 2012

failure is anemia, which typically leads patients to seek medical attention, while neutropenia-associated infection is the most common cause of death. Unlike their normal counterparts, AML blasts can escape into the circulation and infiltrate organs, most notably the lungs and brain, also leading to death. Patients are at high risk of infiltration if they present with high WBC counts, and such patients are those in whom immediate treatment is imperative.

Epidemiology

Aside from a relatively high incidence in infancy, AML is a disease of aging [1]. The median age at diagnosis is approximately 70. The most common known causes of AML are exposure to cytotoxic chemotherapy given for other conditions (therapy-related AML), or an antecedent hematologic disorder (AHD) predisposing to AML. Collectively, patients with therapy-related AML or an AHD are said to have "secondary AML." Secondary AML may comprise up to 30–40% of cases in older patients. The most common AHDs are myelodysplastic syndromes. Myeloproliferative neoplasms (MPN) are less frequent, with myelofibrosis the most common MPN leading to AML and essential thrombocytosis the least common.

Therapy-related AML (t-AML) generally assumes one of two forms [2]. The most usual occurs 5–10 years after exposure to alkylating agents. It is frequently accompanied by monosomies of chromosomes 5 and/or 7 (−5, −7) or deletions of the long arms ("q") of these chromosomes (del 5q, del 7q). The second type of t-AML usually occurs within 5 years of exposure to drugs that interact with the enzyme DNA topoisomerase II. Anthracyclines or etoposide are examples. Here the most common cytogenetic abnormalities are deletions of the long arm of chromosome 11 (del 11q), a pericentric inversion of chromosome 16 (inv 16), and balanced translocations between chromosomes 15 and 17 [t (15; 17)] and between chromosomes 8 and 21 [t (8; 21)].

The incidence of spontaneously arising ("de novo") AML characterized by −5/−7 increases with age, while the incidence of de novo balanced translocation AML does not. These observations suggest that AML in older patients reflects life-long exposure to various environmental carcinogens whose effects are similar to those of alkylating agents. Most of these carcinogens are probably unknown. The chief known culprit is benzene, a principal component of cigarettes.

Pathogenesis

By analogy to cigarettes and lung cancer, the great majority of people who are exposed to carcinogens probably never develop AML. Rather development of AML likely results from interplay between exposure and genetic predisposition, as exemplified by genetic variations (polymorphisms) in enzymes that detoxify benzene and other carcinogens. Polymorphisms are readily assessed in lymphocytes. A single

$609C \rightarrow T$ substitution in the enzyme NAD(P)H:quinone oxidoreductase 1 (NQO1) lowers enzyme activity. If both alleles are mutant, enzyme activity is absent. Studying 45 patients with either therapy-related or de novo AML and $-5/-7$, Larson et al. found that the frequencies of NQO1 heterozygotes and homozygotes were much higher than expected ($p = 0.002$) based on the patients' ethnic distribution [3]. The list of such predisposing polymorphisms is likely to grow and interactions likely to be complex, for example, with predisposition limited by gender or by type of exposure and limited to certain types of AML [4]. For example, an allelic variant of CYP1A1*2B, a member of the cytochrome P450 family, is 16-fold more common in patients with $-5/-7$ and RAS mutations than in other patients with AML [5]. Nonetheless, if a patient about to receive chemotherapy for a solid tumor has a polymorphism predictive of a particularly high risk of developing t-AML, therapy might be changed to one less associated with t-AML, assuming that the risk entailed in this alteration is less than the risk of developing AML.

A crucial question is how carcinogens produce AML blasts. Of particular relevance are differences between abnormal and normal blasts since development of "targeted" therapy is impossible absent such knowledge. The development of "deep sequencing" technology has permitted delineation of the complete DNA sequence of AML genomes. One such effort revealed 750 acquired ("somatic") mutations in a patient with AML, a normal karyotype (NK), and no submicroscopic genomic amplifications or deletions [6]. However, only 64 mutations were located in conserved regions of the genome and thus hypothesized to potentially be involved in pathogenesis. Twelve of the 64 mutations affected genes that code for proteins, but only 7 mutations were predicted to affect protein function, thus plausibly constituting "driver" mutations, a number consistent with previous thoughts on the number of mutations needed to convert a normal cell into a cancer cell [7]. However, it is possible that some of the 52 mutations occurring in noncoding but conserved, and hence perhaps important regulatory, regions were also driver mutations. Furthermore, only 4 of the 64 mutations occurred in at least 1 of 188 NK AML samples that were analyzed specifically for these mutations. Similarly, 8 of the 10 somatic mutations found by deep sequencing another NK patient's genome were previously unknown [8]. Obviously, developing targeted therapies will be more cumbersome if, as these results suggest, there is common little thread in AML genomes. The rapidly increasing ease and rapidly decreasing costs of deep sequencing should provide further insight into this issue.

Adding further complexity is the influence of epigenetic and microRNA (miRNA) dysregulation on gene expression. Current dogma holds that hypermethylation of CpG rich promoter regions of the genome leads to decreased expression of the relevant genes. Figueroa et al. used genome-wise promoter DNA methylation profiling to cluster 344 AML patients into 16 groups, 5 of which had no other distinguishing characteristics, such as mutations in the FLT3 or NPM1 genes [9] (see below); whether the same would apply had deep sequencing been done remains to be seen. The potential interplay between genome and epigenome is illustrated by the observation that mutations in IDH genes in AML, originally discovered via deep sequencing, are associated with a specific hypermethylation signature presumably leading to impaired hematopoietic differentiation [10].

MiRNAs are noncoding RNAs that bind to target messenger RNAs (mRNA), thus inhibiting translation of the RNAs into protein. Characterizing the "microRNAome" of an NK patient, Ramsingh et al. reported a somatic mutation in a gene affecting miRNA binding to mRNA and showed that this alteration resulted in translational repression [11]. No similar mutations were identified in 187 other NK patients.

Which normal hematopoietic cells are affected by these molecular events? Normal hematopoiesis is organized hierarchically such that stem cells are capable of restoring hematopoiesis while their mature progeny, which comprise >99.99% of hematopoietic cells, are not. AML hematopoiesis has been thought similarly organized, with the disease originating in leukemia stem cells (LSC) and being passed on to their differentiated progeny [12]. An alternative hypothesis holds that AML in some cases begins in differentiated cells that acquire stemlike properties. Either scenario implies that cure of AML is impossible, although temporary remissions may occur, unless the AML stem cell is incapacitated. However, LSC are thought to be relatively quiescent and hence less susceptible to chemotherapy than more differentiated cells. Direct proof of this hypothesis is difficult given the difficulty in isolating large numbers of LSC. However, indirect support comes from observations of shorter survival, event-free survival, and relapse-free survival in patients with high expression of a gene signature characteristic of LSC [13]. These findings will likely further encourage development of therapies that may be specifically effective against stem cells.

The hypothesis that AML blasts express different antigens than normal blasts dates back to at least the 1970s; a corollary is that development of AML represents a failure of the immune system to control the transformed cells that lead to clinical AML. The increased frequency of AML in patients receiving immunosuppressive therapies such as azathioprine is consistent with this hypothesis. Perhaps the best support for the hypothesis is the demonstration of a graft-versus-leukemia effect following infusion of T-lymphocytes from normal donors in an attempt to treat relapse after allogeneic hematopoietic cell transplantation (HCT) [14]. The (limited) efficacy of such donor lymphocyte infusions (DLI) has prompted more sophisticated approaches to immunotherapy of AML, some of which are noted below.

Diagnosis

Diagnosis of AML is usually not difficult, requiring demonstration of an excess number of myeloid blasts in blood or marrow. In a minority of cases, the presence of Auer rods establishes the blasts as myeloid in origin. However, multicolor flow cytometry (MFC) is the principal means used for this purpose. Surface antigens detected by MFC and accepted as "myeloid" include CD33, CD13, CD117 (CKIT), CD14, CD64 (these last two detecting blasts of monocytic origin), CD41, and glycophorin A (which respectively detect megakaryoblasts and erythroblasts).

Special cases are those where MFC shows blasts with each expressing both myeloid and lymphoid markers (mixed phenotypic acute leukemia, MPAL) or, even less frequently, a mixture of myeloblasts and lymphoblast. Criteria for MPAL differ [15, 16] as have treatments given patients with this diagnosis, thus complicating analyses. Some believe that MPAL does worse than either AML or ALL [17], while others attribute this to an association with unfavorable prognostic features, such as cytogenetics [18], and still others suggest treating such patients with ALL rather than AML regimens [19].

Excess blasts formerly meant >30% (FAB criteria) [20], but currently >20% suffices [World Health Organization (WHO) criteria] [16]. A formal diagnosis of AML can be made despite the presence of <20% blasts when (a) the marrow contains >50% erythroid cells (glycophorin A positive)(FAB type M6) or if >30% of the nonerythroid cells are myeloblasts, (b) the marrow contains >80% monocytes (CD14 or CD64 positive) (FAB type M5b), or (c) the marrow cannot be aspirated, but biopsy or touch preps show immature CD41 positive cells; here the diagnosis is megakaryoblastic leukemia (FAB type M7) with the difficulty in aspiration a result of fibrosis consequent to release of molecules such as platelet-derived growth factor (PDGF) by megakaryoblasts.

Lysis of red cells is done prior to MFC. Because the total number of cells evaluated with MFC (the denominator) is thus reduced relative to the number of blasts (the numerator), the blast% enumerated by MFC is often somewhat greater than that enumerated by morphology. Although it will be interesting to determine whether cases with an unusually large discordance between MFC and morphology (or where the blast% is higher with morphology) have distinctive characteristics, the currently accepted standard for evaluating blast% is morphology.

Patients with 10–20% blasts by morphology ("high-risk MDS" by IPSS criteria) are often ineligible for "AML protocols." However, it is not clear that this is entirely sensible. Not only are the natural histories of AML and high-risk MDS very similar, but outcome of at least conventional AML therapy appears to depend more on covariates such as cytogenetics, de novo versus secondary AML, and age than on the distinction between "MDS" and "AML," with prognostically unfavorable characteristics more common in MDS [21]. Because they respond so well to AML therapy, the WHO regards patients with <20% blasts but with t (8; 21) or inv (16) as AML (16). Likewise, patients who present with 5–20% blasts but with evidence of infiltration of gums, perianal area, liver, kidney, or lungs should be regarded as AML for treatment purposes even if the blast count is <20%. Such patients often have a preponderance of monocytes.

Acute promyelocytic leukemia (APL) is a distinct type of AML that should be suspected when there are morphologically abnormal promyelocytes regardless of % [22]. As a result of disseminated intravascular coagulation (DIC) and/or excess fibrinolysis, APL is often accompanied by a bleeding diathesis, which can lead to rapid death, thus emphasizing the need for urgent diagnosis. In the great majority of cases, there is an abnormal juxtaposition of the retinoic acid receptor α gene on chromosome 17 and the PML gene on chromosome 15. Definitive diagnosis of APL requires demonstration of the resulting t (15; 17), for example, using fluorescent in situ hybridization (FISH) or, most rapidly, use of immunostaining with anti-PML monoclonal antibodies.

Evaluation

Since it is the principal guide as to the need for urgent treatment, the most important laboratory test in AML is the WBC count. Twenty to twenty five percent of patients presenting with WBC >50,000/μl die within 4 weeks of treatment initiation (vs. 10% for all patients) with death rate increasing as WBC increases above this number [23]. However, although 50,000/μl is often used as a criterion triggering immediate treatment, this number is not inviolate. Rather the criterion should be influenced by how rapidly the WBC is rising, the presence of likely organ infiltration, and a diagnosis of either monocytic AML (AMoL) or acute promyelocytic leukemia (APL). In AMoL, a threshold of 20,000–30,000 should be used while, as discussed later, initiation of treatment is almost always urgent in APL if the WBC is >10,000. If the WBC is judged high enough to warrant immediate treatment, there is no need for bone marrow aspiration. This only delays treatment, and it is very likely that the cytogenetic and molecular genetic information obtained from the marrow (discussed below) is similar to that obtained using blood. Although leukapheresis has some role in reducing tumor lysis syndrome, it should not be allowed to delay start of specific therapy [23].

The principal management decision in newly diagnosed AML is whether to treat the patient and what treatment to employ. Treatment can fundamentally divided into "standard" and "investigational," with the latter preferably given in the context of a clinical trial. Because the results of any ongoing trial are unknown and could in principle be worse than those obtained with standard therapy, the principal reason to recommend a trial is dissatisfaction with results of standard therapy. Hence, evaluation of the AML patient should emphasize assessment of those covariates ("prognostic factors") known to influence outcome of standard therapy [24]. Before pursuing this topic, we will describe standard therapy for AML.

Standard Therapy

Therapy is divided into induction and postremission phases. Induction therapy aims to produce a complete remission (CR), criteria for which are a marrow with <5% recognizable blasts and neutrophil and platelet counts >1,000 and >100,000/μl, respectively. Postremission therapy attempts to prolong the CR. Approximately 60% of relapses occur within 1 year of CR date [25]. However, the rate of relapse does not decline sharply until patients have been in CR for >2–3 years, thus suggesting that patients in CR for this time may be considered "potentially cured" [25].

CR has long been considered an important goal of therapy because it alone was thought to lead to cure and, in the absence of cure, to prolongation of survival. Freireich et al. demonstrated that the difference in survival between patients who achieved and did not achieve CR was entirely due to the time spent in CR, thus suggesting that CR patients lived longer because of the CR and not because they had inherently better prognoses [26].

In the past 10 years, new criteria for response have appeared [27]: CRp referring to a CR but with a platelet count <100,000/μl, CRi referring to marrow that is cellular with <5% blasts but without any minimum levels of blood counts, and hematologic improvement as defined for myelodysplasia [28]. While these responses indicate that a drug has some activity, their effect on lengthening survival has been less clear. Walter et al. showed that potential cure was more likely with CR than CRp [29]. CRp is associated with shorter relapse-free survival ($p < 0.05$) and survival ($p = 0.10$) even after accounting for the poorer underlying prognoses (e.g., worse cytogenetics) of CRp patients. Furthermore, it usually takes longer to reach CRp than CR, suggesting that the longer life expectancy associated with CR does not simply reflect a longer minimum time to reach CR than CRp. However, these results were obtained with standard therapy, and it is plausible that they might not apply with other therapies.

Anthracyclines + Cytarabine (Ara-C)

For 40 years, standard induction therapy has typically consisted of 7 days of Ara-C given by continuous infusion at 100 mg/m^2 daily and 3 days of daunorubicin, idarubicin, or occasionally mitoxantrone. Randomized studies have shown that when used at equitoxic doses, these drugs are very likely therapeutically equivalent. If a bone marrow obtained 14–21 days after treatment begins shows "residual" AML, a second course of this "3+7" (or "7+3") regimen is often given, frequently using 2 days of daunorubicin or idarubicin and 5 days of Ara-C. However, residual AML is variably defined, and in general, the factors governing response to a second course of 3+7 are sufficiently uncertain to make it difficult to know when a change to alternate therapy is advisable.

Over 20 years ago, a randomized trial showed that patients in CR lived longer if therapy continued rather than being stopped once they were in 3+7-induced CR [30]; this has led to widespread use of postremission therapy, with the term "consolidation" referring to doses similar to those given during induction and "maintenance" to lower doses. Patients typically continue daunorubicin or idarubicin and particularly Ara-C consolidation for 2–4 courses, assuming a transplant is not done before this, although a randomized trial in patients aged ≥65 showed superior relapse-free survival and survival with six courses of a low-intensity, outpatient maintenance regimen [31].

Doses of daunorubicin and Ara-C have also been the subject of randomized studies. A trial giving 657 adults age <60 (median age 48) 7 days of standard dose Ara-C while randomizing them to 3 days of daunorubicin at 45 or 90 mg/m^2 daily found a higher CR rate (71% vs. 57%) and, with a median follow-up of 2 years, longer median survival (24 vs. 16 months) with the higher dose [32]. Approximately 40% of the higher and 30% of the lower-dose patients were projected to be alive at 3–4 years and thus potentially cured. A trial similarly randomizing 813 patients age 60–83 (median 67) to standard dose Ara-C + one of the two daunorubicin doses [33] found higher CR rates (64% vs. 54%) with the 90-mg/m^2 dose but similar 30-day death rates (11–12%) and overall survival (median approximately 1 year, with 15% projected to be potentially cured). If anything, grade 3–4 adverse events were less frequent with the higher dose (49% vs. 55%), suggesting a connection between more effective immediate treatment of AML and a decrease in "adverse events." In the 299 patients age 60–65, not only was CR rate superior with the 90-mg/m^2 dose, but survival was as well (medians approximately 18 vs. 12 months, 3 years approximately 35% vs. 15%). These studies might be criticized because the "standard" daunorubicin dose is 60, not 45, mg/m^2 daily × 3. However, I believe there are more profitable subjects of investigation than a trial randomizing large numbers of patients between the 60- and 90-mg/m^2 doses. I believe that, *on average*, in patients under age 65, 90 mg/m^2 daily × 3 should be accepted as the standard anthracycline dose for induction.

Patients under age 60–65 in the USA have typically received Ara-C 3 g/m^2 every 12 h on days 1, 3, and 5 as their first (consolidation) treatment after they achieved CR. However, data from the HOVON/SAKK have cast doubt on the advisability of this dose [34]. These investigators randomized 860 adults under age 60 (median 48) to 3 days of idarubicin and Ara-C at either 200 mg/m^2 continuously for 7 days (intermediate dose) or 1 g/m^2 twice daily on days 1–5 (high dose). As course 2, patients received amsacrine, with intermediate group patients also given Ara-C 1 g/m^2 twice daily on days 1–6 while high-dose patients received Ara-C 2 g/m^2 twice daily on days 1, 2, 4, and 6. Patients in CR after course 2 received a third course: mitoxantrone + etoposide, an autologous transplant, or an allogeneic transplant. CR rates were essentially identical (80–82%) in the intermediate and high-dose groups as, with a median follow-up of 5 years, were relapse-free survival (52–54%) and survival (40–42%). Outcomes were similar in the intermediate and high-dose groups regardless of treatment on course 3 (and were in general similar to those obtained in studies using 3 g/m^2) [35], but the high-dose group experienced more toxicity even with the subsequent mitoxantrone + etoposide. Similarly, the Medical Research Council's AML 15 trial, which randomized 723 patients, found no difference between Ara-C doses of 1.5 and 3.0 g/m^2 during postremission therapy [35]. Finally, a randomized Japanese study involving 822 adults under age 64 found no advantage for three consolidation courses of Ara-C at 2 g/m^2 twice daily on days 1–5 versus four courses using 200 mg/m^2 together with anthracyclines [36].

Prognostic Factors ("Covariates")

Predictors of Treatment-Related Mortality (TRM)

Large randomized studies such as those described above are primarily quoted with reference to a "result." However, a striking feature of AML is the variability of response to standard therapy, questioning the clinical relevance of an "average" result and justifying efforts to identify covariates predictive of outcome with standard therapy in order to advise patients of expected results with such therapy. Covariates include those that predict (a) treatment-related mortality (TRM) and (b) resistance to therapy despite not incurring TRM. At least with standard therapy, the covariates associated with (a) differ from those associated with (b), with resistance being more common than TRM as a cause of therapeutic failure even in patients aged >75 years [37].

TRM has been variably defined as death occurring with the first 28–60 days of start of treatment. However, recent data indicate that the weekly risk of TRM is similar for the first 28 days after which it sharply declines [38]. The same holds true regardless of age, although of course the total TRM rate is higher in older patients. This observation suggested that patients who die within the first 28 days are qualitatively distinct from those who die thereafter and focused efforts on identifying the former patients, who comprise approximately 10% of all newly diagnosed patients. The principal factor associated with TRM is performance status. Others adding to ability to forecast are age, bilirubin, creatinine, and platelet count. The area under the curve (AUC) of receiver operating characteristic curves provides a method to quantify predictive ability An AUC of 1.0 denotes perfect prediction, while an AUC of 0.5 is equivalent to a coin toss. Inclusion of all the covariates listed above results in an AUC of 0.82 for predicting TRM. In contrast, performance status alone has an AUC of 0.65 and age alone an AUC of 0.62, suggesting the unsatisfactory nature of systems that use only a single covariate to predict outcome. Although age is commonly used to determine which treatment protocol a patient is eligible for, removal of age from the "complete" model described above results in reduction of the AUC from 0.82 to only 0.81. The role of comorbidities in predicting TRM remains incompletely explored. Sorror has reported the profound role played by such comorbidities in determining TRM after allogeneic hematopoietic cell transplantation (HCT) [39, 40].

As noted above, the principal cause of treatment failure in AML is resistance to therapy, not TRM, and this is true even in older patients. For example, Appelbaum et al. reported that, following administration of standard 3 + 7 induction therapy, resistance defined as failure to enter complete remission (CR) despite living at least 30 days was responsible for 71% of induction failures in patients younger than age 56, 61% in patients age 66–75, and 54% in patients age >75 [41]. Resistance also encompasses relapse from CR, and when the five- to sixfold higher rates of relapse than of death in remission are accounted for [42], the importance of resistance is even more apparent.

Predictors of Resistance

Cytogenetics, CKIT, NPM1, FLT3, and CEBPA

The principal covariate associated with sensitivity/resistance to standard therapy is leukemia cell cytogenetics. For practical purposes, these are divided into four groups. A "best" group includes patients with pericentric inversion of a chromosome 16 (inv 16), a balanced translocation involving a chromosome 8 and a chromosome 21 [t (8; 21)], or rarely a t (16; 16), but not a del 16q. A "worst group" is defined by the presence of a "monosomal karyotype" (MK) [43, 44], criteria for which are at least two autosomal monosomies, or a single autosomal monosomy together with structural changes (as opposed to gains or losses of whole chromosomes), most commonly a translocation. Some systems consider the better of the two intermediate groups to consist solely of patients with normal karyotype (NK), with the worse intermediate group including patients with abnormalities other than inv (16) t (8; 21) or MK [43]. Other systems regard the worse intermediate group as including patients with −5, −7 (each without MK), del 5q, del 7q, t (3; 3), inv [3], t (6; 9), an abnormality involving 11q or 17p, or a complex karyotype (at least three separate clonal abnormalities but without MK), and the better intermediate group as including patients with other cytogenetic abnormalities including NK [44]. NK requires at least 10 normal metaphases. If there are <10 normal metaphases and no clonal abnormality (defined as at least two cells with the same trisomy or structural abnormality and at least three with the same monosomy), the patient is said to have "insufficient metaphases." These are patients in whom fluorescent in situ hybridization (FISH) is most valuable [45]. FISH routinely examines 500 cells rather than 20–25. Hence, there is much greater probability of detecting an abnormality. However, there is much less data concerning the clinical significance of an abnormality found only using FISH. Patients occasionally have abnormalities on conventional cytogenetics that are shared by relatively few patients. Reference [46] details the prognostic significance of many of these.

CBF AML

Patients with inv (16) or t (8; 21) are said to have "core binding factor" (CBF) AML because each of these results in disruption of a transcription factor (i.e., CBF) that regulates transcription of genes important in normal hematopoiesis. Despite this molecular similarity, inv (16) and t (8; 21) are quite different clinically, although each generally associated with a relatively favorable prognosis. While both are typically found in younger patients (median age 40) and comprise 10–20% of AML in patients under age 60, t (8; 21) is more likely to present with a low WBC, Auer rods, and at a site outside blood or marrow [47]. Likelihood of obtaining CR after relapse is typically better with inv (16), and hence these patients often have better survival [48], although not necessarily better long-term survival. Patients with either inv (16) or t (8; 21) should have CR rates in excess of 90% with standard 3 + 7, and both studies comparing 45 and 90 mg/m^2 daunorubicin found superior survival in CBF patients receiving the higher dose [32, 33]. A CALGB study randomizing patients to four cycles of consolidation therapy with 3 g/m^2 twice daily on days 1, 3, and 5, 400 mg/m^2 daily 5 days by continuous infusion (CI), or 100 mg/m^2 daily × days by CI found at 5 years from CR date 78%, 57%, and 16% of CBF patients remained in CR at the 3-g/m^2, 400-mg/m^2, and 100-mg/m^2 doses, respectively [49]. However, the above quoted HOVON/SAAK study [34] found 5-year survival rates of 64–67%

with both high and intermediate dose Ara-C during both induction and postremission therapy in such patients. While it might be tempting to state that these rates are lower than the rates for remission duration produced by the CALGB [49], the presence of prognostic factors within the CBF group itself (see below) makes such speculation difficult outside a randomized study. The same applies to a report that the FLAG regimen improves outcome in CBF AML [50]. In contrast, two randomized studies [51, 52] have found an advantage for use of gemtuzumab ozogamicin (GO), although this drug is no longer readily available. The role of HCT is described below.

CBF AML itself is not a uniform prognostic entity; differences between inv (16) and t (8; 21) were noted above. It is generally held that the presence of cytogenetic abnormalities other than inv (16) or t (8; 21) does not affect outcome [46]. However, age 65 or above, although uncommon in CBF patients, reduces potential cure rates to 20–25 [53], with age >35 reportedly associated with a relapse rate of 55% versus 29% in younger patients with inv (16) [54]. Nor is it clear that Ara-C at consolidation doses $\geq$500 mg/m^2 is beneficial in patients aged $\geq$60 with inv (16) [55]. A high WBC index defined as WBC count X% marrow blasts/100 is an adverse prognostic factor in t (8; 21) AML; among 151 patients, 3-year relapse-free survival rates were approximately 74%, 57%, and 33% in patients with WBC indices <2.5, 2.5–20, and >20, respectively, with all patients given Ara-C in doses of at least 1 g/m^2 or HCT [56]. More recently, CKIT mutations have been found associated with poorer prognosis in patients with either t (8; 21) or inv (16). Thus, CALGB reported that 10 patients with t (8; 21) and a mutation had a 70% 2-year cumulative incidence of relapse (CIR) versus 36% in 31 patients with wild-type CKIT [57]. Analogous rates were 56% (17 patients) and 29% (40 patients) in inv (16). While this finding has been confirmed [58], it may not be generally applicable [59]. However, since the relevant CKIT mutation(s) is targeted by dasatinib, trials randomizing patients with CBF to receive or not receive this drug during postremission therapy are planned. Absent such a trial, the data suggest that while all patients with CBF may benefit from daunorubicin at 90 mg/m^2 (perhaps unless age >70 or with poor performance status), therapy other than merely Ara-C at 1 g/m^2 as described in the HOVON/SAKK study [34] might be appropriate for CBF patients who (a) are older, particularly those with inv (16); (b) have a WBC index >2.5, and certainly >20, in the presence of t (8; 21); or (c) have a CKIT mutation. HCT might be an option for some of these patients (see below).

Monosomal Karyotype (MK) and Other "Unfavorable Karyotypes"

Previously, complex karyotypes ($\geq$3 distinct clonal abnormalities) were felt associated with a particularly poor prognosis. Recent findings suggest, however, that MK, defined above, confers a uniquely bad prognosis [43, 44] (Fig. 1.1). For example, 4-year survival probabilities with a complex karyotype were 13% without and 0% with MK ($p<0.01$) [44]. The Southwest Oncology Group (SWOG) found CR rates with 3+7 for patients age 31–40, 41–50, 51–60 and >60 of 60%,

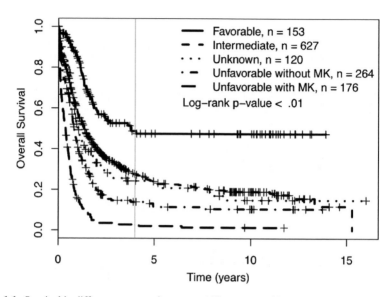

Fig. 1.1 Survival in different cytogenetic groups. *MK* monosomal karyotype [44]

67%, 52%, and 27% in the absence of MK versus 27%, 14%, 24%, and 14% with an MK [44]. The prognostic effect of MK is not substantively different at intermediate and high Ara-C doses [34] and appears impervious to daunorubicin dose (45 vs. 90 mg/m², [33]).

In patients with unfavorable cytogenetics defined as abnormalities other than CBF, the CALGB found 5-year remission rates of 21%, 13%, and 13% at postremission doses of 3 g/m², 400 mg/m², and 100 mg/m², respectively [49]. Defining unfavorable cytogenetics as MK together with the worst intermediate group in reference 44, the ECOG found median survivals of 10.2 months with 45 mg/m² daunorubicin and 10.4 months with 90 mg/m² in patients under age 60 [32]. In patients under age 55 with a complex karyotype and/or −5, −7, del 5q, or del 7q, the SWOG noted CR rates <50% with 3 + 7 [60]. It is difficult not to conclude that patients with MK, and perhaps many of those in the SWOG unfavorable without MK category [44], should be offered induction therapies other than 3 + 7, particularly given data (described below) suggesting that induction therapy can influence duration of remission as well as its achievement.

Intermediate Prognosis Karyotypes: The Role of Molecular Markers

Intermediate prognosis cytogenetics include those other than inv 16, t (8; 21), t (16; 16), −5, −7, del 5q, del 7q, t (3; 3), inv (3), t (6; 9), an abnormality involving 11q or 17p, or a complex karyotype. The most common abnormality in the intermediate group is +8, while the most common finding is NK. The latter patients have traditionally had the most variable prognoses with standard therapy. However, it is now clear that patients with de novo AML can be divided into those with "high" and "low" risks of relapse-free survival (RFS) and survival according to the presence/absence in AML blasts of internal tandem duplications (ITDs) in the Fms-like tyrosine kinase 3 gene (FLT3 ITD), mutations in exon 12 of the nucleophosmin 1 (NPM1) gene, and mutations—particularly double mutations—in the CCAAT enhancer-binding protein (CEBPA) gene [61]. In particular, those of such patients with (a) an NPM1 mutation, but no FLT3 ITD, or (b) a CEBPA mutation are in a "low-risk" group, whereas other patients are in a "high-risk" group (Fig. 1.2). Daunorubicin at 90 rather than 45 mg/m^2 is associated with a median survival improvement of 12 months in patients who are FLT3 ITD negative ($p=0.01$) but of only 5 months in those who are FLT3 ITD positive ($p=0.09$) [32]. Although data are lacking regarding the efficacy of higher doses of Ara-C in FLT3 ITD–positive disease, results in patients with MK [34] suggest that such doses will be of marginal benefit.

Table 1.1 uses the cytogenetic and molecular information described so far in this chapter to place patients in five groups according to risk of resistance to standard therapy, with resistance defined as failure to enter CR despite surviving ≥28 days from start of therapy or relapse from CR. The system differs slightly from that suggested by the European Leukemia Net [24] in that it recognizes a unique significance of MK and weighs FLT3 ITDs somewhat more unfavorably than the ELN.

Most of the data about the prognostic effect of FLT3, NPM1, and CEBPA were obtained in patients aged <60 with de novo AML. However, the CALGB has observed that in patients aged ≥60, lack of an NPM1 mutation, but not age, was a significant predictor of lower CR rate and shorter RFS, and survival, with the favorable effect of an NPM1 mutation even apparent in patients aged ≥70 (Fig. 1.3) [62].

Newer Molecular Markers

Analyses using AUC analogous to those described above for TRM indicate that even accounting for presence/absence of FLT3 ITD, cytogenetics, and clinical parameters such as age, WBC count, etc., our ability to identify resistant patients is closer to a coin flip than certainty (AUC 0.72) [38]. As with TRM, removal of age from models predicting resistance has little effect on AUC. The difficulty forecasting resistance is prima facie evidence for the need of randomization in AML trials.

Beyond this, ability to predict resistance can be improved by including additional analyses of FLT3 beyond the presence/absence of an ITD. FLT3 ITDs differ in their number, length, and insertion site. However, prognosis is most affected by differences in relative levels of abnormal and normal FLT3 protein. Higher levels of abnormal protein correspond to higher "allelic burden," with levels >50% indicating a loss of the wild-type FLT3 allele or a homozygous mutation. Gale et al. [63] found that the difference in cumulative incidence of relapse between patients with allelic burdens >50% and patients with allelic burdens of 1–49% was similar to the difference between patients in the 1–49% group and patients without an ITD (Fig. 1.4).

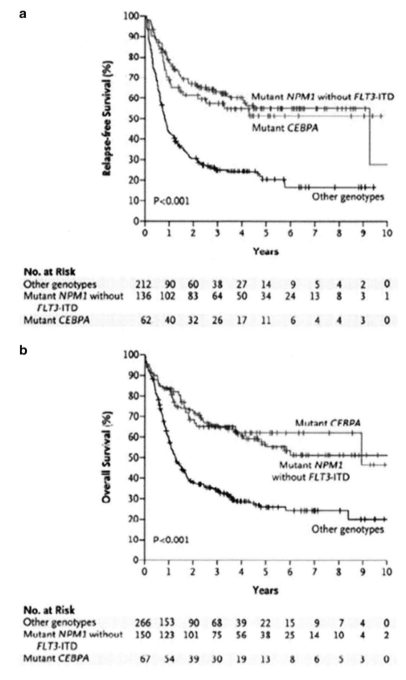

Fig. 1.2 (**a**) Relapse-free survival and (**b**) survival according to NPM1, FLT3, and CEBPA mutation status [61]

Table 1.1 Predictors of resistance to standard therapy

Prognostic group	Subsets
Best	t (8; 21)[a]
	Inv (16)[a] or t (16; 16)
	Mutated NPM1 without FLT3 ITD (NK)
	Double-mutated CEBPA (NK)
Intermediate 1	Wild-type *NPM1* without *FLT3* ITD (NK)
Intermediate 2	*FLT3* ITD (NK)
	Cytogenetic abnormalities other than best or unfavorable (see text)
Intermediate 3	Unfavorable cytogenetics without MK
Worst	MK

MK monosomal karyotype, *NK* normal karyotype
[a]Patients with inv (16) or 6t (8; 21) and CKIT mutations should be considered as belonging to the intermediate 1 group as should patients with t (8; 21) and a WBC index >20 and patients age >65 and possibly patients with inv (16) age >35 (see text)

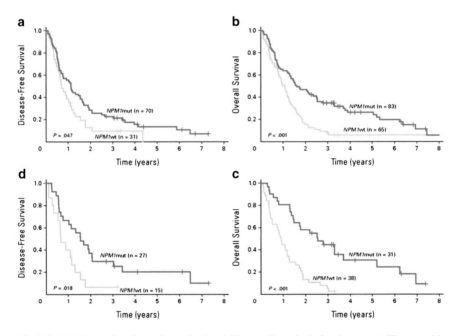

Fig. 1.3 (**a**) Disease-free (i.e., relapse-free) and (**b**) overall survival of patients age ≥60 years with CN de novo AML according to NPM1 mutation status. (**c**) The same as (**a**), but including only patients age < 70. (**d**) The same as (**b**), but including only patients age ≥70

Mutations in other molecular markers have been associated with unfavorable prognoses and noted to add independent prognostic information [64, 65]. These include mutations in WT1 [66, 67], TET2 [68], IDH 1 or IDH 2 [69, 70], and DNMT3a [71]. The latter are found in 10–25% of patients with de novo AML and NK. However, with the exception of DNMT3a, which is perhaps the least studied to

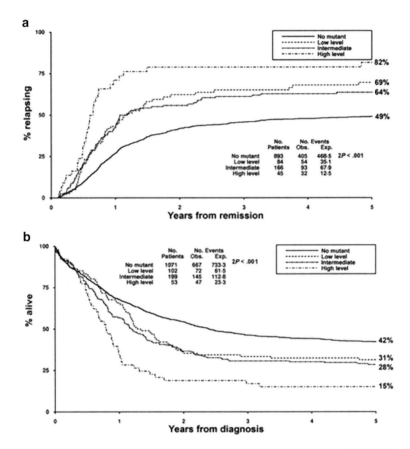

Fig. 1.4 Cumulative incidence of relapse and survival stratified according to total FLT3 ITD level. (**a**) proportion relapsing and (**b**) proportion alive

date, prognostic effects have been inconsistent. There are several possible explanations. Prognostic effect may be treatment-specific, or perhaps more plausibly, limited to a particular subgroup; for example, the unfavorable effect of TET2 mutations appears to occur only in patients who are NPM1 +/FLT3 ITD −, or CEBPA double mutated [68]. Patients in different studies may have had varying incidences of unknown yet prognostic genetic abnormalities. Finally, the downstream effects of a genetic abnormality may depend on whether the abnormality is expressed and ultimately reflected in an abnormal protein. Hence, differences in expression or translation may account for discordant results seen when analysis is limited to presence/ absence of genetic abnormalities such as those noted above. This possibility has motivated interest in comprehensive studies of gene expression, microRNA (miR) expression, DNA methylation, and proteomics. These studies may be particularly useful in the 15% of CN patients who appear to lack the genetic abnormalities described to date. For example, independent of FLT3 or NPM status, shorter relapse-free survival has been found in patients with high expression levels of various genes

(*BAALC, ERG, EVI1*, and *MN1*) [reviewed by Marcucci et al. [65]], setting the stage for generalized gene expression profiling (GEP). Metzeler et al. identified a GEP consisting of 66 genes, each of which was associated with at least a 2.9-fold increase or decrease in the risk of death in NK AML. These genes were weighted according to their effect on survival and incorporated into a continuous score that accurately predicted outcome in two independent sets of NK patients [72]. Although FLT3 ITDs correlated with a worse score, the score replaced FLT3 ITD as a predictor of outcome. Analogous results have been reported with miRNA [73, 74] methylation [9, 75], or proteomic profiling [76].

Secondary AML

Secondary AML refers to either a history of (a) cytotoxic or immunosuppressive chemotherapy (t-AML) or (b) an antecedent hematologic disorder (AHD), most commonly myelodysplasia and less frequently a myeloproliferative neoplasm (MPN) especially myelofibrosis. Secondary AML is well known to be associated with treatment resistance in comparison to de novo AML. Although frequently associated with particularly unfavorable cytogenetic abnormalities, the prognostic effect of secondary AML is independent of this association [77]. What is less clear is the prognostic significance of t-AML relative to that of an AHD. Nor is it known whether the type of AHD (number of affected blood counts, MDS vs. MPN, etc.) has prognostic import.

Use of Prognostic Factors

Given the role of NPM1, FLT3, and CEBPA in predicting response to standard therapy and hence in advising patients as to whether they might be better served by receiving HCT or investigational therapy, NPM1, FLT3, and, where practical, CEBPA status should be determined prior to beginning therapy in much the same way as cytogenetic status. Except in patients requiring emergency treatment (see "Evaluation" above), strong consideration should be given to using cytogenetic and molecular information not only in planning postremission therapy but in planning induction therapy. Several considerations are relevant here. First, it seems useful to avoid giving 3 + 7 to patients in whom the CR rate is likely to be <50% such those even aged <55 with a complex karyotype and/or −5, −7, del 5q, or del 7q [60], and in particular an MK [44]. This is even more the case in older patients in whom not only may the CR rate be <50% with such therapy but who may incur TRM before a second therapy can be given. Second, data from studies assessing the role of higher doses of daunorubicin [32, 33] or Ara-C [34, 49] do not suggest that dose increases will abrogate the effect of unfavorable cytogenetics or a FLT3 ITD. Third, even if patients obtain CR with 3 + 7, induction regimen can influence duration of CR as well as its achievement, and this is true even if HCT is done in CR [78]. Strikingly, the presence of minimal residual disease (MRD, see below) as measured by multicolor flow cytometry (MFC) prior to HCT in CR1 increases relapse rate after HCT, independently of cytogenetics [79]. The presence of such MRD reflects the ineffectiveness of therapy given prior to HCT. Therefore, relapse rates, including those after HCT, might be reduced if even younger high-risk patients receive potentially more effective induction therapies in clinical trials; an example would be use of newer FLT3 inhibitors such as AC220 together with standard 3 + 7. An obvious risk in waiting for cytogenetic and molecular information to become available prior to initiation of treatment is clinical deterioration during this time. Examining the effect on outcome of time from diagnosis to therapy (TDT) in 1,361 patients with newly diagnosed AML and WBC count <50,000, Sekeres et al. found that after accounting for other covariates associated with outcome, TDT (median only 4 days) had no influence on CR or survival in patients age ≥60 and a deleterious effect on survival after 6 months in younger patients, which was much less than that associated with cytogenetics [80]. The negative associated with delaying therapy in younger patients should be weighed against that associated with giving suboptimal induction therapy to patients with unfavorable cytogenetics because of a perceived need to treat the patient promptly.

Posttreatment Monitoring: Minimal Residual Disease (MRD)

Although newer molecular markers measured prior to treatment are likely to increase prognostic accuracy and provide new biologic insights, incorporation of posttreatment data may also be useful. A simple example is the finding reported years ago that the number of courses needed to enter CR is the principal predictor of length of remission [81]. This finding has been questioned [82], and the prognostic role of courses to CR may reflect differing criteria used to begin a second course; confounding would result if a patient who would have entered CR with one course receives a second because of the presence of a relatively small number of blasts in a hypocellular marrow 14 days after beginning treatment.

However, the most valuable posttreatment marker may be the level of MRD. Numerous studies indicate that MFC [83] or PCR for molecules such as WT1 [84] or NPM1 [85] provide a sensitive and specific means to detect impending relapse in patients in CR by morphologic criteria. Hence, patients with such MRD, particularly if persistent, or present at a relatively high level, should be considered a high-risk group and ipso facto candidates for HCT or investigational therapies.

Hematopoietic Cell Transplantation

HCT is done most frequently in patients <age 60 in first CR. Such patients typically receive a "myeloablative HCT." Depending largely on comorbidities as described by Sorror et al. [39, 40], mortality rates in the first 100 days after HCT may be as

Table 1.2 Donor–no donor comparison of survival in patients aged <60

Cytogenetic risk[a]	Patients in donor group	Patients in no donor group	Number of trials	Hazard rate[b] (95% CI)
Best	188	359	10	1.07 (0.83–1.38)
Intermediate	864	1,635	14	0.83 (0.74–0.93)
Worst	226	366	14	0.73 (0.59–0.90)

Note: Patients received myeloablative HCT from human leukocyte antigen (HLA)–matched donors

CI confidence interval

[a]Southwest Oncology Group (SWOG)/Eastern Cooperative Oncology Group (ECOG) criteria [60]

[b]Hazard rate <1.0 favors allogeneic HCT

low as 10%, which nonetheless is considerably higher than seen in patients receiving postremission chemotherapy [42]. However, if the increase in TRM with HCT is more than offset by a decrease in relapse risk (although relapse is the principal cause of failure after HCT as well as chemotherapy), survival should be better with HCT. To avoid bias favoring HCT, comparisons of chemotherapy and HCT typically compare patients with and without donors; if the donor group does better, so would patients actually given HCT, with the results in such patients setting an upper limit on the effectiveness of HCT. However, donor–no donor comparisons are problematic [86], and a preferable technique for avoiding bias would be to consider all patients in the no donor group with those found to have a donor right censored from the no donor group and left censored into the donor group on the date that a match is identified [87]. However, this is logistically difficult compared to the donor–no donor method. Using the latter, Koreth et al. undertook a meta-analysis to assess relapse-free survival and survival in patients receiving an HLA-matched myeloablative transplant in CR1 rather than chemotherapy or an autologous transplant [88]; autologous transplant and chemotherapy are generally held to afford similar survival [89]. The median age of the patients was approximately 40 (all were below 60), and their median follow-up was 4–5 years. In only one trial considered in the meta-analysis did less than 60% of patients with donors receive HCT. The results showed that both relapse-free survival and survival (Table 1.2) were superior in the donor group if patients had intermediate or worse cytogenetics while there was no benefit in patients with inv (16) or t (8; 21). The results are perhaps less significant medically than statistically. For example, assume a patient with unfavorable cytogenetics would survive 1 year after achieving CR if given chemotherapy or an autologous transplant. A reduction in hazard rate to 0.73 (Table 1.2) translates into a survival of 16.4 months. Hence, while the objective should be to perform myeloablative HCT in as many patients aged <60 as possible, means to reduce relapse after HCT are needed; some of these are noted below. An alternative approach to immediate HCT would be to reserve HCT for patients with increasing evidence of MRD [90]; presumably, the criteria for "MRD" would have to be liberal given that immediate HCT is the "default" treatment. An advantage of the delayed strategy might be avoidance of late complications of HCT. In particular, in patients cured of their

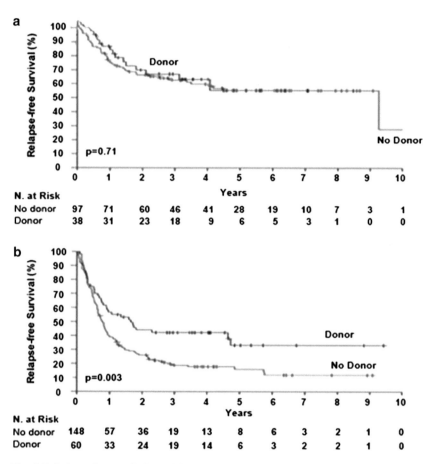

Fig. 1.5 Relapse-free survival according to genotype and donor or no donor. (**a**) Mutant NPM1 without FlT3JTD, (**b**) other genotypes

AML, HCT is associated with a 30% decrease in life expectancy [91]. Of course this is preferable to relapse and consequent more immediate death.

Less is known about the role of HCT in high-risk patients as defined by molecular abnormalities. Schlenk et al. [61] noted longer RFS, but not survival, in normal karyotype patients younger than age 60 who had a sibling donor and were neither CEBPA mutated nor NPM1 mutated/FLT3 wild type (Fig. 1.5) [61]. Although finding a negative effect of FLT3 ITD in both patients who were and were not transplanted, Gale et al. [92] reported a reduced cumulative incidence of relapse, but not improved survival, in the former.

Many patients do not have HLA-matched sibling donors. However, modern typing techniques have allowed matched unrelated donors to be identified for most patients without sibling donors [93]. Although a true comparison of matched sibling and matched unrelated donor HCT would require randomization of patients with sibling donors to receive transplant from the sibling or a matched unrelated donor, such a trial is not feasible. With this constraint and bearing in mind the increased difficulties with donor–no donor analyses in the unrelated setting, data suggest equivalent results with matched sibling and matched unrelated HCT [94, 95] and that if HCT from a (living) matched unrelated donor is not feasible, double cord blood transplants are (at least) their equivalent [96].

The past 20 years have also seen the development of reduced-intensity conditioning (RIC) regimens [97]. These reduce toxicity but permit engraftment and subsequent development of T-cell-mediated graft-versus-AML effects and allow patients in their 70s or with significant comorbidities to receive HCT. Analyzing 274 patients (median age 60, up to age 74) who received RIC-HCT from 1998 to 2008, Gyurkocza et al. [98] noted nonrelapse mortality (NRM) rates of 4%, 16%, and 26% at 100 days, 1 year, and 5 years, with NRM chiefly from graft-versus-host disease (GVHD). Relapse accounted for 60% of the deaths and with a median follow-up of 38 months, the probability of 5-year survival was 37% for patients transplanted in CR1, 34% for those transplanted in CR2, and 18% for patients with more advanced and refractory disease. Five-year survival rates were similar in patients with matched sibling (37%) and matched unrelated donors (33%).

These results certainly suggest that RIC-HCT is superior to chemotherapy in older patients in CR1 or CR2, and indeed a donor–no donor analysis in CR1 has suggested the same [99]. However, related to the inability of such an analysis to completely account for bias is the general applicability of RIC-HCT [100] or of even myeloablative HCT. A forthcoming US Intergroup study will address the latter question. It is also noteworthy that at least some of the covariates that predict relapse after chemotherapy [cytogenetics, CRp rather than CR [29]] do the same after HCT, suggesting that these modalities are not as different as might be hoped. Nonetheless, it is clear that the mortality after HCT is decreasing (41% from 1993 to 1997 vs. 2003 to 2007) [101] after adjustment for covariates such as age and comorbidities. This might motivate interest in greater use of HCT in conjunction, however, with methods to decrease post-HCT relapse.

Newer Therapies

Most new therapies are first tested either in relapsed AML, AML that has not entered CR with initial therapy, or patients aged ≥60 with newly diagnosed AML, many of whom have unfavorable cytogenetics and/or secondary AML. This practice may make it harder to discover effective new therapies, in contrast to examining new treatments in patients in remission (see below). This difficulty has led to the advent of new response categories such as CRp or CRi described above [27, 29]. Many newer induction regimens have been or are being investigated. Any listing would be incomplete and quickly outdated. Hence, we will describe only a few regimens followed by a brief description of some problems attendant in clinical trials of new drugs.

Nucleoside Analogs

The Polish Acute Leukemia Group has reported a randomized study showing that addition of cladribine to 3+7 (daunorubicin 60 mg/m² daily × 3) produced a higher rate of CR after a single course despite similar or less toxicity [102]. This has sparked interest in clofarabine, which is structurally related to cladribine and fludarabine but more active at tolerable doses than the latter. After accounting for prior CR duration, number of salvage treatments, age, and cytogenetics, Becker et al. reported that in patients with relapsed/refractory AML, the combination of clofarabine and Ara-C (2 g/m² daily×5)+G-CSF before during and after chemotherapy appeared superior, to a similar regimen containing fludarabine with (FLAG) or without G-CSF (FA) [103]. The differences largely reflected results in patients with short or no first remissions, or, alternatively, unfavorable cytogenetics. However, a trial (CLASSIC 1) randomizing similar patients age 55 or above to high-dose Ara-C +/− clofarabine found that while CR rates were higher with the combination, survival was not, as a result of more TRM in patients given the combination. It might be possible to identify patients who are at relatively high risk of TRM [38] and exclude them from treatment with the combination. Turning to newly diagnosed patients, Burnett et al. have found that, after adjusting for other covariates, CR and survival rates in 106 patients (median age 71) considered unfit for 3+7 and thus given clofarabine were higher than when similarly unfit patients received low-dose Ara-C (LDAC) and comparable with those observed when fitter older patients received 3+7-like therapy [104]. Of note, CR rates with clofarabine were similar in patients with unfavorable and intermediate cytogenetics (44% vs. 52%). In 70 relatively fit patients (median age 71 years) randomized to clofarabine or clofarabine+LDAC, the combination produced superior CR (63% vs. 31%) and survival rates, but survival remained short (median 11 months), even with the combination [105]. Further information about clofarabine's role in newly diagnosed AML will likely be forthcoming from an ongoing ECOG study randomizing older patients to 3+7 or clofarabine, albeit without Ara-C.

Hypomethylating Agents (HAs): Azacitidine and Decitabine

These drugs were first investigated in patients with MDS, some of whom had 21–30% blasts and were thus reclassified as newly diagnosed AML. In the azacitidine trial, physicians first declared a preference for supportive care only, LDAC, or 3+7 in a given patient. Patients were then randomized to the selected conventional care regimen or azacitidine. Among 113 AML patients (median age 70), median survivals were 24.5 months (azacitidine) and 16.0 months (conventional care) and were 12 months (azacitidine) and 5 months (conventional care) in the patients with unfavorable cytogenetics [106]. Too few patients received LDAC or 3+7 to permit robust comparisons with azacitidine. However, unlike LDAC or 3+7, achievement of CR with azacitidine did not seem a precondition for longer survival.

Decitabine at 20 mg/m^2 daily × 5 days produced a 25% CR rate (similar in intermediate and unfavorable cytogenetics) and median survival 8 months in 55 patients aged >60 with newly diagnosed AML [107]. Results of a trial randomizing patients aged ≥65 between decitabine and physician's choice of LDAC or supportive care only were presented at the 2011 meeting of the American Society of Clinical Oncology (ASCO) [108]. An "updated unplanned analysis" performed after 92% of patients had died showed median survival of 7.7 months for decitabine and 5.0 months for physicians' choice ("nominal $p=0.03$"). The previously planned "final analysis" done after 82% of patients had died showed the same median survivals, but $p=0.10$. As is often the case, there may be a gap between statistical and clinical significance. In particular, it is likely that given the small survival advantage provided by azacitidine or decitabine, many patients would opt for a clinical trial that might, for example, include use of these drugs in combination with other agents.

Because the results noted above likely reflect an average of more and less sensitive patient results, it is important to identify patients who are more likely to respond. Administering decitabine for 10 days, Blum et al. noted a CR rate of 67% in 27 patients with unfavorable cytogenetics, a much higher rate than with the usual 5-day schedule [109]. Although median survival was not reported for these patients, it was 1 year for all 53 patients (median age 74 years). Responders had higher expression of miR-29b, presumably reflecting miR-29b's ability to downregulate enzymes involved in methylation. It remains unclear, however, whether response to HAs correlates with hypomethylation and, in particular, with reexpression of silenced genes. Such a correlation might encourage further studies combining HAs and histone deacetylase inhibitors, which appear to cooperate with HAs in inducing reexpression of silenced genes. It is yet unclear, however, whether the combination is superior to azacitidine or lenalidomide alone.

FLT3 Inhibitors

Midostaurin (formerly PKC412) and lestaurtinib (formerly CEP701) inhibit multiple kinases, among them FLT3, whereas sorafenib and, particularly, AC220, are more specific for FLT3 and much more potent FLT3 inhibitors. Each of the four drugs inhibits wild-type FLT3, but more effectively inhibits FLT3 ITDs, and has been studied essentially exclusively in ITD-positive patients. Midostaurin and lestaurtinib produced minor responses in relapsed disease and are being studied in trials randomizing untreated patients to 3 +7 +/− the FLT3 inhibitor. A similar trial in 224 relapsed patients found no difference in CR or survival between patients given chemotherapy +/− lestaurtinib [110]. However, the ability of patients' serum to inhibit ITD+ cell lines correlated with clinical response, suggesting that response rates might be higher with a more potent inhibitor, such as AC220. This drug has considerably more single-agent activity in relapsed patients than midostaurin or lestaurtinib [111] and is being combined with chemotherapy in untreated patients. Sorafenib, the only one of these drugs currently available commercially, has also been combined with chemotherapy [112], although a randomized trial giving chemotherapy +/– sorafenib suggests that the probability of great benefits in ITD+ disease is unlikely [113]. One issue to consider in combining chemotherapy with FLT3 inhibitors is the ability of the former to induce FLT3 ligand which antagonizes the effect of the FLT3 inhibitor [114]. Cytotoxicity as a result of FLT3 inhibition is greater at high allelic burdens, perhaps because blasts in patients with such burdens are more "addicted" to FLT3 [114]. Because allelic burden is typically higher in relapsed than in untreated patients, the former may benefit more from potent FLT3 specific inhibitors, such as AC220, and the latter from less potent FLT3 inhibitors with, however, a broader spectrum of kinase inhibition [114].

New Therapy for Patients in Remission

The principal problem with HCT is the incidence of relapse following the procedure. This limitation might be overcome by more effective/less toxic conditioning regimens or immunologic augmentation of the post-HCT graft-versus-AML effect. Examples of the former include use of clofarabine or radiolabeled antibodies to CD45 [115]. Immunologic augmentation might be achieved using T cells specific for well-defined AML-associated antigens such as WT1, or for minor histocompatibility antigens expressed on host hematopoietic cells but not cells affected by graft-versus-host disease [116].

Likewise, immunologic approaches might be used as postremission therapy outside the RIC-HCT setting. For example, Brune et al. randomized 320 patients (80% in first, 20% in subsequent, CR) to receive either an IL2-histamine combination or no further treatment after completion of maintenance therapy and typically 4–5 months after entering CR [117]. IL2 + histamine prolonged survival and relapse-free survival by a median of 4–6 months in CR1 patients. Although as often the case the improvement in relapse-free survival but not survival was significant at $p < 0.05$, the data prompted the European Medicines Agency to approve IL2 + histamine for patients in CR1.

With a goal of increasing the chance of discovering effective new drugs, there appears to be some movement toward investigation of new drugs in patients in CR with or without MRD. Examples are ongoing studies of decitabine or bortezomib. Furthermore, the future is likely to see increasing use of agents whose mode of action, such as specifically targeting AML "stem cells," suggests they would be most effective in patients with relatively small amounts of disease, for example, those in CR [118]. It is also probable that, instead of being viewed separately, "HCT" and "non-HCT" approaches will be combined to prolong CR. Examples are the prophylactic use of azacitidine [119], or AC220, in patients at high risk of relapse after HCT.

Issues in New Drug Development

It is well known that the great majority of new drugs reported as "promising" in early phase trials in AML never migrate into clinical practice [120]. This suggests that there are fundamental lesions in the methods used to conduct, analyze, and report early trials. Walter et al. have listed some of these: small sample sizes, lack of a control group, unaccounted for patient heterogeneity, selected (and nonrepresentative) study cohorts, and use of endpoints with an uncertain relation to survival, the principal concern of patients [120]. Another issue is whether the large phase 3 trial has outlived its usefulness and might be replaced with smaller randomized phase 2 trials. Although such trials have less power than conventional phase 3 trials, they may avoid the worst false negative: not investigating a new drug at all.

Management of the Older Patient

Many, if not most, protocols for newly diagnosed AML are open either for older (usually aged ≥60 years) or younger patients but not both. This practice seems clinically dubious since patients aged >65 or even 70 years are not infrequently healthier than patients aged <60. This clinical observation has been verified by finding that addition of covariates other than age considerably improves prediction of TRM and resistance following standard therapy [38]. Removal of age from these models has minimal effect on predictive accuracy, suggesting that age is largely a surrogate for other covariates [38]. These data might be used to support a practice of considering all adults for a given protocol and basing assignment on covariates other than age.

Absent this possibility, the management approach to an older patient should be similar to that in a younger patient. In particular, as described above, the choice is supportive care only, a standard therapy such as 3 + 7 or LDAC (and increasingly HAs), or investigational therapy. Because the results of the latter are perforce unknown, the decision must rest on results of standard therapy. Several prognostic scoring systems have been developed to assess response to standard therapy in patients aged 60 or above using many of the covariates described earlier [121–124]. The author finds the system described by Wheatley et al. [121] convenient (Fig. 1.6), while the Juliusson et al. study makes the point that "intensive therapy," despite the negative connotations attached to "intensive," can be useful in prolonging survival [125]. Experience suggests that the great majority of patients unlikely to do well with standard therapy (e.g., because of MK) will opt for a clinical trial or occasionally supportive care only, rather than standard therapy. Some patients with intermediate prognoses (e.g., a 66-year-old with de novo AML and NK) will prefer standard induction followed by HCT. For the reasons described earlier, others will prefer induction on a clinical trial followed by HCT. As can be inferred from the previous section, it is impossible to know which of the many ongoing trials is best. Hence, the authors advise that patients who prefer investigational therapy to choose a specific trial based on logistics.

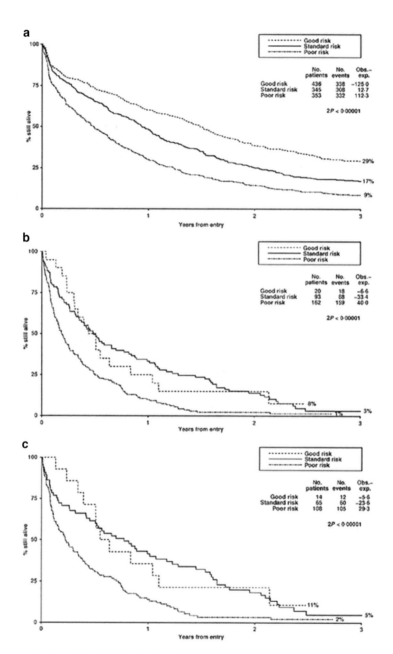

Fig. 1.6 Survival in patients aged ≥60 with newly diagnosed according to risk score calculated as follows: Cytogenetics: 1=favorable/intermediate, 5=unfavorable, 2=unknown WBC: 1=<10, 2=10–49, 3=50–99.9, 4=>100 Performance status: 0, 1, 2, 3, and 4 as per Eastern Cooperative Oncology Group (ECOG) Age: 1=60–64, 2=65–69, 3=70–74, 4=>74 AML type: 1=de novo, 2=secondary Total score: 4–6=better risk, 7–8=standard risk, >8=highest risk System was developed using data from AML11 trial and applied to AML14 trial [121]. (**a**) AML14 intensive: overall survival by AML11 risk group, (**b**) AML14 non-intensive: overall survival by AML11 risk group, (**c**) AML 14 non-intensive (low dose Ara-C patients only): overall survival by AML11 risk group

Management of Relapsed/Refractory AML

Here again the fundamental decision is between a standard (reinduction) regimen such as FLAG or mitoxantrone + etoposide, and an investigational regimen. The principal predictor of response to standard therapy is duration of first CR, with "primary refractory" patients assigned CR duration of 0 [126]. Estey et al. reported that patients about to receive their first reinduction attempt (first salvage) had CR rates of 60% (15 patients), 40% (30 patients), and 15% (160 patients) if their first CR durations were >2 years, 1–2 years, and <1 year, respectively [126]. Patients who were about to receive > first salvage with a first CR <1 year had essentially no chance of attaining a CR (58 patients, 96 salvage attempts, 0 CR). Focusing more on survival, Breems et al. developed a prognostic score based on 667 patients in first relapse [127]. The score accounted for CR duration (>18 months 0 points, 7–18 months 3 points, <7 months 5 points), cytogenetics (inv 16) 0 points, t (8; 21) 3 points, other 5 points, age (<36 0 points, 36–45 1 point, >45 2 points), and prior allogeneic or autologous transplant (no 0 points, yes 2 points). As seen in Fig. 1.7, most patients were in the worst group and clearly are candidates for investigational salvage regimens.

Management of APL

APL is highly curable, although the cure rates of >90% quoted in clinical trials are considerably higher than the rates of 75% reported from large community-hospital databases [128]. The difference, to some extent, reflects patient selection and a

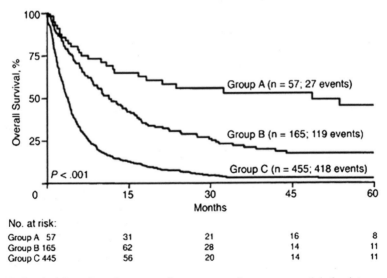

Fig. 1.7 Survival from first relapse according to prognostic score: *group A* 1–6 points, *group B* 7–9 points, *group C* 10–14 points [127]

tendency to exclude patients who die before they can be registered on a trial. Indeed, death from CNS and/or pulmonary hemorrhage within the first few days of presentation is the principal obstacle to curing APL and is particularly common in patients with WBC >10,000. Crucial to prevention of such death is prompt initiation of therapy at earliest suspicion of the diagnosis [129], for example, based on examination of a blood smear, with diagnosis confirmed later by immunostaining with anti-PML monoclonal antibodies or FISH [22]. In addition to specific APL therapy, management consists of redressing the characteristic thrombopenia and deficiencies of coagulation factors, for example, by checking platelet count, INR, and fibrinogen every 8–12 h and administering platelets and blood products to maintain a platelet count >30,000, an INR <1.5, and fibrinogen >150, while avoiding fluid overload. The most commonly used treatment for APL is ATRA + idarubicin ("AIDA") or daunorubicin. However, recent data suggest that in patients presenting with WBC >10,000, addition of Ara-C (200 mg/m^2 daily × 7) to daunorubicin + ATRA improves outcome while patients with WBC <10,000 randomly assigned to Ara-C + daunorubicin + ATRA had superior RFS and survival than similar patients receiving daunorubicin + ATRA [130]. A benefit for Ara-C might have been more difficult to discern with a daunorubicin dose of 90 mg/m^2 (rather than 60 mg/m^2) daily × 3, but benefit/risk calculations argue for adding Ara-C to daunorubicin + ATRA in all patients with APL. It is now established that arsenic trioxide (ATO) is a more effective agent in APL than ATRA; in particular, single agent ATO can cure APL much more frequently than single agent ATRA [131]. The combination of ATO + ATRA appears at least as effective as AIDA in patients with WBC <10,000 and is being compared with AIDA in randomized trials in such patients [132]. For patients with WBC >10,000, consideration should be given to immediate addition of ATO to ATRA + anthracycline + Ara-C. Although routinely unavailable, gemtuzumab ozogamicin is highly effective in APL [133] and is being combined with ATO + ATRA in the current US Intergroup trial for newly diagnosed patients with WBC >10,000. Once in CR, benefit/risk arguments suggest younger patients with initial WBC counts >10,000 should receive postremission therapy with Ara-C in doses of 1–2 g/m^2, which has the added benefit of CSF penetration and hence the potential to prevent CSF relapse, which has a cumulative incidence of 5% 3 years after achievement of CR [134]. Older patients might receive ATO and ATRA (with intrathecal Ara-C if they presented with WBC >10,000) rather than anthracycline + Ara-C; such an approach is being used by several European groups. Finally, MRD monitoring, most sensitively using PCR to detect residual PML-RARα transcripts appears likely to improve outcome, particularly in patients presenting with WBC >10,000 [135].

References

1. Howlader N, Noone AM, Krapcho M, Neyman N, Aminou R, Waldron W, Altekruse SF, Kosary CL, Ruhl J, Tatalovich Z, Cho H, Mariotto A, Eisner MP, Lewis DR, Chen HS, Feuer EJ, Cronin KA, Edwards BK, editors. SEER cancer statistics review, 1975–2008. National Cancer Institute, Bethesda. http://seer.cancer.gov/csr/1975_2008/, based on November 2010 SEER data Submission, posted to the SEER web site, 2011.

2. Smith SM, Le Beau MM, Huo D, et al. Clinical-cytogenetic associations in 306 patients with therapy-related myelodysplasia and myeloid leukemia: the University of Chicago series. Blood. 2003;102:43–52.

3. Larson RA, Wang Y, Banerjee M, et al. Prevalence of the inactivating 609C T polymorphism in the NAD(P)H:quinone oxidoreductase (NQO1) gene in patients with primary and therapy-related myeloid leukemia. Blood. 1999;94:803–7.

4. Bolufer P, Collado M, Barragan E, et al. The potential effect of gender in combination with common genetic polymorphisms of drug-metabolizing enzymes on the risk of developing acute leukemia. Haematologica. 2007;92:308–14.

5. Bowen DT, Frew ME, Rollinson S, et al. CYP1A1*2B (Val) allele is overrepresented in a subgroup of acute myeloid leukemia patients with poor-risk karyotype associated with NRAS mutation, but not associated with FLT3 internal tandem duplication. Blood. 2003;101:2770–4.

6. Mardis ER, Ding L, Dooling DJ, et al. Recurring mutations found by sequencing an acute myeloid leukemia genome. N Engl J Med. 2009;361:1058–66.

7. Downing JR. Cancer genomes – continuing progress. N Engl J Med. 2009;361:1111–2.

8. Ley TJ, Mardis ER, Ding L, Wilson RK, et al. DNA sequencing of a cytogenetically normal acute myeloid leukaemia genome. Nature. 2008;456:66–72.

9. Figueroa ME, Lugthart S, Li Y, et al. DNA methylation signatures identify biologically distinct subtypes in acute myeloid leukemia. Cancer Cell. 2010;17:13–27.

10. Figueroa ME, Abdel-Wahab O, Lu C, et al. Leukemic IDH1 and IDH2 mutations result in a hypermethylation phenotype, disrupt TET2 function, and impair hematopoietic differentiation. Cancer Cell. 2010;18:553–67.

11. Ramsingh G, Koboldt DC, Trissal M, et al. Complete characterization of the microRNAome in a patient with acute myeloid leukemia. Blood. 2010;116:5316–26.

12. Lapidot T, Sirard C, Vormoor J, et al. A cell initiating human acute myeloid leukaemia after transplantation into SCID mice. Nature. 1994;367:645–8.

13. Gentles AJ, Plevritis SK, Majeti R, Alizadeh AA. Association of a leukemic stem cell gene expression signature with clinical outcomes in acute myeloid leukemia. JAMA. 2010;304:2706–15.

14. Kolb HJ. Graft-versus-leukemia effects of transplantation and donor lymphocytes. Blood. 2008;112:4371–83.

15. Matutes E, Morilla R, Farahat N, Carbonell F, Swansbury J, Dyer M, Catovsky D. Definition of acute biphenotypic leukemia. Haematologica. 1997;82:64–6.

16. Bene MC, Castoldi G, Knapp W, et al. Proposals for the immunological classification of acute leukemias. European Group for the Immunological Characterization of Leukemias (EGIL). Leukemia. 1995;9:1783–6.

17. Xu XQ, Wang JM, Lu SQ, et al. Clinical and biological characteristics of adult biphenotypic acute leukemia in comparison with that of acute myeloid leukemia and acute lymphoblastic leukemia: a case series of a Chinese population. Haematologica. 2009;94:919–27.

18. Legrand O, Perrot JY, Simonin G, et al. Adult biphenotypic acute leukaemia: an entity with poor prognosis which is related to unfavourable cytogenetics and P-glycoprotein over-expression. Br J Haematol. 1998;100:147–55.

19. Aribi A, Bueso-Ramos C, Estey E, et al. Biphenotypic acute leukaemia: a case series. Br J Haematol. 2007;138:213–6.

20. Bennett JM, Catovsky D, Daniel MT, et al. Proposals for the classification of the acute leukaemias. French-American-British (FAB) Co-operative Group. Br J Haematol. 1976;33:451–8.

21. Estey E, Thall P, Beran M, Kantarjian H, Pierce S, Keating M. Effect of diagnosis (refractory anemia with excess blasts, refractory anemia with excess blasts in transformation, or acute myeloid leukemia [AML]) on outcome of AML-type chemotherapy. Blood. 1997;90:2969–77.

22. Sanz MA, Grimwade D, Tallman MS, et al. Management of acute promyelocytic leukemia: recommendations from an expert panel on behalf of the European LeukemiaNet. Blood. 2009;113:1875–91.

23. Giles FJ, Shen Y, Kantarjian HM, et al. Leukapheresis reduces early mortality in patients with acute myeloid leukemia with high white cell counts but does not improve long-term survival. Leuk Lymphoma. 2001;42:67–73.

24. Dohner H, Estey EH, Amadori S, et al. Diagnosis and management of acute myeloid leukemia in adults: recommendations from an international expert panel, on behalf of the European LeukemiaNet. Blood. 2010;115:453–74.
25. de Lima M, Strom SS, Keating M, et al. Implications of potential cure in acute myelogenous leukemia: development of subsequent cancer and return to work. Blood. 1997;90:4719–24.
26. Freireich EJ, Gehan EA, Sulman D, Boggs DR, Frei 3rd E. The effect of chemotherapy on acute leukemia in the human. J Chronic Dis. 1961;14:593–608.
27. Cheson BD, Bennett JM, Kopecky KJ, et al. Revised recommendations of the international working group for diagnosis, standardization of response criteria, treatment outcomes, and reporting standards for therapeutic trials in acute myeloid leukemia. J Clin Oncol. 2003;21: 4642–9.
28. Cheson BD, Bennett JM, Kantarjian H, et al. Report of an international working group to standardize response criteria for myelodysplastic syndromes. Blood. 2000;96:3671–4.
29. Walter RB, Kantarjian HM, Huang X, et al. Effect of complete remission and responses less than complete remission on survival in acute myeloid leukemia: a combined Eastern Cooperative Oncology Group, Southwest Oncology Group, and M. D. Anderson Cancer Center Study. J Clin Oncol. 2010;28:1766–71.
30. Cassileth PA, Harrington DP, Hines JD, et al. Maintenance chemotherapy prolongs remission duration in adult acute nonlymphocytic leukemia. J Clin Oncol. 1988;6:583–7.
31. Gardin C, Turlure P, Fagot T, et al. Postremission treatment of elderly patients with acute myeloid leukemia in first complete remission after intensive induction chemotherapy: results of the multicenter randomized Acute Leukemia French Association (ALFA) 9803 trial. Blood. 2007;109:5129–35.
32. Fernandez HF, Sun Z, Yao X, et al. Anthracycline dose intensification in acute myeloid leukemia. N Engl J Med. 2009;361:1249–59.
33. Lowenberg B, Ossenkoppele GJ, van Putten W, et al. High-dose daunorubicin in older patients with acute myeloid leukemia. N Engl J Med. 2009;361:1235–48.
34. Lowenberg B, Pabst T, Vellenga E, et al. Cytarabine dose for acute myeloid leukemia. N Engl J Med. 2011;364:1027–36.
35. Burnett AK, Hills RK, Milligan DW, et al. Attempts to optimize induction and consolidation treatment in acute myeloid leukemia: results of the MRC AML12 trial. J Clin Oncol. 2010;28:586–95.
36. Ohtake S, Miyawaki S, Fujita H, et al. Randomized study of induction therapy comparing standard-dose idarubicin with high-dose daunorubicin in adult patients with previously untreated acute myeloid leukemia: the JALSG AML201 study. Blood. 2011;117:2358–65.
37. Estey E. High cytogenetic or molecular genetic risk acute myeloid leukemia. Hematol Am Soc Hematol Educ Progr. 2010;2010:474–80.
38. Walter R, Othus M, Borthakur G, et al. Quantitative effect of age in predicting empirically-defined treatment-related mortality and resistance in newly diagnosed AML: case against age alone as primary determinant of treatment assignment [ASH abstract 2191]. Blood. 2010;116(21):904.
39. Sorror M. Impacts of pretransplant comorbidities on allogeneic hematopoietic cell transplantation (HCT) outcomes. Biol Blood Marrow Transplant. 2009;15:149–53.
40. Sorror ML. Comorbidities and hematopoietic cell transplantation outcomes. Hematol Am Soc Hematol Educ Progr. 2010;2010:237–47.
41. Appelbaum FR, Gundacker H, Head DR, et al. Age and acute myeloid leukemia. Blood. 2006;107:3481–5.
42. Yanada M, Garcia-Manero G, Borthakur G, Ravandi F, Kantarjian H, Estey E. Relapse and death during first remission in acute myeloid leukemia. Haematologica. 2008;93:633–4.
43. Breems DA, Van Putten WL, De Greef GE, et al. Monosomal karyotype in acute myeloid leukemia: a better indicator of poor prognosis than a complex karyotype. J Clin Oncol. 2008;26:4791–7.
44. Medeiros BC, Othus M, Fang M, Roulston D, Appelbaum FR. Prognostic impact of monosomal karyotype in young adult and elderly acute myeloid leukemia: the Southwest Oncology Group (SWOG) experience. Blood. 2010;116:2224–8.

45. Coleman JF, Theil KS, Tubbs RR, Cook JR. Diagnostic yield of bone marrow and peripheral blood FISH panel testing in clinically suspected myelodysplastic syndromes and/or acute myeloid leukemia: a prospective analysis of 433 cases. Am J Clin Pathol. 2011;135:915–20.
46. Grimwade D, Hills RK, Moorman AV, et al. Refinement of cytogenetic classification in acute myeloid leukemia: determination of prognostic significance of rare recurring chromosomal abnormalities among 5876 younger adult patients treated in the United Kingdom Medical Research Council trials. Blood. 2010;116:354–65.
47. Tallman MS, Hakimian D, Shaw JM, Lissner GS, Russell EJ, Variakojis D. Granulocytic sarcoma is associated with the 8;21 translocation in acute myeloid leukemia. J Clin Oncol. 1993;11:690–7.
48. Marcucci G, Mrozek K, Ruppert AS, et al. Prognostic factors and outcome of core binding factor acute myeloid leukemia patients with t(8;21) differ from those of patients with inv(16): a Cancer and Leukemia Group B study. J Clin Oncol. 2005;23:5705–17.
49. Bloomfield CD, Lawrence D, Byrd JC, et al. Frequency of prolonged remission duration after high-dose cytarabine intensification in acute myeloid leukemia varies by cytogenetic sub-type. Cancer Res. 1998;58:4173–9.
50. Borthakur G, Kantarjian H, Wang X, et al. Treatment of core-binding-factor in acute myelog-enous leukemia with fludarabine, cytarabine, and granulocyte colony-stimulating factor results in improved event-free survival. Cancer. 2008;113:3181–5.
51. Petersdorf S, Kopecky K, Stuart RK, et al. Preliminary results of Southwest Oncology Group Study S0106: an international intergroup phase 3 randomized trial comparing the addition of gemtuzumab ozogamicin to standard induction therapy versus standard induction therapy followed by a second randomization to post-consolidation gemtuzumab ozogamicin versus no additional therapy for previously untreated acute myeloid leukemia [ASH abstract 790]. Blood. 2009;114:326.
52. Burnett AK, Hills RK, Milligan D, et al. Identification of patients with acute myeloblastic leukemia who benefit from the addition of gemtuzumab ozogamicin: results of the MRC AML15 trial. J Clin Oncol. 2011;29:369–77.
53. Appelbaum FR, Kopecky KJ, Tallman MS, et al. The clinical spectrum of adult acute myeloid leukaemia associated with core binding factor translocations. Br J Haematol. 2006;135:165–73.
54. Delaunay J, Vey N, Leblanc T, et al. Prognosis of inv(16)/t(16;16) acute myeloid leukemia (AML): a survey of 110 cases from the French AML Intergroup. Blood. 2003;102:462–9.
55. Prebet T, Boissel N, Reutenauer S, et al. Acute myeloid leukemia with translocation (8;21) or inversion (16) in elderly patients treated with conventional chemotherapy: a collaborative study of the French CBF-AML Intergroup. J Clin Oncol. 2009;27:4747–53.
56. Nguyen S, Leblanc T, Fenaux P, et al. A white blood cell index as the main prognostic factor in t(8;21) acute myeloid leukemia (AML): a survey of 161 cases from the French AML Intergroup. Blood. 2002;99:3517–23.
57. Paschka P, Marcucci G, Ruppert AS, Mrozek K, Chen H, Kittles RA, Vukosavljevic T, Perrotti D, Vardiman JW, Carroll AJ, Kolitz JE, Larson RA, Bloomfield CD. Adverse prog-nostic significance of KIT mutations in adult acute myeloid leukemia with inv(16) and t(8;21): a Cancer and Leukemia Group B study. J Clin Oncol. 2006;24:3904–11.
58. Schnittger S, Kohl TM, Haferlach T, Kern W, Hiddemann W, Spiekermann K, Schoch C. KIT-D816 mutations in AML1-ETO-positive AML are associated with impaired event-free and overall survival. Blood. 2006;107:1791–9.
59. Pollard JA, Alonzo TA, Gerbing RB, Ho PA, Zeng R, Ravindranath Y, Dahl G, Lacayo NJ, Becton D, Chang M, Weinstein HJ, Hirsch B, Raimondi SC, Heerema NA, Woods WG, Lange BJ, Hurwitz C, Arceci RJ, Radich JP, Bernstein ID, Heinrich MC, Meshinchi S. Prevalence and prognostic significance of KIT mutations in pediatric patients with core bind-ing factor AML enrolled on serial pediatric cooperative trials for de novo AML. Blood. 2010;115:2372–9.
60. Slovak ML, Kopecky KJ, Cassileth PA, Harrington DH, Theil KS, Mohamed A, Paietta E, Willman CL, Head DR, Rowe JM, Forman SJ, Appelbaum FR. Karyotypic analysis predicts

outcome of preremission and postremission therapy in adult acute myeloid leukemia: a Southwest Oncology Group/Eastern Cooperative Oncology Group Study. Blood. 2000; 96:4075–83.

61. Schlenk RF, Dohner K, Krauter J, Frohling S, Corbacioglu A, Bullinger L, Habdank M, Spath D, Morgan M, Benner A, Schlegelberger B, Heil G, Ganser A, Dohner H. Mutations and treatment outcome in cytogenetically normal acute myeloid leukemia. N Engl J Med. 2008;358:1909–18.

62. Becker H, Marcucci G, Maharry K, Radmacher MD, Mrozek K, Margeson D, Whitman SP, Wu YZ, Schwind S, Paschka P, Powell BL, Carter TH, Kolitz JE, Wetzler M, Carroll AJ, Baer MR, Caligiuri MA, Larson RA, Bloomfield CD. Favorable prognostic impact of NPM1 mutations in older patients with cytogenetically normal de novo acute myeloid leukemia and associated gene- and microRNA-expression signatures: a Cancer and Leukemia Group B study. J Clin Oncol. 2010;28:596–604.

63. Gale RE, Green C, Allen C, Mead AJ, Burnett AK, Hills RK, Linch DC. The impact of FLT3 internal tandem duplication mutant level, number, size, and interaction with NPM1 mutations in a large cohort of young adult patients with acute myeloid leukemia. Blood. 2008;111:2776–84.

64. Burnett A, Wetzler M, Lowenberg B. Therapeutic advances in acute myeloid leukemia. J Clin Oncol. 2011;29:487–94.

65. Marcucci G, Haferlach T, Dohner H. Molecular genetics of adult acute myeloid leukemia: prognostic and therapeutic implications. J Clin Oncol. 2011;29:475–86.

66. Hou HA, Huang TC, Lin LI, et al. WT1 Mutation in 470 adult patients with acute myeloid leukemia: stability during disease evolution and implication of its incorporation into a survival scoring system. Blood. 2010;115:5222–31.

67. Gaidzik VI, Schlenk RF, Moschny S, et al. Prognostic impact of WT1 mutations in cytogenetically normal acute myeloid leukemia: a study of the German-Austrian AML Study Group. Blood. 2009;113:4505–11.

68. Metzeler KH, Maharry K, Radmacher MD, et al. TET2 Mutations improve the new European LeukemiaNet risk classification of acute myeloid leukemia: a Cancer and Leukemia Group B study. J Clin Oncol. 2011;29:1373–81.

69. Marcucci G, Maharry K, Wu YZ, et al. IDH1 And IDH2 gene mutations identify novel molecular subsets within de novo cytogenetically normal acute myeloid leukemia: a Cancer and Leukemia Group B study. J Clin Oncol. 2010;28:2348–55.

70. Wagner K, Damm F, Gohring G, et al. Impact of IDH1 R132 mutations and an IDH1 single nucleotide polymorphism in cytogenetically normal acute myeloid leukemia: SNP rs11554137 is an adverse prognostic factor. J Clin Oncol. 2010;28:2356–64.

71. Ley TJ, Ding L, Walter MJ, et al. DNMT3A mutations in acute myeloid leukemia. N Engl J Med. 2010;363:2424–33.

72. Metzeler KH, Hummel M, Bloomfield CD, et al. An 86-probe-set gene-expression signature predicts survival in cytogenetically normal acute myeloid leukemia. Blood. 2008;112:4193–201.

73. Marcucci G, Radmacher MD, Maharry K, et al. MicroRNA expression in cytogenetically normal acute myeloid leukemia. N Engl J Med. 2008;358:1919–28.

74. Garzon R, Volinia S, Liu CG, et al. MicroRNA signatures associated with cytogenetics and prognosis in acute myeloid leukemia. Blood. 2008;111:3183–9.

75. Bullinger L, Ehrich M, Dohner K, et al. Quantitative DNA methylation predicts survival in adult acute myeloid leukemia. Blood. 2010;115:636–42.

76. Kornblau SM, Tibes R, Qiu YH, et al. Functional proteomic profiling of AML predicts response and survival. Blood. 2009;113:154–64.

77. Kayser S, Dohner K, Krauter J, et al. The impact of therapy-related acute myeloid leukemia (AML) on outcome in 2853 adult patients with newly diagnosed AML. Blood. 2011;117: 2137–45.

78. Woods WG, Kobrinsky N, Buckley JD, et al. Timed-sequential induction therapy improves postremission outcome in acute myeloid leukemia: a report from the Children's Cancer Group. Blood. 1996;87:4979–89.

79. Walter RB, Gooley TA, Wood BL, et al. Impact of pretransplantation minimal residual disease, as detected by multiparametric flow cytometry, on outcome of myeloablative hematopoietic cell transplantation for acute myeloid leukemia. J Clin Oncol. 2011;29:1190–7.

80. Sekeres MA, Elson P, Kalaycio ME, et al. Time from diagnosis to treatment initiation predicts survival in younger, but not older, acute myeloid leukemia patients. Blood. 2009;113:28–36.

81. Keating MJ, Smith TL, Gehan EA, et al. Factors related to length of complete remission in adult acute leukemia. Cancer. 1980;45:2017–29.

82. Rowe JM, Kim HT, Cassileth PA, et al. Adult patients with acute myeloid leukemia who achieve complete remission after 1 or 2 cycles of induction have a similar prognosis: a report on 1980 patients registered to 6 studies conducted by the Eastern Cooperative Oncology Group. Cancer. 1980;116:5012–21.

83. Kern W, Haferlach C, Haferlach T, Schnittger S. Monitoring of minimal residual disease in acute myeloid leukemia. Cancer. 2008;112:4–16.

84. Cilloni D, Renneville A, Hermitte F, et al. Real-time quantitative polymerase chain reaction detection of minimal residual disease by standardized WT1 assay to enhance risk stratification in acute myeloid leukemia: a European LeukemiaNet study. J Clin Oncol. 2009;27:5195–201.

85. Kronke J, Schlenk RF, Jensen KO, Tschurtz F, Corbacioglu A, Gaidzik VI, Paschka P, Onken S, Eiwen K, Habdank M, Spath D, Lubbert M, Wattad M, Kindler T, Salih HR, Held G, Nachbaur D, von Lilienfeld-Toal M, Germing U, Haase D, Mergenthaler HG, Krauter J, Ganser A, Gohring G, Schlegelberger B, Dohner H, Dohner K. Monitoring of minimal residual disease in NPM1-mutated acute myeloid leukemia: a study from the German-Austrian Acute Myeloid Leukemia Study Group. J Clin Oncol. 2011;29(19):2709–16. Epub 2011 May 9.

86. Wheatley K, Gray R. Commentary: Mendelian randomization – an update on its use to evaluate allogeneic stem cell transplantation in leukaemia. Int J Epidemiol. 2004;33:15–7.

87. Mantel N, Byar DB. Evaluation of response time data involving transient states: an illustration using heart-transplantation data. J Am Stat Assoc. 1974;69:81–6.

88. Koreth J, Schlenk R, Kopecky KJ, et al. Allogeneic stem cell transplantation for acute myeloid leukemia in first complete remission: systematic review and meta-analysis of prospective clinical trials. JAMA. 2009;301:2349–61.

89. Burnett AK, Goldstone AH, Stevens RM, et al. Randomised comparison of addition of autologous bone-marrow transplantation to intensive chemotherapy for acute myeloid leukaemia in first remission: results of MRC AML 10 trial. UK Medical Research Council Adult and Children's Leukaemia Working Parties. Lancet. 1998;351:700–8.

90. Appelbaum FR. Incorporating hematopoietic cell transplantation (HCT) into the management of adults aged under 60 years with acute myeloid leukemia (AML). Best Pract Res Clin Haematol. 2008;21:85–92.

91. Martin PJ, Counts Jr GW, Appelbaum FR, et al. Life expectancy in patients surviving more than 5 years after hematopoietic cell transplantation. J Clin Oncol. 2010;28:1011–6.

92. Gale R, Hills R, Wheatley K, Burnett A, Linch D. Response: still a need for more robust evidence that FLT3/ITD status should influence the decision to proceed to transplantation in AML patients. Blood. 2007;109 (5):2265.

93. Horowitz MM. High-resolution typing for unrelated donor transplantation: how far do we go? Best Pract Res Clin Haematol. 2009;22:537–41.

94. Basara N, Schulze A, Wedding U, et al. Early related or unrelated haematopoietic cell transplantation results in higher overall survival and leukaemia-free survival compared with conventional chemotherapy in high-risk acute myeloid leukaemia patients in first complete remission. Leukemia. 2009;23:635–40.

95. Schlenk RF, Dohner K, Mack S, et al. Prospective evaluation of allogeneic hematopoietic stem-cell transplantation from matched related and matched unrelated donors in younger adults with high-risk acute myeloid leukemia: German-Austrian trial AMLHD98A. J Clin Oncol. 2010;28:4642–8.

96. Wagner JE. Should double cord blood transplants be the preferred choice when a sibling donor is unavailable? Best Pract Res Clin Haematol. 2009;22:551–5.

97. Storb R. Reduced-intensity conditioning transplantation in myeloid malignancies. Curr Opin Oncol. 2009;21 Suppl 1:S3–5.
98. Gyurkocza B, Storb R, Storer BE, et al. Nonmyeloablative allogeneic hematopoietic cell transplantation in patients with acute myeloid leukemia. J Clin Oncol. 2010;28:2859–67.
99. Mohty M, de Lavallade H, Ladaique P, et al. The role of reduced intensity conditioning allogeneic stem cell transplantation in patients with acute myeloid leukemia: a donor vs no donor comparison. Leukemia. 2005;19:916–20.
100. Estey E, de Lima M, Tibes R, et al. Prospective feasibility analysis of reduced-intensity conditioning (RIC) regimens for hematopoietic stem cell transplantation (HSCT) in elderly patients with acute myeloid leukemia (AML) and high-risk myelodysplastic syndrome (MDS). Blood. 2007;109:1395–400.
101. Gooley TA, Chien JW, Pergam SA, et al. Reduced mortality after allogeneic hematopoietic-cell transplantation. N Engl J Med. 2010;363:2091–101.
102. Holowiecki J, Grosicki S, Robak T, et al. Addition of cladribine to daunorubicin and cytarabine increases complete remission rate after a single course of induction treatment in acute myeloid leukemia. Multicenter, phase III study. Leukemia. 2004;18:989–97.
103. Becker PS, Kantarjian H, Appelbaum FR, et al. Multivariate analysis of response and survival after treatment with clofarabine, c and G-CSF priming (BCLAC) in relapsed/refractory acute myeloid leukemia (AML): comparison with prior experience using fludarabine and cytarabine combination regimens [ASH abstract 1065]. Blood. 2010;116(21):466.
104. Burnett AK, Russell NH, Kell J, et al. European development of clofarabine as treatment for older patients with acute myeloid leukemia considered unsuitable for intensive chemotherapy. J Clin Oncol. 2010;28:2389–95.
105. Faderl S, Ravandi F, Huang X, et al. A randomized study of clofarabine versus clofarabine plus low-dose cytarabine as front-line therapy for patients aged 60 years and older with acute myeloid leukemia and high-risk myelodysplastic syndrome. Blood. 2008;112:1638–45.
106. Fenaux P, Mufti GJ, Hellstrom-Lindberg E, et al. Azacitidine prolongs overall survival compared with conventional care regimens in elderly patients with low bone marrow blast count acute myeloid leukemia. J Clin Oncol. 2010;28:562–9.
107. Cashen AF, Schiller GJ, O'Donnell MR, DiPersio JF. Multicenter, phase II study of decitabine for the first-line treatment of older patients with acute myeloid leukemia. J Clin Oncol. 2010;28:556–61.
108. Thomas XG. Results from a randomized phase III trial of decitabine versus supportive care or low-dose cytarabine for the treatment of older patients with newly diagnosed AML [ASCO abstract 6504]. J Clin Oncol. 2011;29.
109. Blum W, Garzon R, Klisovic RB, et al. Clinical response and miR-29b predictive significance in older AML patients treated with a 10-day schedule of decitabine. Proc Natl Acad Sci USA. 2010;107:7473–8.
110. Levis M, Ravandi F, Wang ES, et al. Results from a randomized trial of salvage chemotherapy followed by lestaurtinib for patients with FLT3 mutant AML in first relapse. Blood. 2011;117:3294–301.
111. Cortes J, Foran J, Ghirdaladze D, et al. AC220, a potent, selective, second generation FLT3 receptor tyrosine kinase (RTK) inhibitor, in a first-in-human (FIH) phase 1 AML study [ASH abstract 636]. Blood. 2009;114(22):264.
112. Ravandi F, Cortes JE, Jones D, et al. Phase I/II study of combination therapy with sorafenib, idarubicin, and cytarabine in younger patients with acute myeloid leukemia. J Clin Oncol. 2010;28:1856–62.
113. Serve H, Wagner R, Sauerland C, et al. Sorafenib in combination with standard induction and consolidation therapy in elderly AML patients: results from a randomized, placebo-controlled phase II trial [ASH abstract 333]. Blood. 2010;116(21):151.
114. Levis M. FLT3/ITD AML and the law of unintended consequences. Blood. 2011;117(26):6987–90. Epub 2011 May 17.

115. Pagel JM, Gooley TA, Rajendran J, et al. Allogeneic hematopoietic cell transplantation after conditioning with 131I-anti-CD45 antibody plus fludarabine and low-dose total body irradiation for elderly patients with advanced acute myeloid leukemia or high-risk myelodysplastic syndrome. Blood. 2009;114:5444–53.

116. Warren EH, Fujii N, Akatsuka Y, et al. Therapy of relapsed leukemia after allogeneic hematopoietic cell transplantation with T cells specific for minor histocompatibility antigens. Blood. 2010;115:3869–78.

117. Brune M, Castaigne S, Catalano J, et al. Improved leukemia-free survival after postconsolidation immunotherapy with histamine dihydrochloride and interleukin-2 in acute myeloid leukemia: results of a randomized phase 3 trial. Blood. 2006;108:88–96.

118. Konopleva MY, Jordan CT. Leukemia stem cells and microenvironment: biology and therapeutic targeting. J Clin Oncol. 2011;29:591–9.

119. de Lima M, Giralt S, Thall PF, et al. Maintenance therapy with low-dose azacitidine after allogeneic hematopoietic stem cell transplantation for recurrent acute myelogenous leukemia or myelodysplastic syndrome: a dose and schedule finding study. Cancer. 2010;116: 5420–31.

120. Walter RB, Appelbaum FR, Tallman MS, Weiss NS, Larson RA, Estey EH. Shortcomings in the clinical evaluation of new drugs: acute myeloid leukemia as paradigm. Blood. 2010; 116:2420–8.

121. Wheatley K, Brookes CL, Howman AJ, et al. Prognostic factor analysis of the survival of elderly patients with AML in the MRC AML11 and LRF AML14 trials. Br J Haematol. 2009;145:598–605.

122. Malfuson JV, Etienne A, Turlure P, et al. Risk factors and decision criteria for intensive chemotherapy in older patients with acute myeloid leukemia. Haematologica. 2008;93:1806–13.

123. Kantarjian H, Ravandi F, O'Brien S, et al. Intensive chemotherapy does not benefit most older patients (age 70 years or older) with acute myeloid leukemia. Blood. 2010;116:4422–9.

124. Krug U, Rollig C, Koschmieder A, et al. Complete remission and early death after intensive chemotherapy in patients aged 60 years or older with acute myeloid leukaemia: a web-based application for prediction of outcomes. Lancet. 2010;376:2000–8.

125. Juliusson G, Antunovic P, Derolf A, et al. Age and acute myeloid leukemia: real world data on decision to treat and outcomes from the Swedish Acute Leukemia Registry. Blood. 2009;113:4179–87.

126. Estey E, Kornblau S, Pierce S, Kantarjian H, Beran M, Keating M. A stratification system for evaluating and selecting therapies in patients with relapsed or primary refractory acute myelogenous leukemia. Blood. 1996;88:756.

127. Breems DA, Van Putten WL, Huijgens PC, et al. Prognostic index for adult patients with acute myeloid leukemia in first relapse. J Clin Oncol. 2005;23:1969–78.

128. Park JH, Qiao B, Panageas KS, Schymura MJ, Jurcic JG, Rosenblat TL, Altman JK, Douer D, Rowe JM, Tallman MS. Early death rate in acute promyelocytic leukemia remains high despite all-trans retinoic acid. Blood. 2011;118(5):1248–54. Epub 2011 Jun 8.

129. Breccia M, Latagliata R, Cannella L, Minotti C, Meloni G, Lo-Coco F. Early hemorrhagic death before starting therapy in acute promyelocytic leukemia: association with high WBC count, late diagnosis and delayed treatment initiation. Haematologica. 2010;95:853–4.

130. Ades L, Raffoux E, Chevret S, et al. Is AraC required in the treatment of standard risk APL? Long term results of a randomized trial (APL 2000) from the French Belgian Swiss APL Group [ASH abstract 13]. Blood. 2010;116(21):11.

131. Ghavamzadeh A, Alimoghaddam K, Shahrbano R, et al. Phase II study of single agent arsenic trioxide for the frontline therapy of acute promyelocytic leukemia. J Clin Oncol. 2011; 29(20):2753–7.

132. Ravandi F, Estey EH, Cortes JE, et al. Phase II study of all-trans-retinoic acid and arsenic trioxide, with or without gemtuzumab ozogamicin, for the front-line therapy of patients with acute promyelocytic leukemia [ASH abstract 1080]. Blood. 2010;116(21):473.

133. Estey EH, Giles FJ, Beran M, et al. Experience with gemtuzumab ozogamicin ("mylotarg") and all-trans retinoic acid in untreated acute promyelocytic leukemia. Blood. 2002;99: 4222–4.
134. de Botton S, Sanz MA, Chevret S. Extramedullary relapse in acute promyelocytic leukemia treated with all-trans retinoic acid and chemotherapy. Leukemia. 2006;20:35–41.
135. Lo-Coco F, Cimino G, Breccia M, et al. Gemtuzumab ozogamicin (Mylotarg) as a single agent for molecularly relapsed acute promyelocytic leukemia. Blood. 2004;104:1995–9.

Chapter 2
The Treatment of Adult Acute Lymphoblastic Leukemia (ALL): Risk Stratification and Strategies

Andrei R. Shustov

Abstract Acute lymphoblastic leukemia (ALL) is a highly aggressive neoplasm of precursor cells (lymphoblasts) committed to the lymphoid B-cell or T-cell lineage. It is significantly more prevalent in children, representing nearly 25% of all childhood cancers, but accounting for only 1% of all adult malignancies. The peak prevalence of ALL falls between the ages of 2 and 5 years, and 75% of all cases occur in children under the age of 6 years. The estimated number of new cases in the United States in 2008 was approximately 5,400, and 1,460 people died of their disease.

Keywords Acute lymphoblastic leukemia • Chemotherapy • Bone marrow transplantation

Introduction

Acute lymphoblastic leukemia (ALL) is a highly aggressive neoplasm of precursor cells (lymphoblasts) committed to the lymphoid B-cell or T-cell lineage. It is significantly more prevalent in children, representing nearly 25% of all childhood cancers, but accounting for only 1% of all adult malignancies. The peak prevalence of ALL falls between the ages of 2 and 5 years, and 75% of all cases occur in children under the age of 6 years. The estimated number of new cases in the United States in 2008 was approximately 5,400, and 1,460 people died of their disease. Precursor B-cell type comprised 80–85% of these cases. In 2008, World Health Organization (WHO) Classification of Hematologic Malignancies, lymphoblastic lymphoma (LBL) is merged with ALL underscoring the unity between the two entities in

A.R. Shustov, M.D. (✉)
Division of Hematology, University of Washington School of Medicine,
825 Eastlake Ave E, Seattle, WA 98109, USA
e-mail: ashustov@fhcrc.org

E.H. Estey and F.R. Appelbaum (eds.), *Leukemia and Related Disorders: Integrated Treatment Approaches*, Contemporary Hematology,
DOI 10.1007/978-1-60761-565-1_2, © Springer Science+Business Media, LLC 2012

Table 2.1 World Health Organization (*WHO*) and European Group for Immunological Characterization of Leukemias (*EGIL*) classification of acute lymphoblastic leukemia

2008-WHO (B-ALL)	EGIL (T-ALL)
t(9;22)(q34;q11.2); BCR-ABL1	TI, pro-T-ALL; CD7+
t(v;11q23); MLL-rearranged	TII, pre-T-ALL; CD7+ CD2+ CD5±
t(12;21)(p13;q22); TEL-AML1	TIII, cortical T-ALL; CD7+ CD2+ CD1a+
B-ALL with hyperploidy >50	TIV, mature T-ALL; CD7+ CD2+ CD3+ CD1a–
B-ALL with hypoploidy	
t(5;14)(q31;q32); IL3-IGH	

MLL myeloid lymphoid leukemia

biology, natural history, and outcomes. By convention, the term lymphoma is used when the process is confined to nodal or extranodal sites with no or minimal peripheral blood (PB) and bone marrow (BM) involvement. If the patient presents with both, nodal masses and lymphoblasts in the BM, the distinction is arbitrary. The term B-cell ALL/LBL should not be used to define Burkitt leukemia/lymphoma despite its histologic similarities and historic association. The latter is a highly aggressive mature B-cell neoplasm.

Morphologically, both, B-cell and T-cell ALL/LBL blasts can vary from small-/medium-sized cells with scant cytoplasm, moderately condensed nuclear chromatin and indistinct nucleoli, to larger cells with a moderate amount of cytoplasm, occasionally vacuolated, dispersed nuclear chromatin, and multiple prominent nucleoli. Under light microscopy, B-cell and T-cell lymphoblasts are indistinguishable, and immunophenotyping is necessary to establish correct histologic diagnosis.

Overall, ALL/LBL is a heterogeneous group of malignancies with regard to immunophenotype, cytogenetics, molecular genetic abnormalities, clinical features, response to therapy, and prognosis, comprising several clinical-biological entities. The WHO Classification of hematologic malignancies recognizes several distinct subtypes of B-cell ALL, based on recurrent cytogenetic abnormalities; while the European EGIL classification is most commonly used to define the variants of T-cell ALL, based predominantly on immunophenotype, reflecting the stage of thymic maturation of lymphoblasts (Table 2.1). This chapter will examine the evidence supporting current risk stratification, modern treatment strategies for Ph⁻ and Ph⁺ ALL, novel chemotherapeutic and biologic agents under development, and the role of allogeneic HCT in adult ALL, as well as comment on special clinical challenges.

Trends in Treatment Outcomes

ALL has a good prognosis in children, but a much less favorable one in adults. Complete remission (CR) can be expected in >95% of pediatric patients, and approximately 80% of children appear to be cured. Initial response rates to modern combination chemotherapy in adults are almost as high as those seen in children.

However, chance of relapse and the risk of treatment-related mortality are both considerably higher in adults than in children [1]. The pressing question is whether different outcomes in childhood and adult ALL are determined by differences in disease biology or result from a different approach to or tolerance of therapy. There are evident changes in biology of the disease with age; most notably, the incidence of "high-risk" cytogenetic categories, such as Philadelphia-chromosome-positive (Ph+) ALL, accounts for 20–30% of adult ALL cases [2], while it is uncommon (3–4%) in children [3]. Conversely, there is an accumulating body of evidence suggesting that a "pediatric approach" to therapy might give superior survival than an "adult approach" in adolescents and young adults with ALL [4–6]. Prospective non-randomized studies evaluating "pediatric approaches" in adult patients up to 30 years of age (Cancer and Leukemia Group B, CALG-B) or even 50 years (Dana-Farber Cancer Institute, DFCI) have been initiated. In addition, there is a great paucity of evidence regarding appropriate therapy of elderly ALL patients (>65 years) since very few studies have included this age group. Hence, the most appropriate therapy for older adults with ALL is unknown.

Despite the relatively low incidence of ALL in adults, substantial progress in outcomes has been made in the late twentieth and early twenty-first century in large part due to large national and international collaborations. Recent reports indicate positive trends in survival with an age-dependent increase of 14–20% in the years 2000–2004 compared with 1980–1984 (Fig. 2.1) [7, 8]. Improvement in up-front risk stratification, intensification of induction phase of treatment protocols, aggressive management of central nervous system (CNS) disease, early referral for allogeneic hematopoietic cell transplantation (HCT) for high-risk ALL, improvements in supportive care, as well as introduction of new targeted therapy have all contributed to continuous progress in adult ALL patients. In addition, a multitude of new chemotherapeutic and targeted biologic agents have entered human clinical trials fostering further improvement in adult ALL care. These changes, as well as the multitude of ongoing clinical trials, bring hope to both ALL patients and treating oncologists that in the foreseeable future, adult ALL will join the list of cancers that have succumbed to effective treatment.

Prognostic Factors and Risk Stratification

Careful assessment of the risk of relapse in individual ALL patients ensures that very intensive and, hence, potentially detrimental treatments are given only to high-risk cases, thus avoiding undue excessive toxicities and treatment-related mortality. Although intensified treatment protocols have abolished the prognostic strength of many clinical and biologic factors identified in the past, e.g., the prognostic significance of T-cell phenotype, it is important to stress that even "standard-risk" or "low-risk" patients need a certain degree of treatment intensification to avoid unacceptable rates of relapse. Prognostic models for ALL have been continuously refined since the 1980s [9, 10].

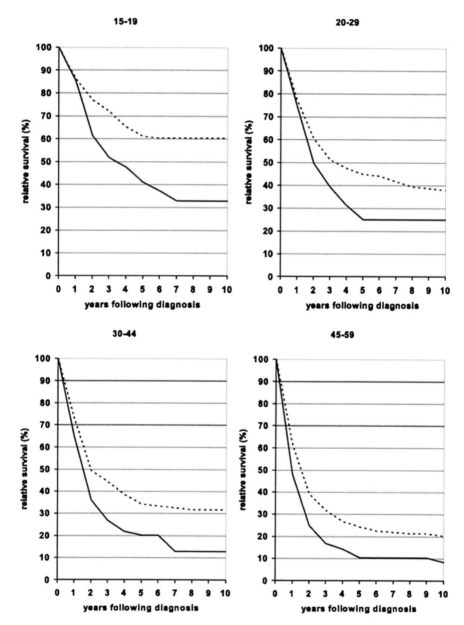

Fig. 2.1 Ten-year relative survival curves of patients with ALL by major age groups. Period estimates for 1980–1984 (*solid curves*) and 2000–2004 (*dashed curves*) (With permission from American Society of Hematology @ 2009)

Increasing age, higher white blood cell count, slow response to initial therapy, presence of minimal residual disease, and, most importantly, presence of adverse cytogenetic aberrations are all associated with poor outcomes [11]. The presence of CNS disease at diagnosis is also associated with adverse outcome and requires specific therapy [12]. Overall, prognostic factors in ALL can be divided into several groups.

Presenting Clinical Features

White blood cell (WBC) at initial diagnosis has a significant prognostic effect. Although the WBC is a continuum, for statistical stratification purposes, cutoffs for poor prognosis have been drawn at $30 \times 10^9/L$ for patients with pre-B-cell ALL and $100 \times 10^9/L$ for those with pre-T-cell ALL [13]. Elevated WBC above these thresholds have a prognostic impact on all clinical outcomes including initial response, event-free survival (EFS), disease-free survival (DFS), and overall survival (OS). In addition, in T-cell ALL, WBC above $100 \times 10^9/L$ is associated with increased risk of relapse in the central nervous system (CNS). Patients with extreme leukocytosis/blastemia ($>400 \times 10^9/L$) are at high risk for early complications and mortality from CNS hemorrhage, pulmonary, and neurologic events due to leukostasis; and tumor lysis syndrome [14]. Elevated WBC is frequently associated with other high-risk features, especially unfavorable cytogenetic aberrations like t(4;11) and t(9;22).

Age is a continuous prognostic variable, with outcomes becoming steadily worse with advancing age [15]. This effect is observed throughout the pediatric, adolescent, adult, and elderly range. Several observations might explain this correlation. These include (1) evident changes in disease biology, i.e., incidence of "high-risk" cytogenetic abnormalities [Philadelphia-chromosome-positive (Ph+) ALL accounts for 25% of adult cases, while seen only in 3% of pediatric cases]; and higher presenting WBC with age; and (2) clear differences in tolerance of treatment between younger and older patients, resulting in higher rate of TRM (particularly during remission induction) and frequent compromises in treatment intensity due to significant adverse events.

CNS involvement has significant impact on OS in ALL [13, 16]. Approximately 5% of adults have CNS involvement at initial diagnosis. Among 1,508 patients enrolled in UKALL/ECOG2993 clinical trial, 5-year OS was 29% for those with CNS disease versus 38% for those without CNS involvement [17].

Presenting Biologic Features

The immunophenotype of malignant lymphoblasts has been associated with treatment outcomes. However, modern intensified treatment protocols have abrogated some of the previously significant prognostic markers. T-cell and mature B-cell immunophenotypes, once linked to poor prognosis, are actually considered favorable features in adult ALL in the context of contemporary treatments [13, 18]. In B-cell ALL, a CD10-negative pro-B-cell phenotype or pre-B-cell phenotype with expression of cytoplasmic μ heavy chains portends poor prognosis, especially if associated with translocations or abnormality in 11q23.

CD20 antigen is expressed in approximately 40% of B-cell ALL and may have negative prognostic impact on the CR rate, OS [19], as well as the relapse rate and DFS [20]. Studies of targeted therapy with anti-CD20 monoclonal antibody, rituximab, in CD20+ ALL represent recent attempts to overcome this adverse factor, and the results are eagerly awaited.

P-glycoprotein-encoding multidrug resistance gene (*MRD1*) is detectable in more than 20% of patients with ALL (more frequently in pro-T ALL) and confers increased risk of induction treatment failure [21, 22]. In the same study, expression of CD33 adversely affected CR rate during induction therapy in T-ALL.

A recent study of folate pathway gene expression in ALL patients found much lower levels of folylpolyglutamate synthetase (FPGS) that determine cytosolic glutamation of methotrexate (MTX>MTXPG), a critical step in MTX antitumor activity, in T-ALL compared to all other ALL subtypes [23]. Suboptimal accumulation of MTXPG in T-ALL blasts might be responsible for reduced antileukemic activity of MTX. Consistent with these findings, recent clinical trials suggested improved outcomes in pediatric T-ALL patients with the use of very high doses of MTX [24, 25].

Molecular Genetic Alterations

Genetic aberrations in leukemia cells have important prognostic significance in predicting outcomes in adult ALL and play an important role in up-front risk stratification [26]. The prevalence of high-risk chromosomal translocations and epigenetic lesions increases with age and are partially responsible for inferior outcomes in adults when compared to pediatric patients. In addition, DNA-array technology and global gene expression profiling have identified a growing number of genetically silent deregulations of signaling, cell cycle, and apoptotic pathways that correlate with treatment outcomes [27, 28].

A reciprocal t(9;22) fuses *BCR* (breakpoint cluster region) gene on chromosome 22 to *ABL* (Abelson) gene on chromosome 9, i.e., Philadelphia (Ph) chromosome. The BCR-ABL fusion protein is a constitutive protein kinase that alters multiple signaling pathways, controlling proliferation, survival, and self-renewal of hematopoietic stem cells [29]. The incidence of this translocation increases from 3% in children to 20% in adults and more than 50% in patients older than 50 years [30, 31]. Irrespective of the breakpoint, Ph positivity is associated with the high-risk clinical features of older age and higher WBC and predicts poor treatment outcomes, including lower chance of initial treatment response (68.4% versus 84.6%) and lower probability of 3-year disease-free survival (0.13 versus 0.47). This bad outcome is not influenced by post-induction high-dose treatment stratification. The recent introduction of tyrosine kinase inhibitors into treatment protocols have started to positively affect outcomes in this patient population.

MLL gene rearrangements, including t(4;11); t(11;19); t(9;11); and a few others, are found in approximately 10% of adult ALL patients [32, 33]. This genetic feature is also associated with older age of patients and high presenting WBC. Mixed-lineage leukemia (MLL) protein is a nuclear factor that maintains the expression of particular members of the *HOX* family. Translocation of the *MLL gene* can involve more than 40 molecular partners, resulting in a gain-of-function effect that enhances their transcriptional activity and deregulates normal pattern of expression of *HOX* genes, causing a change in self-renewal and growth of hematopoietic stem cells and committed progenitors. Patients harboring *MLL* alterations, especially those with t(4;11), have compromised prognoses with median disease-free survival (DFS) of 7 months and 5-year DFS of 25% or less [2, 26, 34].

Another *HOX* family regulator, PBX1, is affected by t(1;19) translocation that fuses PBX1 with E2A transcription factor and affects 3–5% of adults with ALL. E2A-PBX1 fusion protein disrupts both the expression of *HOX* genes and other targets of the E2A [35]. A finding of t(1;19) might convey a poor prognosis with a 5-year DFS of 30% or less resulting from early treatment failure despite high initial CR rates [36].

Hypodiploidy (<45 chromosomes) and near triploidy represents a single clinically distinct subtype of adult ALL and is found in 3–5% of cases [37]. Patients tend to have significantly lower WBC at diagnosis compared with other Ph patients and are less likely to have T-ALL. These karyotypes negatively impact prognosis with a 5-year OS of approximately 20% [2]. Outcomes appear even worse in rare cases of low hypodiploidy (33–39 chromosomes) or near haploidy (23–29 chromosomes). Hyperdiploidy (>50 chromosomes) is the most common chromosomal abnormality in Ph- adult ALL patients occurring in 7–10% of diagnoses. It confers a highly favorable prognosis with one large study reporting 5-year EFS and OS of 50% and 53%, respectively, and a 5-year freedom from relapse rate of 66% [2]. Similar results have been reported by another group of investigators [26].

Approximately 5% of adult ALL patients will have a complex karyotype (≥5 chromosomal alterations) at diagnosis (not due to chemotherapy-induced genetic instability). While not associated with any particular sex, age, WBC or phenotype, it has significant negative impact on outcomes with inferior 5-year EFS and OS (21% and 28%, respectively) [2].

Patients with normal karyotype are considered to have standard-risk ALL and have significantly improved outcomes with contemporary intensive treatment protocols, unless prognosis is affected by other biologic or clinical risk factors. For those adult ALL patients who are able to tolerate necessary intensity and duration of induction, consolidation, and maintenance therapy, 5-year DFS should be expected to be between 45% and 65% and 5-year OS between 45% and 50% [2, 34].

Based on comprehensive analysis of common genetic aberrations and clinical outcomes observed in 325 patients treated on GIMEMA 0496-protocol, Mancini et al. suggested stratifying adult ALL into three cytogenetic-molecular risk categories [26]. Patients with normal karyotype and isolated 9p/*p15-p-16* deletions are considered a "standard-risk" group (median DFS >3 years); patients with t(9;22), t(4;11), and t(1;19) compose an "adverse-risk" group (median DFS 7 months); and patients with miscellaneous abnormalities, deletion 6q, and hyperdiploidies represent an "intermediate-risk" group (median DFS 19 months). Table 2.2 summarizes the prognostic impact of the more common selected chromosomal aberration on outcome in adult T-cell and B-cell ALL.

Table 2.2 Prognostic significance of selected chromosomal aberrations in adult acute lymphoblastic leukemia

Genetic aberration	Frequency in adult ALL (%)	Effect on prognosis
T-cell ALL		
t(5;14)(q35;q32) *HOX11L2*	18–23	Poor [38]/Neutral [39]
t(10;14)(q24;q11) *HOX11(TLX1)*	31	Favorable [40]
t(7;10)(q34;q24) del(6q) Unknown	20–31	Poor [41]
TAL1/LYL1	45	Poor [42]
t(11;19)(q23;p13) *MLL/ENL*	8 (all *MLL*)	Favorable [43]
Other 11q23/*MLL*		Poor [26, 44]
t(10;11)(p13;q14) *CALM/AF10*	10	Favorable [45]
del(9p) *p15-p16*	65	[a]Poor [46]
B-cell ALL		
t(9;22) *BCR-ABL*	25	Poor [30]
t(4;11), other *MLL*	10	Poor [2, 26]
t(1;19) *E2A-PBX1*	3–5	Poor [36]
t(12;21) *TEL-AML1*	2	[a]Favorable [47]
del(9p)/del p14-p16	12%/45	Neutral [26, 48]
Hypodiploidy	2	Poor [2]
Hyperdiploidy	7	Favorable [2, 26]

[a] Pediatric patients, less evidence in adult ALL

Pharmacodynamic Factors

Host factors can significantly influence treatment efficacy and outcomes [49, 50]. Examples include genetic polymorphisms of drug-metabolizing enzymes, specifically the hepatic P450 system, drug transporters, receptors, and targets. Concomitant medications can severely impact clearance or metabolism of the antileukemic agents. Anticonvulsant drugs (phenytoin, phenobarbital, etc.) can significantly increase cytochrome P450 activity in the liver thereby enhancing clearance and reducing efficacy of chemotherapeutic agents and adversely affecting outcomes [51]. Also, delayed administration or undue reduction in treatment intensity, especially during the induction phase, is an underestimated adverse risk factor. Adherence to the treatment plan is essential for successful ALL therapy. Inability to deliver required intensity and density of therapy has significant negative impact on ALL cure rates in older adults and, especially, elderly patients.

Kinetics of Early Response and Change in Risk Stratification

Response to treatment is determined by the entire constellation of biological features of leukemic cells, pharmacodynamics and pharmacogenomics of the host, the intensity of administered regimens, and treatment compliance. Hence, it is not surprising that the rapidity and the degree of reduction in leukemic cell burden during initial therapy are independent and powerful predictors of outcome in both low-risk and high-risk patients, as defined by clinical and biologic features at diagnosis. Patients achieving CR after the first cycle of chemotherapy and showing a rapid peripheral blood (within 7 days) or bone marrow (within 14 days) blast cell clearance show superior outcomes [9, 52, 53]. It seems logical to use all available prognostic markers at diagnosis, such as age, WBC, immunophenotype, cytogenetics, and an increasing number of emerging molecular markers for initial risk stratification. This is of practical importance, i.e., immediate HLA-typing and stem cell donor search for high-risk patients. However, after induction/early consolidation, response kinetics and depth of response gain a much higher prognostic value and should drive ultimate treatment decisions.

The assessment of *minimal residual disease* (*MRD*) provides the best evaluation of response kinetics. This term defines microscopic disease in remission patients, whose bone marrow may still contain up to 10^{10} leukemic blasts. Accumulating evidence suggests that persistence of MRD after induction/early consolidation (weeks 4–22) at the level of $\geq 10^{-4}$ is reflective of intrinsic drug resistance and predicts early overt hematologic relapse [53–56]. The methodology of MRD detection has been standardized by a recent joint expert panel consensus [57]. Molecular and flow-cytometric methods, which are at least 1,000-fold more sensitive than morphological determinations, allow detection of MRD at very low levels of $\leq 0.01\%$. Patients with $\geq 0.1\%$ of leukemic blasts at the end of 4–6-week remission induction therapy have outcomes as poor as those who fail to achieve clinical remission by morphologic assessment (>5% blasts), whereas patients with <0.01% of leukemic blasts have an excellent outcome. In addition, prospective monitoring of MRD can be used for early detection of imminent hematologic relapse and therefore facilitate early treatment intervention [58]. A major challenge of current and future trials in adult ALL is to determine whether MRD could replace the traditional risk factors in the individual risk assessment and treatment stratification. While this has not been conclusively proven for high-risk patients, standard-risk patients should be routinely managed with MRD-based treatment programs. In this way, standard-risk patients are confirmed as such if MRD-negative and are "upgraded" to high-risk if MRD-positive (Table 2.3). It is provocative but more controversial to state that high-risk patients can be "downgraded" to standard-risk if MRD-negative.

Treatment Outcomes

Improved treatments in the last decade have abolished the adverse prognostic influence of multiple prognostic factors. Complete response rates as high as 85–90% and 5-year leukemia-free survival rates of 45–50% can be obtained with modern therapies in adults with both T-cell and B-cell ALL and standard-intermediate-risk category [8]. Children with ALL fare even better after contemporary pediatric treatment protocols with a 5–8-year event-free survival rate reaching 85–90% [59].

Table 2.3 Clinical significance of MRD in predicting outcomes in adult ALL

Study	MRD method/timing	DFS (MRD+ vs MRD−)
GMALL, 2006/2009 [53]	RT-PCR; negative/$<10^{-4}$ post-induction I–II and first consolidation	SR: 5-year OS 67% vs 38% HR: 5-year OS 66% vs 42% MRD+ until week 16→94% risk of relapse
PETHEMA, 2009	IF; <0.1% post-consolidation	HR: 4-year DFS 54% vs 31%
NILG, 2009 [54]	RT-PCR; $<10^{-4}$, week 16/negative, week 22	SR/HR: 5-year DFS 72% vs 14%
PALG, 2008 [55]	IF, <0.1% post-induction	SR/HR: 3-year DFS 61% vs 17%
MRC, 2010 [56]	RT-PCR; $<10^{-4}$ 1–9 months	SR/HR: 5-year DFS 74% vs 30%
GRAALL, 2009 [75]	RT-PCR; $<10^{-4}$ post-induction/ first consolidation	SR/HR: 3-year DFS 82% vs 3-year RR 56%

DFS disease-free survival, *GMALL* German Multicenter ALL, *GRAALL* Group for Research on Adult Lymphoblastic Leukemia, *HR* high risk, *IF* immunofluorescence, *MRC* Medical Research Council, *MRD* Minimal Residual Disease, *NILG* Northern Italy Leukemia Group, *PALG* Polish Adult Leukemia Group, *PETHEMA* Programa Español de Tratamientos en Hematologia, *RT-PCR* Real time polymerase chain reaction, *SR* standard risk

Outcomes of selected clinical trials are presented in Table 2.4 [60–75]. Pediatric trials are listed for comparative overview.

Several conclusions can be drawn from these studies. *First*, pediatric ALL patients have significantly better survival rates than adults. Factors influencing this difference are likely to include but are not limited to a higher intensity of pediatric protocols; more rigorous adherence to treatment doses and schedules in children compared to adult patients due to higher tolerance of treatment toxicities by pediatric oncologists, "treatment culture," and lack of autonomy in children; presence of comorbidities in older adults precluding the use of intensive regimens required for cure; higher proportions of children being treated on clinical protocols at academic centers versus by community adult oncologists; and higher rates of adverse prognostic features in adult ALL, most notably cytogenetic aberrations compared to childhood ALL [76]. *Second*, more recent trials report better survival in both pediatric and adult ALL when compared to trials two to three decades ago [8, 59]. This is most pronounced in patients treated within the same cooperative groups and single institutions over the span of several decades when outcomes are compared between different time periods [61, 65, 74]. Analyses of changes in clinical protocols might suggest what specific interventions led to improvement in outcomes. *Third*, in contradiction to earlier reports assigning a poor prognosis to ALL patients with T-cell phenotype, survival of both pediatric and adult T-ALL patients appears to be at least comparable if not superior to patients with B-cell ALL, when treated with modern protocols, with the exception of small proportion of T-ALL patients harboring adverse chromosomal aberrations discussed earlier in this review.

Table 2.4 Clinical outcomes in selected pediatric and adult ALL trials according to disease phenotype

Study group		B-lineage	T-lineage (reference)	P value
Childhood ALL (EFS%)				
ALL-BFM 86	(6-year)	77	73 [60]	0.096
ALL-BFM 90	(6-year)	82	61 [24]	NR
AIEOP-ALL 82	(8-year)	63	55 [61]	NR
AIEOP-ALL 87	(8-year)	68	78 [61]	NR
AIEOP-ALL 88	(8-year)	73	83 [61]	NR
AIEOP-ALL 91	(8-year)	78	65 [61]	NR
CCG 1989-95	(8-year)	78	79 [62]	NR
DCLSG ALL-8	(5-year)	73	83 [63]	0.31
CLCG-EORTC	(8-year)	69	62 [64]	NR
NOPHO	(5-year)	85	75 [65]	<0.01
DFCI-91-01	(5-year)	84	79 [66]	0.34
SJCRH XIIIB	(5-year)	83	72 [67]	0.17
UKALL XI	(10-year)	65	52 [68]	0.04
Adult ALL (OS%)				
MDACC	(5-year)	45	48 [16]	0.18
CALGB-8811	(3-year)	36	67 [69]	0.004
LALA 94	(5-year)	34	32 [70]	NR
GIMEMA	(8-year)	30	27 [71]	NR
JALSG-ALL93	(6-year)	36	42 [72]	0.85
UCSF	(5-year)	66	48 [73]	NR
EHH	(8-year)	17	36 [74]	0.05
GRAALL-2003	(4-year)	52	62 [75]	0.09

AIEOP Italian Association of Pediatric Hematology Oncology, *BFM* Berlin-Frankfurt-Munster study group, *CALGB* Cancer and Leukemia Group B, *CCG* Children Cancer Group, *CLCG-EORTC* Children Leukemia Cooperative Group–European Organization for Research and treatment of Cancer, *DCLSG* Dutch Childhood Leukemia Study Group, *DFCI* Dana-Farber Cancer Institute, *EFS* Event-free survival, *EHH* Edouard Herriot Hospital, *GIMEMA* Gruppo Italiano Malattie Ematologiche dell'Adulto, *GRAALL* Group for Research on Adult Lymphoblastic Leukemia, *JALSG* Japan Adult Leukemia Study Group, *LALA* Leucemie Aigue Lymphoblastique de l'Adulte, *MDACC* MD Anderson Cancer Center, *NOPHO* Nordisk Forening for Pediatrisk Hematologi og Oncologi, *NR* not reported, *OS* overall survival, *SJCRH* St. Jude Cancer Research Hospital, *UCSF* University of California at San Francisco, *UKALL* United Kingdom ALL Study Group

Treatment of Newly Diagnosed ALL

Typical treatment of newly diagnosed adult ALL consists of a remission induction phase, an intensification (or consolidation) phase, and continuation (or maintenance) phase. Early prophylactic chemotherapy directed to the CNS to prevent relapses attributable to sequestration of leukemic blasts at this sanctuary site is critical for successful cure. The agents currently used in all treatment phases were developed and tested several decades ago, but growing efforts are introducing new antileukemic agents into early clinical trials that are expected to affect outcomes in both standard- and high-risk ALL.

Supportive care, including use of hematopoietic growth factors, transfusion of blood products, monitoring, prophylaxis, and aggressive early therapy of infectious events, is an important part of comprehensive patient care and facilitates delivery of necessary treatment intensity.

Remission Induction

The goal of remission induction therapy is to eradicate more than 99% of the initial leukemic cell burden and symptoms of the disease in as many patients, as early, and with as few toxic side effects as possible and to restore normal hematopoiesis and restore adequate performance status. Induction is the most critical phase of ALL therapy, carrying the highest risk of serious and potentially fatal toxicities and requiring a high level of supportive care. Tumor lysis syndrome, intracranial hemorrhage, serious infections, adult respiratory distress syndrome (ARDS), and disseminated intravascular coagulation (DIC) syndrome are leading causes of early mortality of initial ALL therapy.

Most standard induction protocols typically include vincristine, glucocorticoid (prednisone or dexamethasone), and anthracycline, with or without L-asparaginase (three- or four-drug induction) [69, 73]. Cyclophosphamide, cytarabine, methotrexate, and 6-mercaptopurine are frequently added to adult induction protocols [7, 16]. The majority of contemporary protocols are expected to produce clinical complete remission in 75–85% of high-risk and in 85–95% of standard-risk ALL patients [1].

Although no one induction protocol is clearly superior to another, specific features of selected protocols might have benefited subgroups of patients with ALL. Addition of cyclophosphamide, use of very high-dose methotrexate, and intensive L-asparaginase schedules are broadly considered to have improved outcomes in patients with T-cell ALL [18, 25, 77–79]. Introduction of imatinib mesylate into induction regimens has significantly improved the remission induction rate in Philadelphia-chromosome-positive ALL [80–83].

Additional observations from numerous adult ALL clinical trials suggested advantages of using specific preparations of antileukemic drugs. Presumably because of its longer half-life increased penetration into the CNS, dexamethasone might be more effective than either prednisone or prednisolone in treatment of ALL [84, 85]. The pharmacodynamics of different formulations of L-asparaginase might affect both antileukemic activity and toxicity. However, in terms of clinical efficacy, the dose intensity and duration of asparagines depletion are far more important than the type of L-asparaginase used. Pegylated asparaginase, with superior activity due to longer periods of asparagines depletion and less potential for allergic reactions, may be preferable and has replaced the native products in some induction protocols [78, 86–88]. It has to be noted that excessive complications were observed in adult and elderly ALL patients with concomitant use of glucocorticoids and L-asparaginase. Physicians need to be aware that in the context of multiagent induction therapy, minimal increases in the doses of dexamethasone and/or L-asparaginase can lead to serious and potentially fatal toxicities.

Expression of CD20 antigen is observed in approximately 40% of precursor B-ALL patients and predicts shorter duration of remission after initial therapy and inferior overall survival when compared to CD20 patients (49% versus 61%) [19]. Similarly, CD20+ predicts higher relapse rate (1.9-fold increase) resulting in inferior DFS [20]. A recent study demonstrated significantly superior outcomes in younger patients (<60 years) with CD20+ ALL when rituximab was added to multiagent chemotherapy with 3-year CR rate of 70% (versus 38%) and 3-year OS of 75% (versus 47%) [89]. These results support the addition of rituximab to induction regimens in CD20+ ALL patients.

Consolidation/Intensification Treatment

The role of intensified post remission therapy is to eradicate drug-resistant residual leukemic cells, thereby reducing the risk of relapse and improving outcomes, especially in high-risk patients. Frequently used strategies include high-dose methotrexate, high-dose cytarabine, mercaptopurine, etoposide, and high-dose L-asparaginase. Patients typically receive six to eight courses of consolidative therapy. Protocols developed in the last two decades produce on average 35–50% cure rate in unselected patient analyses from multicentric prospective trials [16, 69–73, 90, 91].

High-dose cytarabine is usually administered for 4–12 doses during consolidation at 1–3 g/m^2. The best dose of methotrexate depends on the leukemic cell phenotype and host pharmacokinetic variables. Methotrexate at 1–2 g/m^2 is adequate for standard-risk B-cell ALL; higher doses of 4–5 g/m^2 might benefit patients with T-cell or high-risk B-cell ALL [24, 92]. Patients whose leukemia cells harbor t(12;21) or t(1;19) translocations (*TEL-AML1* or *E2A-PBX1* fusion genes, respectively) might also benefit from increased doses of methotrexate due to low accumulation of polyglutamated methotrexate in blast cells [23]. It is noteworthy that while leucovorin rescue is necessary after high-dose methotrexate therapy, it must not be given too early or at too high of a dosage because it might counteract the antileukemic effect of the latter [23, 93].

Long-Term Maintenance

Patients with ALL require long-term continuation treatment to prevent or delay relapses. Daily 6-mercaptopurine and weekly low-dose methotrexate are continued for 2.0–2.5 years. Omission of maintenance worsens outcomes significantly in B-cell ALL, but probably less so in T-cell ALL [94]. Many experts advocate that drug doses be adjusted to maintain neutrophil counts between 0.5 and 1.0 K/um to ensure adequate dose intensity during the continuation phase [95]. Overzealous use of 6-mercaptopurine might be counterproductive since it can result in severe neutropenia necessitating dose interruption and reducing overall intensity of maintenance. Elevation of liver transaminases is a common finding during 6-mercaptopurine therapy; it appears to be caused by the methylated metabolites of the drug, resolves promptly upon completion of therapy, and might correlate with treatment compliance and therefore favorable outcome [96]. In some protocols, intensification pulses of vincristine and dexamethasone/prednisone are added to two-drug regimen (POMP). However, in randomized trial, addition of six such pulses to during early maintenance treatment failed to improve outcomes in children with intermediate-risk ALL [97]. There were no definitive randomized trials in adults to identify risk groups that would benefit the most from prolonged chemotherapy; hence, all patients should be offered this approach. As a general statement, the role of chemotherapy maintenance after stem cell transplantation has not been evaluated and cannot be recommended for routine use. In the future studies, newer biologic/targeted agents should studied in maintenance schedules with the goal of improving efficacy, reducing toxicity and possibly affecting biology of both leukemic clone and leukemia stem cells. To address this hypothesis, classes of agents to consider should include histone deacetylase inhibitors (HDACi), hypomethylating drugs, proteosome inhibitors, monoclonal antibodies, and antibody-drug conjugates, among others. First attempts to introduce this approach are ongoing clinical trials of imatinib and nilotinib maintenance after allogeneic HCT for Philadelphia-chromosome-positive ALL (*FHCRC 2223.00*).

Allogeneic Hematopoietic Stem Cell Transplantation

Allogeneic hematopoietic stem cell transplantation (Allo-HSCT) is the most intensive form of treatment of ALL and represents an important part of post-remission strategy. It relies on high-dose chemo(radio)therapy to eradicate any residual chemo-refractory leukemia cells as well as an immunologic graft-versus-leukemia response mediated by donor lymphocytes to reestablish immune surveillance and immunologic control of potential future relapses. For patients with high-risk ALL (i.e., Ph+, t(4;11) etc.), those with MRD-positive status after induction therapy, and patients with relapsed ALL, allo-HSCT provides the only chance of cure or long-term leukemia control [98]. The curative potential of this approach must be balanced against the disadvantages of mortality of 20–30%, morbidity, debilitating late complications such as chronic graft-versus-host disease (GVHD) and reduced quality of life. It is unequivocal that the relapse rate after allo-HSCT is significantly reduced compared to chemotherapy alone or autologous HCT owing to powerful antileukemic activity of the allogeneic graft. However, the OS is hindered by significant rate of non-relapse mortality that increases with age of the patients and can be as high as 36% [99].

Appropriate selection of patients and timing of allo-HCT in ALL remains a matter of debate [99–101]. Recently reported analysis of a large international Medical Research Council (MRC) UKALL/Eastern Cooperative Oncology Group (ECOG) E2993 trial suggested that standard-risk patients in first complete remission benefit more from allo-HCT than from chemotherapy alone (5-year OS rates 62% versus 52%, $p=0.02$) [99]. However, several other studies contradict these results indicating that except for high-risk patients, allo-HCT was not advantageous for standard-risk patients [70, 102, 103]. The discrepancies between the trials might be partly explained by differences in definition of high-risk population. Given current data, the majority of experts would agree that patients with Ph+ disease, those with t(4;11), and older patients (>40 years) constitute high-risk and that among younger (<40 years) standard-risk patients approximately 60% will be cured by modern chemotherapy regimens sparing toxicity and mortality of allo-HSCT.

One of the evolving risk stratification paradigms is based on evaluation of MRD after induction chemotherapy. Rapidity and depth of the response to treatment is determined by the entire constellation of biological features of leukemic cells, pharmacodynamics and pharmacogenomics of the host, the intensity of administered regimens, and treatment compliance. Given the complexity of known and still unidentified risk factors at diagnosis, presence or absence of MRD at determined points after induction therapy might be a more reliable clinical predictor of the treatment failure risk and could become a main tool to stratify patients to consolidative allo-HCT. Increasing number of modern clinical trials confirm that presence of MRD after initial cycle(s) of therapy predicts significantly higher risk of relapse and inferior PFS compared to MRD-negative patients (Table 2.4).

The benefit of allo-HCT could be extended to older ALL patients (>60 years) or patients with comorbidities with utilization of reduced-intensity conditioning (RIC). European Group for Blood and Marrow Transplantation reported DFS, TRM, and relapse risk (RR) of 18%, 24%, and 58%, respectively for 91 adult patients with median age 40 years [104]. In the study conducted by the Fred Hutchinson Cancer Research Center, 51 adult ALL patients (median age, 56 years) underwent RIC-HSCT with 3-year probabilities of OS, TRM, and RR of 34%, 28%, and 40%, respectively [105]. Results were significantly superior for patients who underwent transplantation in first versus second remission. Strikingly, for patients with Philadelphia-chromosome-positive ALL in first remission who received post-grafting imatinib, the 3-year OS rate was 62%; for the subgroup without evidence of minimal residual disease at transplantation, the overall survival was 73%. Another report describes 22 ALL patients with median age of 49 years (range 24–68 years) who received RIC-HSCT at the University of Minnesota. OS, TRM and RR at 3 years were 50%, 27%, and 36%, respectively [106].

In summary, one sensible option in selecting patients for allo-HSCT consolidative therapy and containing the risk of treatment-related mortality (TRM) is to reserve this approach for high-risk patients (those with Ph+, t(4;11)+ ALL, other adverse cytogenetics (Table 2.2), and WBC > 100 K/ul) and standard-risk patients with MRD+ status early after induction therapy (testing time vary by treatment protocol) [70, 71, 91, 107, 108]. MRD- standard-risk patients would be treated with chemotherapy alone [53–56, 109]. This approach would reduce the risk of TRM for standard-risk patients who have real chance of cure without allo-HCT. The provocative idea that high-risk patients with MRD- status after induction therapy might avoid the necessity of allo-HCT should be a topic of evaluation in current clinical trials.

Special Situations

Philadelphia-Chromosome-Positive ALL

Treatment of Ph+ ALL deserves special consideration. Translocation t(9;22) resulting in uninhibited transcription of *BCR-ABL* fusion protein with constitutive activity of ABL-kinase until recently projected the most unfavorable prognosis with dismal historical survival in adult ALL patients. Although CR rates could be obtained in 70–75% of patients, overall survival was only 10–20%, with minimal improvement after consolidative allo-HSCT (up to 30%) [29–31]. Introduction of tyrosine kinase inhibitors (TKI) substantially changed the outcomes in Ph+ ALL and opened a whole new paradigm in managing these patients. Even single agent TKIs can produce remarkably high rates of CRs (71–96%) in previously untreated patients that in some studies were even higher when compared to chemotherapy [110–112]. In addition, dasatinib and nilotinib, second generation TKIs, exhibit antileukemic effect through inhibition of multiple signaling pathways and are active in patients with imatinib-resistant Ph+ ALL [113, 114].

There are several approaches to using TKIs in Ph+ ALL therapy. First, TKI monotherapy provides a rare opportunity to significantly prolong survival and improve quality of life in elderly patients that historically have extremely poor outcomes. Imatinib, with or without corticosteroids, produces remarkable CR rates of 90–100%, which in one study were superior to chemotherapy (93% versus 54%) [110–112]. Survival was improved not only due to higher response rate but also due to significantly lower treatment-related mortality in the imatinib arm. Unfortunately, majority of patients would eventually relapse, likely due to emergence of imatinib-resistant mutations. Dasatinib has also been studied as a monotherapy in Ph+ ALL. In one study, patients were treated with dasatinib with or without steroids regardless of their age. Response rate was astonishing at 100%. Based on these data, TKI therapy with or without glucocorticoids might be preferred approach for elderly or debilitated patients who are not candidates for aggressive induction protocols and/ or allo-HCT. Second, combination of TKIs and aggressive chemotherapy induction and consolidation has increased CR rates to above 90% and molecular remission rates to above 50% in majority of studies. This approach also increased number of patients able to proceed to consolidative allo-HSCT without significant increase in overall toxicity [80, 82, 83, 115–118]. These improvements significantly changed overall outcomes for Ph+ adult ALL patients, and use of TKIs during induction and consolidation therapy should routinely be utilized in this patient cohort. Specific dosing and duration varies by published treatment regimens. Third, the role of

TKIs in post-chemotherapy and post-transplant maintenance is being evaluated in ongoing clinical trials and is likely to further reduce relapse rates and improve survival [119].

Despite high remission rates and favorable disease-free survival data, how to continue in CR patients remains open. Consolidative allo-HSCT might not be necessary or advantageous for patients achieving molecular remissions on TKI therapy. While this idea is provocative, until survival benefit is clearly documented in future clinical trials, younger and eligible patients, especially those with HLA-matched siblings or high-resolution- matched unrelated donors, should strongly consider allo-HSCT in first CR as definitive cure-oriented approach.

Central Nervous System Involvement

Central nervous system (CNS) involvement occurs in 1–10% of patients with ALL at diagnosis and represents approximately 6% of disease relapses [17, 110]. Diagnosis of CNS leukemia is made/confirmed by presence of ALL cells in the cerebral-spinal fluid (CSF), cranial nerve palsies, neurologic dysfunction, findings on computed tomography (CT), or magnetic resonance (MRI) imaging. Factors associated with high risk of CNS involvement or relapse include high-risk cytogenetics, T-cell immunophenotype, a large leukemia cell burden, and elevated lactate dehydrogenase level at diagnosis (>3 times upper limit norm) [111]. Treatment and prophylaxis of CNS leukemia usually consist of intrathecal (IT) methotrexate administration alone or in combination with cytarabine and hydrocortisone (triple therapy), use of high-dose cytarabine during induction and consolidation cycles, allowing for blood-brain barrier penetration, and in some cases cranial irradiation.

Patients with CNS disease at diagnosis are sometimes considered high-risk group with inferior outcomes and candidates for consolidative allo-HSCT [70, 75]. They are generally treated with triple IT therapy twice a week until clearance of CSF, then weekly for four more doses, and then variably per treatment protocol. This therapy might be combined with cranial irradiation (18–30 Gy), intensive systemic therapy (preferably containing high-dose cytarabine), and followed by allo-HSCT. Spinal radiation (12 Gy) can be added, but its role is controversial [17].

Patients with CSF-negative initial status receive aggressive IT chemoprophylaxis with total number of treatments dependent on clinical risk of CNS involvement (see risk factors above) and specific protocol. Usually, prophylactic therapy consists of 8–16 IT doses. This practice is supported by the observation of the reduction in the risk of CNS relapse from 30% when prophylaxis is not used to below 5% with prophylactic therapy [110, 112].

Treatment of CNS relapse is largely unsuccessful because it is frequently followed by systemic relapse and requires therapy combining aggressive CNS-directed measures (i.e., intensive IT therapy, craniospinal irradiation) and high-dose systemic treatment posing a real risk of acute leukoencephalopathy and patient demise. Hence, alternative therapies, including the use of liposomal cytarabine and

IT-administered monoclonal antibodies, should be evaluated in future trials. Allo-HSCT is the only curative option for very select patients with isolated CNS relapse.

Relapsed and Refractory ALL

Patients who fail to achieve response to induction therapy or have relapsed disease have generally poor prognosis, and despite variety of protocols, salvage therapy in ALL remains challenging [113–115]. In recent studies, the CR rates vary between 40% and 45%, and OS was <10%. Allo-HSCT provides the best curative chance for patients achieving second CR with long-term leukemia-free survival rates between 14% and 43% [113]. Therefore, the general goal is to achieve second CR or very good PR (preferably <5% of abnormal lymphoblasts in the bone marrow), to search immediately for a donor, and proceed to allo-HSCT. However, the lack of suitable HLA-matched donor, comorbidities, and inability to achieve second CR are frequent barriers. Predictors of failure after salvage allo-HSCT are high-risk ALL at diagnosis, duration of initial CR less than 12 months, and inadequate response to salvage therapy (>5% leukemic blasts in the bone marrow); patients with these characteristic are unlikely to survive long-term and best treated on experimental protocols with new agents.

Future studies in relapsed and refractory ALL should focus on increasing the rates of CR or CR without hematologic recovery to facilitate transition to allo-HSCT. This could be accomplished by incorporating new chemotherapeutic and biologic agents into salvage protocols. Among those, nelarabine, a pro-drug for 9-β-arabinofuranosylguanine (ara-G) has shown remarkable single agent activity in prospective CALG-B/SWOG clinical trial in patients with relapsed and refractory T-cell ALL. Twenty-six patients were treated, and 41% achieved a response while 31% of patients had a CR [116]. Even higher activity was reported in pediatric trial [117]. These results were very encouraging in this difficult patient population and lead to the approval of nelarabine by the FDA for treatment of adult relapsed/refractory T-cell ALL [118].

In addition, prospective monitoring of MRD and early detection of molecular or subclinical relapses may improve the outcomes by eliminating the necessity of prolonged salvage therapy, allowing for use of biologic or targeted agents, and enabling early definitive treatment with HSCT. The use of the anti-CD19 monoclonal antibody, blinatumomab, in this low tumoral mass setting was one example of successful application of this strategy [119].

Outside clinical trials, conventional treatment regimens mainly incorporate drug combinations used in known induction protocols, with focus on avoiding cross-resistant agents if possible: (1) FLAG (fludarabine, high-dose cytarabine, G-CSF) with anthracycline [120, 121], (2) very high-dose methotrexate with L-asparaginase [122], (3) high-dose cytarabine with mitoxantrone [123], and (4) combination of ifosfamide, mitoxantrone, and etoposide [124]; to name a few frequently used salvage regimens. In general, patients who had initial CR lasting >12 months could be treated with original induction protocol as first attempt of salvage.

Elderly Patients

Elderly patients (>60 years of age) have a worse prognosis than younger patients when treated with the same intensive regimens in the majority of studies. Although, remission can be achieved in more than half of elderly patients, their long-term survival probability is usually less than 20% [125]. Specifically designed reduced-intensity protocols are more successful than unmodified regimens for younger adults that produce unacceptably high treatment-associated mortality in complete remission from myelosuppression-related complications. European Working Group for Adult ALL reported very provocative results with moderate dose intensity treatment protocol, showing remission rate of 85% and probability of 1-year survival of 61%. Even more encouraging was a low rate of treatment-related mortality of less than 10% (personal communication). Recent development and continuous improvement in reduced-intensity conditioning allo-HSCT have made it feasible to consider this previously prohibitive consolidative therapy for older patients and those with comorbidities, providing a chance for further improvement in outcomes for this high-risk population. In elderly ALL cohort with median age of 62 years, recent study reported survival rate of 40% after RIC-allo-HSCT [104].

Novel Therapies and Future Directions

A number of normal biochemical and molecular processes are deregulated in the process of leukemogenesis. These complex pathways involve the intrinsic control of cellular proliferation, cell cycle, apoptosis, angiogenesis, and many others. In lymphoid leukemias, the malignant cells rely on certain signaling pathways that are pathologically altered to provide the leukemic clone with a continuous survival and proliferation advantage. Intracellular pathways known to be pathologically upregulated in ALL include mTOR (mammalian target of rapamycin), AKT, PI3K (phosphoinositide-3-kinase), MAPK/ERK signaling, among others (Fig. 2.2). While these pathways are also utilized by non-malignant cells, it is the reliance of the leukemic clone on these pathways for survival that makes them suitable targets for therapeutic approaches.

The understanding of intrinsic mechanisms in leukemogenesis and advances in biopharmaceutical technologies opened a new era in the development of novel chemotherapeutic and targeted/biologic agents for both B-cell and T-cell ALL (Table 2.5). Numerous agents targeting specific intracellular pathways have entered pediatric and adult ALL trials [126]. Given the heterogeneity and complexity of both newly diagnosed and relapsed/refractory ALL, it is unlikely that a single drug

Table 2.5 Novel agents in trials for treatment of adult acute lymphoblastic leukemia

Agent	Mechanism of action	Agent type/route
Imatinib (STI571)	ABL, cKIT inhibition	SM/oral
Dasatinib (BMS-354825)	ABL, SRC, cKIT, EPHA2, PDGFβ	SM/oral
Nilotinib (AMN107)	ABL, cKIT	SM/oral
MK0752	β-secretase inhibition (interference with NOTCH signaling)	SM/oral
Midostaurin (PKC412)	FLT3 inhibition	SM/oral
Lestaurtanib (CEP701)		SM/oral
Tipifarnib	Farnesyltransferase inhibition	SM/oral
Rapamycin	mTOR inhibition	SM/oral
Temsirolimus (CCI-779)		SM/IV
MLN8237	Aurora-kinase inhibition	SM/oral
Sorafenib (BAY439006)	Muti-kinase inhibition (RAF; FLT3; VEGFR; PDGFR; cKIT)	SM/oral
Obatoclax (GX 15-070)	BCL2 inhibition	SM/IV
Decitabine 5-azacitidine	DNA demethylation	SM/IV
Vorinostat MS-275	Histone deacetylase inhibition	SM/oral
Bortezomib	Ubiquitin proteosome inhibition	SM/IV
Clofarabine	Deoxyadenosine analogue	SM/IV
Forodesine	PNP inhibition	SM/oral
Alemtuzumab	Anti-CD52	mAb/IV
Rituximab	Anti-CD20	mAb/IV
Epratuzimab	Anti-CD22	mAb/IV
Blinatumomab	Anti-CD19	mAb/IV
CAT8015	Anti-CD22-PSA-E	ADC/IV
DT2219ARL	Anti-CD19/22-DT	ADC/IV
BU-12	Anti-CD19-Y90	ADC/IV

ADC antibody-drug conjugate, *IV* intravenous, *SM* small molecule *PNP* purine nucleoside phosphorylase

alone will make a crucial difference (with rare exceptions like BCR-ABL kinase inhibitors). Rather, it is a painstaking endeavor of filtering out the agents with the most prominent activity in early studies and learning how to use those agents best in combination regimens that might eventually make significant impact on outcomes in adult ALL [127–136].

Conclusions

Adult ALL remains a challenging hematologic malignancy. Despite the high rate of complete remissions in current protocols, durable disease control and cure remain elusive. The challenge is to maintain the remissions and, for patients with relapsed and refractory disease, to provide effective salvage therapy with acceptable toxicity. First, there is a need to design a mechanism to quickly screen the increasing number

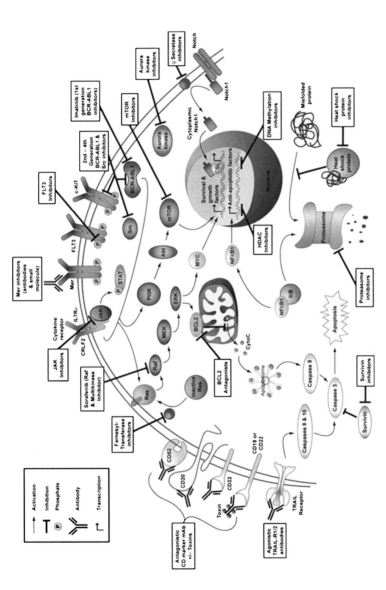

Fig. 2.2 Cellular pathways under investigation as potential therapeutic targets in pediatric ALL. With the exception of aurora kinase, which is required for mitotic spindle assembly, all other kinases included here are *purple* and activate the PI3K-Akt and/or Ras-MAPK pro-survival pathways. Cluster of differentiation (*CD*) surface marker proteins are *pink*. Proteins in the apoptotic pathway are *yellow*. Molecules involved in protein degradation are *green*. Transcription factors are *blue*. Compounds in development as targeted therapeutics are described in *black boxes* (With permission from John Wiley and Sons @ 2010)

of new biologic agents and incorporate the most promising of them into induction, maintenance, and salvage protocols. A recent successful example of this approach is the introduction of ABL-kinase inhibitors into treatment regimens of Ph+ ALL. Second, there should continue to be focus on improving risk stratification of adult ALL patients and selection of most appropriate candidates for allo-HSCT with goal of increasing cure rate for high-risk patients utilizing potent graft-versus-leukemia effect and improving survival for non-high-risk patients by reducing treatment-related mortality. A recent large step forward in this direction is the introduction and refinement of MRD monitoring and inclusion of MRD assessment into treatment decision paradigms. Prospective MRD monitoring has already made an impact on clinical outcomes in recent trials. Finally, designing and testing therapeutic strategies for elderly patients will make further improvement in overall cure rates of adult ALL.

Therapy for adult ALL remains a therapeutic challenge. Progress ultimately will depend on successful integration of drug development with adult ALL biology and fine-tuning of risk stratification/prognostic systems.

References

1. Pui CH, Evans WE. Treatment of acute lymphoblastic leukemia. N Engl J Med. 2006;354(2): 166–78.
2. Moorman AV, Harrison CJ, Buck GA, Richards SM, Secker-Walker LM, Martineau M, et al. Karyotype is an independent prognostic factor in adult acute lymphoblastic leukemia (ALL): analysis of cytogenetic data from patients treated on the medical research council (MRC) UKALLXII/Eastern Cooperative Oncology Group (ECOG) 2993 trial. Blood. 2007;109(8): 3189–97.
3. Jones LK, Saha V. Philadelphia positive acute lymphoblastic leukaemia of childhood. Br J Haematol. 2005;130(4):489–500.
4. Ramanujachar R, Richards S, Hann I, Goldstone A, Mitchell C, Vora A, et al. Adolescents with acute lymphoblastic leukaemia: outcome on UK national paediatric (ALL97) and adult (UKALLXII/E2993) trials. Pediatr Blood Cancer. 2007;48(3):254–61.
5. Boissel N, Auclerc MF, Lheritier V, Perel Y, Thomas X, Leblanc T, et al. Should adolescents with acute lymphoblastic leukemia be treated as old children or young adults? Comparison of the French FRALLE-93 and LALA-94 trials. J Clin Oncol. 2003;21(5):774–80.
6. Hallbook H, Gustafsson G, Smedmyr B, Soderhall S, Heyman M, Swedish Adult Acute Lymphocytic Leukemia Group, et al. Treatment outcome in young adults and children >10 years of age with acute lymphoblastic leukemia in Sweden: a comparison between a pediatric protocol and an adult protocol. Cancer. 2006;107(7):1551–61.
7. Gokbuget N, Hoelzer D. Treatment of adult acute lymphoblastic leukemia. Semin Hematol. 2009;46(1):64–75.
8. Pulte D, Gondos A, Brenner H. Improvement in survival in younger patients with acute lymphoblastic leukemia from the 1980s to the early 21st century. Blood. 2009;113(7):1408–11.
9. Hoelzer D, Thiel E, Loffler H, Buchner T, Ganser A, Heil G, et al. Prognostic factors in a multicenter study for treatment of acute lymphoblastic leukemia in adults. Blood. 1988;71(1):123–31.
10. Kaneko Y, Rowley JD, Variakojis D, Chilcote RR, Check I, Sakurai M. Correlation of karyotype with clinical features in acute lymphoblastic leukemia. Cancer Res. 1982;42(7):2918–29.
11. Faderl S, O'Brien S, Pui CH, Stock W, Wetzler M, Hoelzer D, et al. Adult acute lymphoblastic leukemia: concepts and strategies. Cancer. 2010;116(5):1165–76.

12. Jabbour E, Thomas D, Cortes J, Kantarjian HM, O'Brien S. Central nervous system prophylaxis in adults with acute lymphoblastic leukemia: current and emerging therapies. Cancer. 2010; 116(10):2290–300.
13. Rowe JM, Buck G, Burnett AK, Chopra R, Wiernik PH, Richards SM, et al. Induction therapy for adults with acute lymphoblastic leukemia: results of more than 1500 patients from the international ALL trial: MRC UKALL XII/ECOG E2993. Blood. 2005;106(12):3760–7.
14. Lowe EJ, Pui CH, Hancock ML, Geiger TL, Khan RB, Sandlund JT. Early complications in children with acute lymphoblastic leukemia presenting with hyperleukocytosis. Pediatr Blood Cancer. 2005;45(1):10–5.
15. Chessells JM, Hall E, Prentice HG, Durrant J, Bailey CC, Richards SM. The impact of age on outcome in lymphoblastic leukaemia; MRC UKALL X and XA compared: a report from the MRC paediatric and adult working parties. Leukemia. 1998;12(4):463–73.
16. Kantarjian H, Thomas D, O'Brien S, Cortes J, Giles F, Jeha S, et al. Long-term follow-up results of hyperfractionated cyclophosphamide, vincristine, doxorubicin, and dexamethasone (hyper-CVAD), a dose-intensive regimen, in adult acute lymphocytic leukemia. Cancer. 2004;101(12):2788–801.
17. Lazarus HM, Richards SM, Chopra R, Litzow MR, Burnett AK, Wiernik PH, et al. Central nervous system involvement in adult acute lymphoblastic leukemia at diagnosis: results from the international ALL trial MRC UKALL XII/ECOG E2993. Blood. 2006;108(2):465–72.
18. Landau H, Lamanna N. Clinical manifestations and treatment of newly diagnosed acute lymphoblastic leukemia in adults. Curr Hematol Malig Rep. 2006;1(3):171–9.
19. Thomas DA, O'Brien S, Jorgensen JL, Cortes J, Faderl S, Garcia-Manero G, et al. Prognostic significance of CD20 expression in adults with de novo precursor B-lineage acute lymphoblastic leukemia. Blood. 2009;113(25):6330–7.
20. Maury S, Huguet F, Leguay T, Lacombe F, Maynadie M, Girard S, et al. Adverse prognostic significance of CD20 expression in adults with Philadelphia-chromosome-negative B-cell precursor acute lymphoblastic leukemia. Haematologica. 2010;95(2):324–8.
21. Tafuri A, Gregorj C, Petrucci MT, Ricciardi MR, Mancini M, Cimino G, et al. MDR1 protein expression is an independent predictor of complete remission in newly diagnosed adult acute lymphoblastic leukemia. Blood. 2002;100(3):974–81.
22. Vitale A, Guarini A, Ariola C, Mancini M, Mecucci C, Cuneo A, et al. Adult T-cell acute lymphoblastic leukemia: biologic profile at presentation and correlation with response to induction treatment in patients enrolled in the GIMEMA LAL 0496 protocol. Blood. 2006; 107(2):473–9.
23. Kager L, Cheok M, Yang W, Zaza G, Cheng Q, Panetta JC, et al. Folate pathway gene expression differs in subtypes of acute lymphoblastic leukemia and influences methotrexate pharmacodynamics. J Clin Invest. 2005;115(1):110–7.
24. Schrappe M, Reiter A, Ludwig WD, Harbott J, Zimmermann M, Hiddemann W, et al. Improved outcome in childhood acute lymphoblastic leukemia despite reduced use of anthracyclines and cranial radiotherapy: results of trial ALL-BFM 90. German-Austrian-Swiss ALL-BFM Study Group. Blood. 2000;95(11):3310–22.
25. Pui CH, Sallan S, Relling MV, Masera G, Evans WE. International childhood acute lymphoblastic leukemia workshop: Sausalito, CA, 30 November-1 December 2000. Leukemia. 2001;15(5):707–15.
26. Mancini M, Scappaticci D, Cimino G, Nanni M, Derme V, Elia L, et al. A comprehensive genetic classification of adult acute lymphoblastic leukemia (ALL): analysis of the GIMEMA 0496 protocol. Blood. 2005;105(9):3434–41.
27. Ferrando AA, Neuberg DS, Staunton J, Loh ML, Huard C, Raimondi SC, et al. Gene expression signatures define novel oncogenic pathways in T-cell acute lymphoblastic leukemia. Cancer Cell. 2002;1(1):75–87.
28. Graux C, Cools J, Michaux L, Vandenberghe P, Hagemeijer A. Cytogenetics and molecular genetics of T-cell acute lymphoblastic leukemia: from thymocyte to lymphoblast. Leukemia. 2006;20(9):1496–510.

29. Pane F, Intrieri M, Quintarelli C, Izzo B, Muccioli GC, Salvatore F. BCR/ABL genes and leukemic phenotype: from molecular mechanisms to clinical correlations. Oncogene. 2002;21(56):8652–67.

30. Gleissner B, Gokbuget N, Bartram CR, Janssen B, Rieder H, Janssen JW, et al. Leading prognostic relevance of the BCR-ABL translocation in adult acute B-lineage lymphoblastic leukemia: a prospective study of the German Multicenter Trial Group and confirmed polymerase chain reaction analysis. Blood. 2002;99(5):1536–43.

31. Rambaldi A, Attuati V, Bassan R, Neonato MG, Viero P, Battista R, et al. Molecular diagnosis and clinical relevance of t(9;22), t(4;11) and t(1; 19) chromosome abnormalities in a consecutive group of 141 adult patients with acute lymphoblastic leukemia. Leuk Lymphoma. 1996;21(5–6):457–66.

32. Ayton PM, Cleary ML. Molecular mechanisms of leukemogenesis mediated by MLL fusion proteins. Oncogene. 2001;20(40):5695–707.

33. Ernst P, Wang J, Korsmeyer SJ. The role of MLL in hematopoiesis and leukemia. Curr Opin Hematol. 2002;9(4):282–7.

34. Pullarkat V, Slovak ML, Kopecky KJ, Forman SJ, Appelbaum FR. Impact of cytogenetics on the outcome of adult acute lymphoblastic leukemia: results of Southwest Oncology Group 9400 study. Blood. 2008;111(5):2563–72.

35. Aspland SE, Bendall HH, Murre C. The role of E2A-PBX1 in leukemogenesis. Oncogene. 2001;20(40):5708–17.

36. Foa R, Vitale A, Mancini M, Cuneo A, Mecucci C, Elia L, et al. E2A-PBX1 fusion in adult acute lymphoblastic leukaemia: biological and clinical features. Br J Haematol. 2003;120(3):484–7.

37. Charrin C, Thomas X, Ffrench M, Le QH, Andrieux J, Mozziconacci MJ, et al. A report from the LALA-94 and LALA-SA groups on hypodiploidy with 30 to 39 chromosomes and near-triploidy: 2 possible expressions of a sole entity conferring poor prognosis in adult acute lymphoblastic leukemia (ALL). Blood. 2004;104(8):2444–51.

38. Ballerini P, Blaise A, Busson-Le Coniat M, Su XY, Zucman-Rossi J, Adam M, et al. HOX11L2 Expression defines a clinical subtype of pediatric T-ALL associated with poor prognosis. Blood. 2002;100(3):991–7.

39. Cave H, Suciu S, Preudhomme C, Poppe B, Robert A, Uyttebroeck A, et al. Clinical significance of HOX11L2 expression linked to t(5;14)(q35;q32), of HOX11 expression, and of SIL-TAL fusion in childhood T-cell malignancies: results of EORTC studies 58881 and 58951. Blood. 2004;103(2):442–50.

40. Ferrando AA, Neuberg DS, Dodge RK, Paietta E, Larson RA, Wiernik PH, et al. Prognostic importance of TLX1 (HOX11) oncogene expression in adults with T-cell acute lymphoblastic leukaemia. Lancet. 2004;363(9408):535–6.

41. Burkhardt B, Bruch J, Zimmermann M, Strauch K, Parwaresch R, Ludwig WD, et al. Loss of heterozygosity on chromosome 6q14–q24 is associated with poor outcome in children and adolescents with T-cell lymphoblastic lymphoma. Leukemia. 2006;20(8):1422–9.

42. Ferrando AA, Armstrong SA, Neuberg DS, Sallan SE, Silverman LB, Korsmeyer SJ, et al. Gene expression signatures in MLL-rearranged T-lineage and B-precursor acute leukemias: dominance of HOX dysregulation. Blood. 2003;102(1):262–8.

43. Rubnitz JE, Camitta BM, Mahmoud H, Raimondi SC, Carroll AJ, Borowitz MJ, et al. Childhood acute lymphoblastic leukemia with the MLL-ENL fusion and t(11;19)(q23;p13.3) translocation. J Clin Oncol. 1999;17(1):191–6.

44. Pui CH, Gaynon PS, Boyett JM, Chessells JM, Baruchel A, Kamps W, et al. Outcome of treatment in childhood acute lymphoblastic leukaemia with rearrangements of the 11q23 chromosomal region. Lancet. 2002;359(9321):1909–15.

45. Asnafi V, Radford-Weiss I, Dastugue N, Bayle C, Leboeuf D, Charrin C, et al. CALM-AF10 is a common fusion transcript in T-ALL and is specific to the TCRgammadelta lineage. Blood. 2003;102(3):1000–6.

46. Ramakers-van Woerden NL, Pieters R, Slater RM, Loonen AH, Beverloo HB, van Drunen E, et al. In vitro drug resistance and prognostic impact of p16INK4A/P15INK4B deletions in childhood T-cell acute lymphoblastic leukaemia. Br J Haematol. 2001;112(3):680–90.

47. Loh ML, Goldwasser MA, Silverman LB, Poon WM, Vattikuti S, Cardoso A, et al. Prospective analysis of TEL/AML1-positive patients treated on Dana-Farber cancer institute consortium protocol 95-01. Blood. 2006;107(11):4508–13.

48. Faderl S, Kantarjian HM, Manshouri T, Chan CY, Pierce S, Hays KJ, et al. The prognostic significance of p16INK4a/p14ARF and p15INK4b deletions in adult acute lymphoblastic leukemia. Clin Cancer Res. 1999;5(7):1855–61.

49. Evans WE, McLeod HL. Pharmacogenomics – drug disposition, drug targets, and side effects. N Engl J Med. 2003;348(6):538–49.

50. Evans WE, Relling MV. Moving towards individualized medicine with pharmacogenomics. Nature. 2004;429(6990):464–8.

51. Relling MV, Pui CH, Sandlund JT, Rivera GK, Hancock ML, Boyett JM, et al. Adverse effect of anticonvulsants on efficacy of chemotherapy for acute lymphoblastic leukaemia. Lancet. 2000;356(9226):285–90.

52. Gaynor J, Chapman D, Little C, McKenzie S, Miller W, Andreeff M, et al. A cause-specific hazard rate analysis of prognostic factors among 199 adults with acute lymphoblastic leukemia: the memorial hospital experience since 1969. J Clin Oncol. 1988;6(6):1014–30.

53. Bruggemann M, Raff T, Flohr T, Gokbuget N, Nakao M, Droese J, et al. Clinical significance of minimal residual disease quantification in adult patients with standard-risk acute lymphoblastic leukemia. Blood. 2006;107(3):1116–23.

54. Bassan R, Spinelli O, Oldani E, Intermesoli T, Tosi M, Peruta B, et al. Improved risk classification for risk-specific therapy based on the molecular study of minimal residual disease (MRD) in adult acute lymphoblastic leukemia (ALL). Blood. 2009;113(18):4153–62.

55. Holowiecki J, Krawczyk-Kulis M, Giebel S, Jagoda K, Stella-Holowiecka B, Piatkowska-Jakubas B, et al. Status of minimal residual disease after induction predicts outcome in both standard and high-risk ph-negative adult acute lymphoblastic leukaemia. The Polish Adult Leukemia Group ALL 4-2002 MRD study. Br J Haematol. 2008;142(2):227–37.

56. Patel B, Rai L, Buck G, Richards SM, Mortuza Y, Mitchell W, et al. Minimal residual disease is a significant predictor of treatment failure in non T-lineage adult acute lymphoblastic leukaemia: final results of the international trial UKALL XII/ECOG2993. Br J Haematol. 2010;148(1):80–9.

57. Bruggemann M, Schrauder A, Raff T, Pfeifer H, Dworzak M, Ottmann OG, et al. Standardized MRD quantification in European ALL trials: proceedings of the second international symposium on MRD assessment in Kiel, Germany, 18-20 September 2008. Leukemia. 2010;24(3):521–35.

58. Raff T, Gokbuget N, Luschen S, Reutzel R, Ritgen M, Irmer S, et al. Molecular relapse in adult standard-risk ALL patients detected by prospective MRD monitoring during and after maintenance treatment: data from the GMALL 06/99 and 07/03 trials. Blood. 2007;109(3):910–5.

59. Pui CH, Pei D, Campana D, Bowman WP, Sandlund JT, Kaste SC, et al. Improved prognosis for older adolescents with acute lymphoblastic leukemia. J Clin Oncol. 2011;29(4):386–91.

60. Reiter A, Schrappe M, Ludwig WD, Hiddemann W, Sauter S, Henze G, et al. Chemotherapy in 998 unselected childhood acute lymphoblastic leukemia patients. Results and conclusions of the multicenter trial ALL-BFM 86. Blood. 1994;84(9):3122–33.

61. Conter V, Arico M, Valsecchi MG, Basso G, Biondi A, Madon E, et al. Long-term results of the Italian association of pediatric hematology and oncology (AIEOP) acute lymphoblastic leukemia studies, 1982-1995. Leukemia. 2000;14(12):2196–204.

62. Gaynon PS, Trigg ME, Heerema NA, Sensel MG, Sather HN, Hammond GD, et al. Children's Cancer Group trials in childhood acute lymphoblastic leukemia: 1983–1995. Leukemia. 2000;14(12):2223–33.

63. Kamps WA, Bokkerink JP, Hakvoort-Cammel FG, Veerman AJ, Weening RS, van Wering ER, et al. BFM-oriented treatment for children with acute lymphoblastic leukemia without cranial irradiation and treatment reduction for standard risk patients: results of DCLSG protocol ALL-8 (1991–1996). Leukemia. 2002;16(6):1099–111.

64. Vilmer E, Suciu S, Ferster A, Bertrand Y, Cave H, Thyss A, et al. Long-term results of three randomized trials (58831, 58832, 58881) in childhood acute lymphoblastic leukemia: a CLCG-EORTC report. Children Leukemia Cooperative Group. Leukemia. 2000;14(12):2257–66.

65. Gustafsson G, Schmiegelow K, Forestier E, Clausen N, Glomstein A, Jonmundsson G, et al. Improving outcome through two decades in childhood ALL in the Nordic countries: the impact of high-dose methotrexate in the reduction of CNS irradiation. Nordic society of pediatric Haematology and oncology (NOPHO). Leukemia. 2000;14(12):2267–75.
66. Silverman LB, Gelber RD, Dalton VK, Asselin BL, Barr RD, Clavell LA, et al. Improved outcome for children with acute lymphoblastic leukemia: results of Dana-Farber consortium protocol 91-01. Blood. 2001;97(5):1211–8.
67. Pui CH, Sandlund JT, Pei D, Campana D, Rivera GK, Ribeiro RC, et al. Improved outcome for children with acute lymphoblastic leukemia: results of total therapy study XIIIB at St Jude Children's research hospital. Blood. 2004;104(9):2690–6.
68. Hill FG, Richards S, Gibson B, Hann I, Lilleyman J, Kinsey S, et al. Successful treatment without cranial radiotherapy of children receiving intensified chemotherapy for acute lymphoblastic leukaemia: results of the risk-stratified randomized central nervous system treatment trial MRC UKALL XI (ISRC TN 16757172). Br J Haematol. 2004;124(1):33–46.
69. Larson RA, Dodge RK, Burns CP, Lee EJ, Stone RM, Schulman P, et al. A five-drug remission induction regimen with intensive consolidation for adults with acute lymphoblastic leukemia: Cancer and Leukemia Group B Study 8811. Blood. 1995;85(8):2025–37.
70. Thomas X, Boiron JM, Huguet F, Dombret H, Bradstock K, Vey N, et al. Outcome of treatment in adults with acute lymphoblastic leukemia: analysis of the LALA-94 trial. J Clin Oncol. 2004;22(20):4075–86.
71. Annino L, Vegna ML, Camera A, Specchia G, Visani G, Fioritoni G, et al. Treatment of adult acute lymphoblastic leukemia (ALL): long-term follow-up of the GIMEMA ALL 0288 randomized study. Blood. 2002;99(3):863–71.
72. Takeuchi J, Kyo T, Naito K, Sao H, Takahashi M, Miyawaki S, et al. Induction therapy by frequent administration of doxorubicin with four other drugs, followed by intensive consolidation and maintenance therapy for adult acute lymphoblastic leukemia: the JALSG-ALL93 study. Leukemia. 2002;16(7):1259–66.
73. Linker C, Damon L, Ries C, Navarro W. Intensified and shortened cyclical chemotherapy for adult acute lymphoblastic leukemia. J Clin Oncol. 2002;20(10):2464–71.
74. Thomas X, Danaila C, Le QH, Sebban C, Troncy J, Charrin C, et al. Long-term follow-up of patients with newly diagnosed adult acute lymphoblastic leukemia: a single institution experience of 378 consecutive patients over a 21-year period. Leukemia. 2001;15(12):1811–22.
75. Huguet F, Leguay T, Raffoux E, Thomas X, Beldjord K, Delabesse E, et al. Pediatric-inspired therapy in adults with Philadelphia chromosome-negative acute lymphoblastic leukemia: the GRAALL-2003 study. J Clin Oncol. 2009;27(6):911–8.
76. Stock W, La M, Sanford B, Bloomfield CD, Vardiman JW, Gaynon P, et al. What determines the outcomes for adolescents and young adults with acute lymphoblastic leukemia treated on cooperative group protocols? A comparison of Children's Cancer Group and Cancer and Leukemia Group B studies. Blood. 2008;112(5):1646–54.
77. Amylon MD, Shuster J, Pullen J, Berard C, Link MP, Wharam M, et al. Intensive high-dose asparaginase consolidation improves survival for pediatric patients with T cell acute lymphoblastic leukemia and advanced stage lymphoblastic lymphoma: a Pediatric Oncology Group Study. Leukemia. 1999;13(3):335–42.
78. Wetzler M, Sanford BL, Kurtzberg J, DeOliveira D, Frankel SR, Powell BL, et al. Effective asparagine depletion with pegylated asparaginase results in improved outcomes in adult acute lymphoblastic leukemia: Cancer and Leukemia Group B Study 9511. Blood. 2007;109(10): 4164–7.
79. Bassan R, Pogliani E, Lerede T, Fabris P, Rossi G, Morandi S, et al. Fractionated cyclophosphamide added to the IVAP regimen (idarubicin-vincristine-L-asparaginase-prednisone) could lower the risk of primary refractory disease in T-lineage but not B-lineage acute lymphoblastic leukemia: first results from a phase II clinical study. Haematologica. 1999;84(12):1088–93.
80. Yanada M, Takeuchi J, Sugiura I, Akiyama H, Usui N, Yagasaki F, et al. High complete remission rate and promising outcome by combination of imatinib and chemotherapy for newly diagnosed BCR-ABL-positive acute lymphoblastic leukemia: a phase II study by the Japan Adult Leukemia Study Group. J Clin Oncol. 2006;24(3):460–6.

81. Towatari M, Yanada M, Usui N, Takeuchi J, Sugiura I, Takeuchi M, et al. Combination of intensive chemotherapy and imatinib can rapidly induce high-quality complete remission for a majority of patients with newly diagnosed BCR-ABL-positive acute lymphoblastic leukemia. Blood. 2004;104(12):3507–12.

82. de Labarthe A, Rousselot P, Huguet-Rigal F, Delabesse E, Witz F, Maury S, et al. Imatinib combined with induction or consolidation chemotherapy in patients with de novo Philadelphia chromosome-positive acute lymphoblastic leukemia: results of the GRAAPH-2003 study. Blood. 2007;109(4):1408–13.

83. Thomas DA, Faderl S, Cortes J, O'Brien S, Giles FJ, Kornblau SM, et al. Treatment of Philadelphia chromosome-positive acute lymphocytic leukemia with hyper-CVAD and imatinib mesylate. Blood. 2004;103(12):4396–407.

84. Bostrom BC, Sensel MR, Sather HN, Gaynon PS, La MK, Johnston K, et al. Dexamethasone versus prednisone and daily oral versus weekly intravenous mercaptopurine for patients with standard-risk acute lymphoblastic leukemia: a report from the Children's Cancer Group. Blood. 2003;101(10):3809–17.

85. Mitchell CD, Richards SM, Kinsey SE, Lilleyman J, Vora A, Eden TO, et al. Benefit of dexamethasone compared with prednisolone for childhood acute lymphoblastic leukaemia: results of the UK medical research council ALL97 randomized trial. Br J Haematol. 2005; 129(6):734–45.

86. Avramis VI, Sencer S, Periclou AP, Sather H, Bostrom BC, Cohen LJ, et al. A randomized comparison of native Escherichia coli asparaginase and polyethylene glycol conjugated asparaginase for treatment of children with newly diagnosed standard-risk acute lymphoblastic leukemia: a Children's Cancer Group Study. Blood. 2002;99(6):1986–94.

87. Rizzari C, Valsecchi MG, Arico M, Conter V, Testi A, Barisone E, et al. Effect of protracted high-dose L-asparaginase given as a second exposure in a Berlin-Frankfurt-Munster-based treatment: results of the randomized 9102 intermediate-risk childhood acute lymphoblastic leukemia study – a report from the Associazione Italiana Ematologia Oncologia Pediatrica. J Clin Oncol. 2001;19(5):1297–303.

88. Douer D, Yampolsky H, Cohen LJ, Watkins K, Levine AM, Periclou AP, et al. Pharmacodynamics and safety of intravenous pegaspargase during remission induction in adults aged 55 years or younger with newly diagnosed acute lymphoblastic leukemia. Blood. 2007;109(7):2744–50.

89. Thomas DA, O'Brien S, Faderl S, Garcia-Manero G, Ferrajoli A, Wierda W, et al. Chemoimmunotherapy with a modified hyper-CVAD and rituximab regimen improves outcome in de novo Philadelphia chromosome-negative precursor B-lineage acute lymphoblastic leukemia. J Clin Oncol. 2010;28(24):3880–9.

90. Petersdorf SH, Kopecky KJ, Head DR, Boldt DH, Balcerzak SP, Wun T, et al. Comparison of the L10M consolidation regimen to an alternative regimen including escalating methotrexate/L-asparaginase for adult acute lymphoblastic leukemia: a Southwest Oncology Group Study. Leukemia. 2001;15(2):208–16.

91. Bassan R, Pogliani E, Casula P, Rossi G, Fabris P, Morandi S, et al. Risk-oriented postremission strategies in adult acute lymphoblastic leukemia: prospective confirmation of anthracycline activity in standard-risk class and role of hematopoietic stem cell transplants in high-risk groups. Hematol J. 2001;2(2):117–26.

92. Pui CH, Relling MV, Evans WE. Is mega dose of methotrexate beneficial to patients with acute lymphoblastic leukemia? Leuk Lymphoma. 2006;47(12):2431–2.

93. Skarby TV, Anderson H, Heldrup J, Kanerva JA, Seidel H, Schmiegelow K, et al. High leucovorin doses during high-dose methotrexate treatment may reduce the cure rate in childhood acute lymphoblastic leukemia. Leukemia. 2006;20(11):1955–62.

94. Marks DI, Paietta EM, Moorman AV, Richards SM, Buck G, DeWald G, et al. T-cell acute lymphoblastic leukemia in adults: clinical features, immunophenotype, cytogenetics, and outcome from the large randomized prospective trial (UKALL XII/ECOG 2993). Blood. 2009;114(25):5136–45.

95. Arico M, Baruchel A, Bertrand Y, Biondi A, Conter V, Eden T, et al. The seventh international childhood acute lymphoblastic leukemia workshop report: Palermo, Italy, January 29–30, 2005. Leukemia. 2005;19(7):1145–52.

96. Nygaard U, Toft N, Schmiegelow K. Methylated metabolites of 6-mercaptopurine are associated with hepatotoxicity. Clin Pharmacol Ther. 2004;75(4):274–81.

97. Conter V, Valsecchi MG, Silvestri D, Campbell M, Dibar E, Magyarosy E, et al. Pulses of vincristine and dexamethasone in addition to intensive chemotherapy for children with intermediate-risk acute lymphoblastic leukaemia: a multicentre randomised trial. Lancet. 2007; 369(9556):123–31.

98. Doney K, Gooley TA, Deeg HJ, Flowers ME, Storb R, Appelbaum FR. Allogeneic hematopoietic cell transplantation with full-intensity conditioning for adult acute lymphoblastic leukemia: results from a single center, 1998-2006. Biol Blood Marrow Transplant. 2011;17(8):1187–95.

99. Goldstone AH, Richards SM, Lazarus HM, Tallman MS, Buck G, Fielding AK, et al. In adults with standard-risk acute lymphoblastic leukemia, the greatest benefit is achieved from a matched sibling allogeneic transplantation in first complete remission, and an autologous transplantation is less effective than conventional consolidation/maintenance chemotherapy in all patients: final results of the international ALL trial (MRC UKALL XII/ECOG E2993). Blood. 2008;111(4):1827–33.

100. Lee S, Cho BS, Kim SY, Choi SM, Lee DG, Eom KS, et al. Allogeneic stem cell transplantation in first complete remission enhances graft-versus-leukemia effect in adults with acute lymphoblastic leukemia: antileukemic activity of chronic graft-versus-host disease. Biol Blood Marrow Transplant. 2007;13(9):1083–94.

101. Sebban C, Lepage E, Vernant JP, Gluckman E, Attal M, Reiffers J, et al. Allogeneic bone marrow transplantation in adult acute lymphoblastic leukemia in first complete remission: a comparative study. French group of Therapy of Adult Acute Lymphoblastic Leukemia. J Clin Oncol. 1994;12(12):2580–7.

102. Horowitz MM, Messerer D, Hoelzer D, Gale RP, Neiss A, Atkinson K, et al. Chemotherapy compared with bone marrow transplantation for adults with acute lymphoblastic leukemia in first remission. Ann Intern Med. 1991;115(1):13–8.

103. Messerer D, Neiss A, Horowitz MM, Hoelzer D, Gale RP. Comparison of chemotherapy and bone marrow transplants using two independent clinical databases. J Clin Epidemiol. 1994;47(10):1119–26.

104. Mohty M, Labopin M, Tabrizzi R, Theorin N, Fauser AA, Rambaldi A, et al. Reduced intensity conditioning allogeneic stem cell transplantation for adult patients with acute lymphoblastic leukemia: a retrospective study from the European Group for Blood and Marrow Transplantation. Haematologica. 2008;93(2):303–6.

105. Ram R, Storb R, Sandmaier BM, Maloney DG, Woolfrey A, Flowers ME, et al. Nonmyeloablative conditioning with allogeneic hematopoietic cell transplantation for the treatment of high-risk acute lymphoblastic leukemia. Haematologica. 2011;96(8):1113–20.

106. Bachanova V, Verneris MR, DeFor T, Brunstein CG, Weisdorf DJ. Prolonged survival in adults with acute lymphoblastic leukemia after reduced-intensity conditioning with cord blood or sibling donor transplantation. Blood. 2009;113(13):2902–5.

107. Ribera JM, Oriol A, Bethencourt C, Parody R, Hernandez-Rivas JM, Moreno MJ, et al. Comparison of intensive chemotherapy, allogeneic or autologous stem cell transplantation as post-remission treatment for adult patients with high-risk acute lymphoblastic leukemia. Results of the PETHEMA ALL-93 trial. Haematologica. 2005;90(10):1346–56.

108. Gokbuget N, Hoelzer D, Arnold R, Bohme A, Bartram CR, Freund M, et al. Treatment of adult ALL according to protocols of the German Multicenter Study Group for Adult ALL (GMALL). Hematol Oncol Clin North Am. 2000;14(6):1307, 25, ix.

109. Bassan R, Hoelzer D. Modern therapy of acute lymphoblastic leukemia. J Clin Oncol. 2011;29(5):532–43.

110. Vignetti M, Fazi P, Cimino G, Martinelli G, Di Raimondo F, Ferrara F, et al. Imatinib plus steroids induces complete remissions and prolonged survival in elderly philadelphia chromosome-positive patients with acute lymphoblastic leukemia without additional chemotherapy: results of the gruppo italiano malattie ematologiche dell'Adulto (GIMEMA) LAL0201-B protocol. Blood. 2007;109(9):3676–8.

111. Delannoy A, Delabesse E, Lheritier V, Castaigne S, Rigal-Huguet F, Raffoux E, et al. Imatinib and methylprednisolone alternated with chemotherapy improve the outcome of elderly patients with Philadelphia-positive acute lymphoblastic leukemia: results of the GRAALL AFR09 study. Leukemia. 2006;20(9):1526–32.

112. Ottmann OG, Wassmann B, Pfeifer H, Giagounidis A, Stelljes M, Duhrsen U, et al. Imatinib compared with chemotherapy as front-line treatment of elderly patients with Philadelphia chromosome-positive acute lymphoblastic leukemia (Ph+ ALL). Cancer. 2007;109(10):2068–76.

113. Ottmann O, Dombret H, Martinelli G, Simonsson B, Guilhot F, Larson RA, et al. Dasatinib induces rapid hematologic and cytogenetic responses in adult patients with Philadelphia chromosome-positive acute lymphoblastic leukemia with resistance or intolerance to imatinib: interim results of a phase 2 study. Blood. 2007;110(7):2309–15.

114. Kantarjian H, Giles F, Wunderle L, Bhalla K, O'Brien S, Wassmann B, et al. Nilotinib in imatinib-resistant CML and Philadelphia chromosome-positive ALL. N Engl J Med. 2006;354(24):2542–51.

115. Bassan R, Rossi G, Pogliani EM, Di Bona E, Angelucci E, Cavattoni I, et al. Chemotherapy-phased imatinib pulses improve long-term outcome of adult patients with Philadelphia chromosome-positive acute lymphoblastic leukemia: Northern Italy Leukemia Group protocol 09/00. J Clin Oncol. 2010;28(22):3644–52.

116. Lee KH, Lee JH, Choi SJ, Lee JH, Seol M, Lee YS, et al. Clinical effect of imatinib added to intensive combination chemotherapy for newly diagnosed Philadelphia chromosome-positive acute lymphoblastic leukemia. Leukemia. 2005;19(9):1509–16.

117. Ribera JM, Oriol A, Gonzalez M, Vidriales B, Brunet S, Esteve J, et al. Concurrent intensive chemotherapy and imatinib before and after stem cell transplantation in newly diagnosed Philadelphia chromosome-positive acute lymphoblastic leukemia. Final results of the CSTIBES02 trial. Haematologica. 2010;95(1):87–95.

118. Wassmann B, Pfeifer H, Goekbuget N, Beelen DW, Beck J, Stelljes M, et al. Alternating versus concurrent schedules of imatinib and chemotherapy as front-line therapy for Philadelphia-positive acute lymphoblastic leukemia (Ph+ ALL). Blood. 2006;108(5):1469–77.

119. Wassmann B, Pfeifer H, Stadler M, Bornhauser M, Bug G, Scheuring UJ, et al. Early molecular response to posttransplantation imatinib determines outcome in MRD + Philadelphia-positive acute lymphoblastic leukemia (Ph+ ALL). Blood. 2005;106(2):458–63.

120. Sancho JM, Ribera JM, Oriol A, Hernandez-Rivas JM, Rivas C, Bethencourt C, et al. Central nervous system recurrence in adult patients with acute lymphoblastic leukemia: frequency and prognosis in 467 patients without cranial irradiation for prophylaxis. Cancer. 2006;106(12):2540–6.

121. Pui CH. Central nervous system disease in acute lymphoblastic leukemia: Prophylaxis and treatment. Hematol Am Soc Hematol Educ Progr. 2006;142–6.

122. Cortes J, O'Brien SM, Pierce S, Keating MJ, Freireich EJ, Kantarjian HM. The value of high-dose systemic chemotherapy and intrathecal therapy for central nervous system prophylaxis in different risk groups of adult acute lymphoblastic leukemia. Blood. 1995;86(6):2091–7.

123. Fielding AK, Richards SM, Chopra R, Lazarus HM, Litzow MR, Buck G, et al. Outcome of 609 adults after relapse of acute lymphoblastic leukemia (ALL); an MRC UKALL12/ECOG 2993 study. Blood. 2007;109(3):944–50.

124. O'Brien S, Thomas D, Ravandi F, Faderl S, Cortes J, Borthakur G, et al. Outcome of adults with acute lymphocytic leukemia after second salvage therapy. Cancer. 2008;113(11):3186–91.

125. Oriol A, Vives S, Hernandez-Rivas JM, Tormo M, Heras I, Rivas C, et al. Outcome after relapse of acute lymphoblastic leukemia in adult patients included in four consecutive risk-adapted trials by the PETHEMA Study Group. Haematologica. 2010;95(4):589–96.

126. DeAngelo DJ, Yu D, Johnson JL, Coutre SE, Stone RM, Stopeck AT, et al. Nelarabine induces complete remissions in adults with relapsed or refractory T-lineage acute lymphoblastic leukemia or lymphoblastic lymphoma: Cancer and Leukemia Group B Study 19801. Blood. 2007;109(12):5136–42.

127. Berg SL, Blaney SM, Devidas M, Lampkin TA, Murgo A, Bernstein M, et al. Phase II study of nelarabine (compound 506U78) in children and young adults with refractory T-cell malignancies: a report from the Children's Oncology Group. J Clin Oncol. 2005;23(15):3376–82.

128. Cohen MH, Johnson JR, Massie T, Sridhara R, McGuinn Jr WD, Abraham S, et al. Approval summary: nelarabine for the treatment of T-cell lymphoblastic leukemia/lymphoma. Clin Cancer Res. 2006;12(18):5329–35.

129. Topp MS, Kufer P, Gokbuget N, Goebeler M, Klinger M, Neumann S, et al. Targeted therapy with the T-cell-engaging antibody blinatumomab of chemotherapy-refractory minimal residual disease in B-lineage acute lymphoblastic leukemia patients results in high response rate and prolonged leukemia-free survival. J Clin Oncol. 2011;29(18):2493–8.

130. Yavuz S, Paydas S, Disel U, Sahin B. IDA-FLAG regimen for the therapy of primary refractory and relapse acute leukemia: a single-center experience. Am J Ther. 2006;13(5):389–93.

131. Specchia G, Pastore D, Carluccio P, Liso A, Mestice A, Rizzi R, et al. FLAG-IDA in the treatment of refractory/relapsed adult acute lymphoblastic leukemia. Ann Hematol. 2005;84(12): 792–5.

132. Rijneveld AW, van der Holt B, Daenen SM, Biemond BJ, de Weerdt O, Muus P, et al. Intensified chemotherapy inspired by a pediatric regimen combined with allogeneic transplantation in adult patients with acute lymphoblastic leukemia up to the age of 40. Leukemia. 2011;25(11):1697–703.

133. Hiddemann W, Buchner T, Heil G, Schumacher K, Diedrich H, Maschmeyer G, et al. Treatment of refractory acute lymphoblastic leukemia in adults with high dose cytosine arabinoside and mitoxantrone (HAM). Leukemia. 1990;4(9):637–40.

134. Schiller G, Lee M, Territo M, Gajewski J, Nimer S. Phase II study of etoposide, ifosfamide, and mitoxantrone for the treatment of resistant adult acute lymphoblastic leukemia. Am J Hematol. 1993;43(3):195–9.

135. O'Brien S, Thomas DA, Ravandi F, Faderl S, Pierce S, Kantarjian H. Results of the hyperfractionated cyclophosphamide, vincristine, doxorubicin, and dexamethasone regimen in elderly patients with acute lymphocytic leukemia. Cancer. 2008;113(8):2097–101.

136. Lee-Sherick AB, Linger RM, Gore L, Keating AK, Graham DK. Targeting paediatric acute lymphoblastic leukaemia: novel therapies currently in development. Br J Haematol. 2010;151(4):295–311.

Chapter 3
Chronic Lymphocytic Leukemia (CLL)

Jonathan A. Gutman, Kelly M. Smith, and John M. Pagel

Abstract Chronic lymphocytic leukemia is the most common leukemia affecting adults in Western countries, accounting for about 30% of all leukemias. It is a clonal malignancy of mature CD5$^+$ B-lymphocytes involving the peripheral blood, bone marrow, and lymphoid organs and has a distinct immunophenotype that allows differentiation from other B-cell lymphomas. Most patients with CLL present with a lymphocytosis at diagnosis; however, some patients present with lymphadenopathy alone. CLL is predominantly a disease of the elderly as the median age at diagnosis is 72 years. The clinical course of CLL is quite variable, with survival times from initial diagnosis ranging from 2 to 20 years.

Keywords Chronic lymphocytic leukemia • Leukemia • Peripheral blood • Bone marrow • Lymphoid organs • B-cell lymphoma • Lymphocytosis • Lymphadenopathy • Elderly

J.A. Gutman, M.D.
Department of Medical Oncology, University of Colorado School of Medicine,
1665 Aurora Court, Room 2251A, Aurora, CO 80045, USA
e-mail: jonathan.gutman@ucdenver.edu

K.M. Smith, M.D.
Divisions of Hematology and Oncology, University of Washington School of Medicine,
Seattle, WA, USA
e-mail: kmsmith@seattlecca.org

J.M. Pagel, M.D., Ph.D. (✉)
Associate Professor, Department of Medicine, University of Washington
School of Medicine, Seattle, WA, USA

Associate Member, Fred Hutchinson Cancer Research Center, 1100 Fairview Ave N,
D5-380, Seattle, WA 98109, USA
e-mail: jpagel@fhcrc.org

E.H. Estey and F.R. Appelbaum (eds.), *Leukemia and Related Disorders:*
Integrated Treatment Approaches, Contemporary Hematology,
DOI 10.1007/978-1-60761-565-1_3, © Springer Science+Business Media, LLC 2012

Introduction

Chronic lymphocytic leukemia (CLL) is the most common leukemia affecting adults in Western countries, accounting for about 30% of all leukemias [1]. It is a clonal malignancy of mature CD5$^+$ B-lymphocytes involving the peripheral blood, bone marrow, and lymphoid organs and has a distinct immunophenotype that allows differentiation from other B-cell lymphomas. Most patients with CLL present with a lymphocytosis at diagnosis; however, some patients present with lymphadenopathy alone.

The incidence of CLL increases proportionately by decade. CLL is predominantly a disease of the elderly as the median age at diagnosis is 72 years [2]. The clinical course of CLL is quite variable with survival times from initial diagnosis ranging from 2 to 20 years with a median of 10 years. Some patients may die quickly, within several years of diagnosis, from complications or causes directly related to their CLL. There are other patients that follow a benign course and do not require treatment for many years and may have a relatively normal life span. Recent insight into the molecular biology of CLL has led to the development of important prognostic factors that are helpful in risk stratifying patients. Although there are no known chemotherapeutic regimens that can cure CLL, newer treatment regimens incorporating purine nucleoside analogs and monoclonal antibodies are improving response rates and prolonging survival for the first time in the natural history of this disease. Importantly, results from studies using reduced-intensity stem cell transplantation are promising for a potential cure. To further improve outcomes, there are a number of investigative agents, such as monoclonal antibodies, CDK inhibitors, Bcl-2 inhibitors, and vaccines that are currently under development.

Epidemiology

CLL is the most common leukemia in adults in the West. This disease affects 3–5 per 100,000 persons. SEER estimates for 2010 indicate that approximately 14,990 patients (8,870 men and 6,120 women) will be diagnosed in the United States and that 4,390 people (2,650 men and 1,740 women) will die from CLL-related complications [3]. For unclear reasons, the incidence of CLL is 70–90% higher in men than women [4]. The risk of developing CLL increases progressively with age without reaching a plateau [5]. CLL is largely a disease of the elderly with a median age of diagnosis of 72 [1]. While most patients are elderly, there are still a large number of younger patients affected. Between 20% and 30% of patients are 60 or younger, and 5–10% are 50 or younger [6]. The incidence of CLL also varies among ethnic backgrounds and geographic location. The incidence of CLL is highest in Caucasians, intermediate in African Americans, and lowest in Asians and Pacific islanders [7]. In addition, there is a higher incidence of CLL in North America and Europe when compared to the rest of the world [7].

Etiology

The etiology of CLL is elusive. Ionizing radiation has been linked to other leukemias; however, most studies of individuals exposed to medical, occupational, or environmental sources of ionizing radiation have not found a link between radiation exposure and CLL [4]. Survivors of Hiroshima and Chernobyl do not appear to have an increased incidence of CLL [8, 9]. Furthermore, there is no strong evidence to associate CLL with exposure to nonionizing radiation, such as power lines [4]. There may, however, be a role between chemical exposure and CLL as there are reports of an increased risk of CLL in farmers exposed to certain agricultural chemicals [4]. In addition, CLL is recognized as a service-connected illness among Vietnam War veterans who were exposed to Agent Orange [10].

There is no known association between CLL and viruses, including human T-cell lymphotrophic viruses I and II (HTLV-I and HTLV-II) and Epstein-Barr virus (EBV) [11]. In addition, there is no known link between tobacco use, physical activity, diet, and body mass index and CLL [4].

There are, however, several lines of evidence to suggest that genetic factors may play an important role in this disease. First, the incidence of CLL varies among different ethnicities. CLL is most common in Caucasians and less common in African Americans, Asians, and Pacific islanders [7]. The low incidence of CLL in Asians is maintained in immigrants and their offspring after they move to the United States suggesting that genetics, more than environmental factors, may play an important part in the pathogenesis of this disease [7]. This finding is in stark contrast to breast cancer rates which have increased in Asians who have migrated to Western countries [12]. Secondly, CLL has a strong familial tendency which has been described in many reports of familial clustering, case control, and cohort studies [13]. Six percent of patients with CLL have one or more affected family members [14]. First-degree family members of patients with CLL have a relative risk of 7.5 of developing CLL compared to the general population [1]. Family members also have a higher risk of developing other lymphoproliferative disorders. The relative risk of developing non-Hodgkin lymphoma and Hodgkin disease is 1.45 and 2.35, respectively. This increased risk is similar in parents, siblings, and children of affected individuals [1].

Familial CLL is accompanied by the anticipation phenomenon with subsequent generations developing the disease at an earlier age [1]. The age of onset has been reported to be reduced by approximately 20 years between generations. In addition, some studies indicate that the disease was more severe in the offspring generation [14]. Otherwise, familial CLL does not seem to differ from sporadic CLL in terms of prognostic markers and clinical outcomes [1]. An analysis of 1,449 patients demonstrated that familial and sporadic cases had a similar percentage of advanced stages (10.8% vs 7.1%), patients needing treatment (55% vs 60%), and 10-year overall survival (67% vs 66%) [13].

Research on familial CLL has not led to the discovery yet of any obvious gene or group of genes that are clearly related to the development of CLL. Moreover, there are currently no genetic tests that are available to determine if one has inherited an increased risk of disease. While relatives of affected patients are at increased risk, patients should be reassured that their family members' absolute risk of developing CLL is still very small at about 3% [15, 16].

Pathophysiology

In the past, CLL was thought to be a homogenous disease of immature, immune-incompetent B-cells which were arrested in the G0 phase of the cell cycle and accumulated due to defective apoptotic mechanisms. Recent discoveries about the biology of these leukemic cells have transformed our understanding of CLL. CLL is now thought to arise from antigen-stimulated mature B-lymphocytes that differ in the level of immunoglobulin V gene mutations. New data indicate that antigenic stimulation, in addition to interactions with accessory cells and cytokines, promotes proliferation of CLL cells and enables them to avoid apoptosis [17]. In vivo studies have demonstrated that there is a higher level of proliferation than previously understood. Between 0.1% and 1% of neoplastic cells are actively dividing and contributing to the accumulation of B-lymphocytes. Patients that have leukemic cells with a proliferative rate of 0.35% and greater have been found to have more aggressive disease [18].

Clinical Presentation

Symptoms

Patients can present with a wide range of symptoms related to expansion of the clonal B-cell population in their bone marrow, lymph nodes, and organs. Between 5% and 10% of patients present with constitutional B symptoms, such as fatigue, fevers, night sweats, and weight loss. Patients may also present with infections due to an acquired immunodeficiency disorder or symptoms related to an autoimmune-mediated cytopenia. Approximately 25% of patients, however, are asymptomatic at diagnosis and are discovered to have CLL based on a blood cell count during routine blood work [19].

Physical Examination Findings

The most common abnormal finding on physical examination in patients with CLL is lymphadenopathy, affecting 50–90% of patients. Palpable lymph nodes are typically firm, nontender, round, and mobile and are most often located in the cervical, supraclavicular, and axillary areas. Approximately 25–55% of patients have a palpable spleen on examination. Hepatomegaly is detected in about 15–25% of patients [20]. Skin is the most commonly affected nonlymphoid area, and these skin lesions, known as leukemia cutis, often involve the face [21]. Advanced stage CLL can involve non-lymphoid organs, such as the gastrointestinal tract, prostate, lungs, pleura, and bones; however, involvement of these organs is usually clinically insignificant.

Laboratory Findings

Most patients have a lymphocytosis in the peripheral blood with a median value of $30–50 \times 10^9$/L. The bone marrow is usually hypercellular with at least 30% mature lymphocytes [22]. Patients may also have mild degrees of neutropenia, anemia, and thrombocytopenia. Autoimmune-mediated cytopenias are also common in CLL; autoimmune hemolytic anemia affects 10–25% of patients with advanced stage CLL. It should be suspected when there is an abrupt drop in the hemoglobin with a positive Coombs test, elevated bilirubin, elevated reticulocyte count, elevated lactate dehydrogenase (LDH), and undetectable haptoglobin. Immune thrombocytopenia affects about 2% of patients and is diagnosed when there is a decrease in the platelet count without evidence of bone marrow failure due to leukemic infiltration or hyper-splenism. Pure red cell aplasia affects 6% of patients. It is suspected when there is worsening anemia with a low reticulocyte count and absence of erythroid precursors in the bone marrow. Viral infections, such as cytomegalovirus, Epstein-Barr virus, and parvovirus, need to be excluded before attributing red cell aplasia to an autoimmune process. Unlike typical autoimmune hemolytic anemia, immune thrombocytopenia and pure red cell aplasia can present early in the disease course. Autoimmune neutropenia is rare in CLL unless related to a therapeutic intervention [23, 24].

Hypogammaglobulinemia is a common complication that affects over 50% of CLL patients. Serum immunoglobulin levels tend to decline with increasing disease duration and predispose CLL patients to serious bacterial infections. Up to 10% of patients have a monoclonal gammopathy [20]. In addition, patients may also have elevated levels of serum LDH and beta$_2$ microglobulin [22].

Diagnosis

According to the World Health Organization (WHO), CLL and small lymphocytic lymphoma (SLL) are different manifestations of the same disease. CLL is diagnosed when there are circulating cells in the peripheral blood with certain morphologic and immunophenotypic characteristics. SLL, on the other hand, is diagnosed when lymph nodes or other tissues are infiltrated by these characteristic cells without evidence of these cells circulating in the blood. CLL is much more common with only 5% of patients presenting with SLL. In order to diagnose CLL, one should obtain a complete blood count, peripheral smear, and immunophenotypic analysis by flow cytometry [25]. Standard criteria for the diagnosis of CLL are shown in Table 3.1.

Table 3.1 Criteria for the diagnosis of chronic lymphocytic leukemia[a]

Peripheral blood B-lymphocytes
  $>5 \times 10^9$/L
Morphology
  Small mature lymphocytes
Clonality
  Needs to be confirmed by flow cytometry
Immunophenotype
  Light chain restriction
  Coexpression of T-cell antigen CD5 together with B-cell surface antigens CD19, CD20, and CD23
  Low expression of surface immunoglobulin (sIg) and absent or low expression of CD79b

[a]Based on criteria from National Cancer Institute-Working group (NCI-WG) [25]

Table 3.2 Immunophenotype of chronic lymphocytic leukemia and other chronic B-cell lymphoproliferative disorders [11]

Disease	sIg	CD5	CD10	CD19	CD20	CD22	CD23	CD79b
CLL	Dim	++	–	++	Dim	–/+	++	–
Follicular lymphoma	++	–	++	++	++	++	–	++
Mantle cell lymphoma	++	++	–	++	++	++	–	++
Marginal zone lymphoma	++	–	–	++	++	+/–	+/–	++
Prolymphocytic leukemia	+++	–/+	–/+	++	+++	++	–/+	++
Splenic lymphoma	++	–/+	–/+	++	++	++	+/–	++

sIg surface immunoglobulin; –=not expressed; –/+=usually is not expressed; +/–=usually is expressed; + to +++=varying degrees of strength of expression

The diagnosis of CLL requires that there are at least 5,000 B-lymphocytes/μL in the peripheral blood. Morphologically, these leukemic cells are usually small, mature lymphocytes with a dense nucleus with clumped chromatin without discernible nucleoli and small amounts of cytoplasm. These cells may also be found with larger cells, cleaved cells known as prolymphocytes; however, the presence of more than 55% of prolymphocytes is consistent with a diagnosis of prolymphocytic leukemia (B-cell PLL) instead of CLL. In addition, Gumprecht nuclear shadows, otherwise known as smudge cells, are a characteristic finding in the peripheral smear [25].

Flow cytometry is needed to demonstrate the presence of a clonal B-cell population and determine the immunophenotype of these cells. In CLL, leukemic cells express the T-cell antigen CD5 as well as B-cell surface antigens CD19, CD20, and CD23. The levels of surface immunoglobulin, CD20, and CD79b are low compared to those of normal B-cells [25].

It is crucial to confirm that a patient has CLL and not another lymphoproliferative disorder that can mimic CLL such as hairy cell leukemia or leukemic manifestations of follicular lymphoma, mantle cell lymphoma, marginal zone lymphoma, or splenic marginal zone lymphoma with circulating villous lymphocytes (Table 3.2). Differentiating CLL/SLL from mantle cell lymphoma is essential as they are both CD5[+] B-cell malignancies. While CD23 is often useful, cyclin D1 negativity and the absence of the t(11;14) chromosomal translocation by fluorescence in situ hybridization (FISH) can help distinguish the two entities [26]. There are other tests that are not necessary for diagnosis but may be helpful to assess tumor burden and predict prognosis. These tests will be described in the "Prognostic Factors" section of this chapter.

Monoclonal B-Lymphocytosis

Some individuals have a small clonal population of B-lymphocytes with a lymphocyte count up to 5,000/µL without features of a lymphoproliferative disorder. These patients should not have lymphadenopathy, splenomegaly, or B symptoms such as drenching fatigue, night sweats, unexplained fever, or unintentional weight loss. These patients are diagnosed with "monoclonal B-lymphocytosis" (MBL). MBL is immunophenotypically similar to CLL. Most cases of MBL share a similar expression pattern of markers CD5, CD20, CD23, and CD79b with CLL [27].

MBL is a common finding of unclear clinical significance. The prevalence of MBL is several hundred times greater than the prevalence of CLL with 3–7% of all adults and 9% of elderly individuals having an abnormal B-cell clone detectable by flow cytometry. There is increased detection of MBL in some CLL families. MBL is found in over 10% of individuals with more than two first-degree relatives with CLL [28].

Data on the natural history of MBL are sparse. MBL can have a variable course; it may regress, remain stable, or progress to clinical CLL or another lymphoproliferative disease. Screening usually entails a complete blood count and physical exam every 6–12 months [29]. Most patients will not develop CLL. The chance of progressing to CLL and requiring treatment is 1–2% per year, which is similar to the rate of progression of monoclonal gammopathy of unclear significance (MGUS) to multiple myeloma. Based on a published series, over 15% of MBL patients developed progressive CLL, 7% required chemotherapy, and 2% died due to CLL [27].

In one cohort study, the absolute B-cell count was the only independent prognostic factor associated with worsening lymphocytosis [27]. In a retrospective analysis of hematopathology records from the Mayo Clinic, both absolute B-cell count and CD38 status were related to time to treatment. In another study, the presence of trisomy 12 or deletion 17p13 was the only independent predictors of treatment requirement [28]. Similar to MGUS, most deaths are not due to CLL but to unrelated causes. Age and hemoglobin are the only independent prognostic factors associated with death [27].

There are multiple clinically important differences between MBL and Rai stage 0 CLL that validates the distinction between these entities. Patients with MBL have a more preserved immune function with a lower risk of infection. They also have slower disease kinetics as demonstrated by a longer doubling time [28]. MBL is associated with a more favorable genetic profile compared to CLL. A similar percentage of patients with MBL have favorable chromosomal abnormalities such as 13q14 deletion (48%) and trisomy 12 (20%) compared to patients with CLL. Eighty-seven percent of patients have a mutated IgV$_H$ gene, another favorable finding.

Chromosomal abnormalities associated with a poor prognosis, such as deletions of 11q and 17p, are rare in MBL [27]. In addition, patients with MBL were less likely to need treatment compared to patients with Rai stage 0. Ten-year treatment-free survival was 68.7% in patients with MBL compared to 51.3% in patients with stage 0 CLL [29].

Staging

The Ann Arbor staging system is of limited utility in CLL since almost all patients have lymph node and bone marrow involvement. Instead, there are two other staging systems, the Rai system and the Binet system, which are used worldwide. The original Rai classification was modified to decrease the number of prognostic groups from 5 to 3. Now both staging systems include three major subgroups and are inexpensive and simple to use. They both rely on laboratory findings as well as the physical exam. Imaging such as ultrasound, computed tomography (CT), or magnetic resonance imaging is not necessary.

The Rai staging system is based on the concept that CLL follows a predictable course with a progressive increase in the tumor burden starting in the blood and bone marrow (causing a lymphocytosis), then involving the lymph nodes, spleen, and liver (causing lymphadenopathy and organomegaly) before finally leading to bone marrow failure (causing anemia and thrombocytopenia) [30].

The modified Rai classification defines low-risk disease as patients who have lymphocytosis with leukemia cells in the blood and/or marrow (formerly called Rai stage 0; Table 3.3). Patients with lymphocytosis, enlarged nodes in any site, and splenomegaly and/or hepatomegaly have intermediate-risk disease (formerly considered Rai stage I or stage II). Patients with disease-related anemia (defined by hemoglobin of 11 g/dL or less) and/or thrombocytopenia (defined by a platelet count of less than 100,000/dL) have high-risk disease (formerly classified as stage III and IV disease, respectively) [31].

Table 3.3 Modified Rai staging system [30]

Risk level	Stage	Clinical features	Median survival (years)
Low	0	Lymphocytosis[a] only	10
Intermediate	I	Lymphocytosis[a] with lymphadenopathy	7
	II	Lymphocytosis[a] with splenomegaly and/or hepatomegaly with or without lymphadenopathy	7
High	III	Lymphocytosis[a] with anemia (hemoglobin <11 g/dL) with or without lymphadenopathy, splenomegaly, or hepatomegaly	1.5–4
	IV	Lymphocytosis[a] with thrombocytopenia (platelets <100×10⁹/L) with or without anemia and/or lymphadenopathy, splenomegaly, or hepatomegaly	1.5–4

[a]Lymphocytes $>5 \times 10^9$/L in the peripheral blood and >30% of nucleated cells in the bone marrow

Table 3.4 Binet classification [32]

Stage	Clinical features	Rai staging	Median survival (years)
A	Lymphocytosis[a] with <3 areas of nodal involvement[b]	0–II	12
B	Lymphocytosis[a] with 3 or more areas of nodal involvement[b], with or without splenomegaly and/or hepatomegaly	I–II	7
C	Lymphocytosis[a] with anemia (hemoglobin <11 g/dL in men and <10 g/dL in women) or thrombocytopenia (platelets <100×10^9/L) regardless of the number of areas of nodal involvement, splenomegaly, or hepatomegaly	III–IV	2–4

[a]Lymphocytes >5×10^9/L in the peripheral blood and comprising >30% of total nucleated cells in the bone marrow
[b]Each cervical, axillary, and inguinal area (whether unilateral or bilateral) and spleen and liver count as one area

The Binet staging system is based on the number of involved areas and includes five potential areas of involvement: the head and neck, including the Waldeyer ring; axillae; groin; spleen and liver (Table 3.4). Patients with up to two areas of lymphadenopathy or organomegaly have stage A disease. Patients with three or more areas of lymphadenopathy or organomegaly have stage B disease. All patients that have a hemoglobin of 10 g/dL or less and/or a platelet count of 100,000/dL or less have stage C disease regardless of the number of involved lymph nodes and organs [32].

The Binet staging system may need to be modified in the future as CT scans are becoming more routine and identifying mediastinal and retroperitoneal lymphadenopathy that are not currently included among the five areas of involvement. Furthermore, it may be helpful to differentiate cytopenias due to bone marrow failure from those due to autoimmune phenomena since patients with autoimmune-related anemia and thrombocytopenia have a more favorable prognosis compared to those with anemia and thrombocytopenia due to bone marrow infiltration.

Prognostic Factors

Disease stage is a powerful predictor of survival in CLL. Median survival according to the Rai clinical staging system is over 10 years for stage 0, 9 years for stage I, 7 years for stage II, and 5 years for stage III and stage IV. Median survival according to the Binet clinical staging system is 7–10 years for stage A, 5–7 years for stage B, and 2–5 years for stage C [2]. Although staging is an important prognostic factor, there are multiple limitations to using the staging system by itself. First, the majority of patients (80%) are categorized as early stage at diagnosis. Second, CLL is a very heterogeneous disease and there is tremendous variability in outcomes between individuals in the same stage. The staging system does not help differentiate between indolent and aggressive forms of disease. Third, the tumor burden and mechanism for cytopenias are not taken into consideration. Fourth, the response to therapy is not predicted [18]. Fortunately, there are multiple other variables, both traditional prognostic markers and novel biomarkers, which are predictive of survival in CLL and can be used in conjunction with staging.

Univariate and multivariate analyses were performed on 1,674 previously untreated CLL patients who presented to MD Anderson, and multiple patient characteristics that impacted survival were identified. Women had a superior median survival compared to men (12 vs 10 years). Age was an important predictive factor; the median survival was 13.3 years for individuals less than 50, 11.0 years for individuals aged 50–65, and 7.5 years for individuals over the age of 65. Patients with a performance status of 0 or 1 did better than those with a performance status of 2 or 3 (10.8 years vs 6 years). The number of involved lymph node sites corresponded to survival with a median survival of about 11 years with 0–2 nodal sites and 8.5 years with 3 or more nodal sites [33].

There are a number of laboratory values that are valuable prognostically. Among patients with Binet A stage disease, individuals with a beta$_2$ microglobulin less than 3.5 mg/dL have a progression-free survival (PFS) of over 75 months compared to 13 months for those with a beta$_2$ microglobulin of 3.5 mg/dL or more. A rapid lymphocyte doubling time of 12 months or less is linked to worse PFS (20 vs 75 months). An absolute lymphocyte count (ALC) of greater than 30×10^9/L is associated with PFS of 19 months versus 88 months for an ALC of less than 30×10^9/L [34]. Other adverse prognostic factors include atypical lymphocyte morphology, diffuse bone marrow involvement, high LDH, high levels of soluble CD23, and elevated serum thymidine kinase levels [11].

Chromosomal abnormalities are commonly found in CLL patients. Between 40% and 50% of patients have chromosomal abnormalities detected by karyotype alone, and more than 80% of patients have chromosomal abnormalities found by FISH. The most common recurrent chromosomal abnormalities observed include deletion 13q, deletion 11q, trisomy 12, deletion 17p, and deletion 6q. Certain abnormalities are favorable, while others are unfavorable. Deletion 17 p, which is found in 7% of patients, involves the *p53* locus and is the most unfavorable chromosomal abnormality with a median survival of 32 months and resistance to standard chemotherapy regimens using alkylating agents, purine analogs, and rituximab. Deletion 11q, which involves the ataxia-telangiectasia (ATM) gene, is another unfavorable mutation that is found in 18% of patients and is associated with a median survival of 79 months. These patients are often younger men with bulky lymphadenopathy. Patients with 17p deletions and 11q deletions present with more advanced disease and tend to have rapid disease progression with short treatment-free intervals of 9 and 13 months, respectively. Trisomy 12 is detected in 16% of patients and does not seem to impact survival as it is associated with a median survival of 114 months compared to 111 months for a normal karyotype. Deletion 13q, which is present in 55% of patients, is favorable when it is the sole chromosomal abnormality and is associated with a median survival of 133 months. Patients with 13q deletions have the longest treatment-free interval of 92 months [35].

Patients often have multiple chromosomal abnormalities at once. In this case, there is a hierarchy with the presence of *p53* mutations, deletion 17p, and deletion 11q being associated with poor-risk disease and the presence of deletion 13q as the sole abnormality being associated with better-risk disease. Some of these chromosomal abnormalities may be present at diagnosis; however, others may be acquired during the course of the disease so repeating FISH analyses prior to subsequent therapy may be informative [36].

In CLL, the leukemia cells express immunoglobulin that may have undergone somatic mutations in the immunoglobulin heavy chain variable region genes (also known as IgV_H genes). The cutoff value to identify mutated subtypes is less than 98% homology to germ line sequences [18]. Unmutated IgV_H genes are associated with high-risk cytogenetics and shortened survival of 8 years compared to 25 years in patients with mutated IgV_H genes [37]. Since it is technically difficult to routinely sequence IgV_H genes in clinical practice, surrogate markers for IgV_H mutational status are used instead [18].

CD38 expression correlates with unmutated IgV_H genes and is used as an independent prognostic factor. CD38-positive CLL patients do poorly with a shorter time to progression and overall survival of 3 years and 8–10 years, respectively [38]. The use of CD38 as a marker has several limitations. First of all, the optimal cutoff level for CD38 positivity is not yet known, although most studies use values equal to or greater than 20–30% as being CD38 positive. In addition, there is debate about the stability of the marker during the course of the disease, particularly after patients have been treated [18].

70-kDa zeta-associated protein (ZAP-70) is a tyrosine kinase normally expressed by natural killer and T-cells which is required for normal T-cell receptor signaling. ZAP-70 is not usually expressed in B-lymphocytes; however, it has been found in a subset of CLL patients. ZAP-70 expression of >20% correlates with IgV_H gene expression and worse outcomes including more rapid disease progression and shorter survival [39]. Patients with high ZAP-70 CLL have a median survival of 8–9 years from the time of diagnosis compared with 24 years among patients with low ZAP-70 [38]. Using ZAP-70 expression as a prognostic factor can be problematic; however, because 8–25% of cases show discordance between ZAP-70 expression and IgV_H mutational status [18].

In addition to being prognostic, certain molecular markers are predictive of outcomes (Table 3.5). Patients with 17p deletions have a poorer response as well as shorter PFS and overall survival among patients with CLL treated with first-line fludarabine-containing regimens. On the other hand, treatment with single-agent alemtuzumab has been shown to be effective in patients with 17p or p53 mutations, even those with fludarabine-refractory CLL [39].

Evaluating both traditional and novel prognostic factors can be very useful in patient management. One can risk stratify patients with early stage CLL into three categories: low risk, intermediate risk, and high risk. Low-risk patients have mutated IgV_H and a normal karyotype or deletion 13q by FISH. Intermediate-risk patients have mutated IgV_H and trisomy 12 by FISH. High-risk patients have any of the following: unmutated IgV_H, deletion 17p and/or deletion 11q by FISH. Asymptomatic patients with early stage disease who are in the low-risk category can be reassured that their disease will likely have an indolent course and that their median survival may be over 15–20 years. Many of these patients may never require treatment for their CLL. Patients in the intermediate-risk category often do not need treatment for 3–4 years and have a median survival of about 10 years. These patients should be seen every 6–12 months for a physical exam and complete blood count. Approximately 30–50%

Table 3.5 Prognostic factors for chronic lymphocytic leukemia

Prognostic variable	Clinical risk	
	Low	High
Clinical features		
Sex	Female	Male
Stage	Binet A/Rai 0	Binet C/Rai III–IV
Morphology		
Lymphocyte morphology	Typical	Atypical
Pattern of marrow involvement	Nodular or interstitial	Diffuse
Markers of tumor burden		
Lymphocyte doubling time	>12 months	≤12 months
B2-microglobulin levels	Low to normal	High
Thymidine kinase	Low to normal	High
Lactate dehydrogenase	Low to normal	High
Soluble CD23 levels	Low to normal	High
Chromosomal abnormalities		
	Normal	17p-
	Trisomy 12	11q-
	13q-	
Genetic markers		
CD38 expression	<20–30%	>20–30%
ZAP-70 expression	<20–30%	>20–30%
IgV_H gene status	Mutated	Unmutated
Tumor suppressors or oncogene p53	Normal	Loss, mutation, or dysfunction

of patients with early stage CLL will have aggressive disease with a high risk for early disease progression. These patients with high-risk, early stage disease usually require treatment within 1–4 years and have a median survival of only 3–8 years [6].

Instead of providing a blanket reassurance to newly diagnosed patients with CLL, health care providers can now equip themselves with information about an individual's risk which can help them personalize their counseling. Patients with early stage disease with unfavorable features are at high risk for having disease progression and requiring treatment compared to those with favorable features. These high-risk patients may benefit from closer monitoring compared to those with low-risk features or immediate treatment in the context of a clinical trial [6].

CLL Treatment

Indications for Treatment

CLL is a heterogeneous disease that demonstrates a highly variable clinical course and is traditionally considered, with the exception of allogeneic hematopoietic cell transplantation (HCT), to be incurable using standard treatment options.

Table 3.6   Criteria for treatment[a]

1. Evidence of progressive marrow failure
   Manifested by the development of, or worsening of, anemia and/or thrombocytopenia
2. Massive (i.e., at least 6 cm below the left costal margin) or progressive or symptomatic splenomegaly
3. Massive nodes (i.e., at least 10 cm in longest diameter) or progressive or symptomatic lymphadenopathy
4. Progressive lymphocytosis with an increase of more than 50% over a 2-month period or lymphocyte doubling time (LDT) of less than 6 months
   - LDT can be obtained by linear regression extrapolation of absolute lymphocyte counts obtained at intervals of 2 weeks over an observation period of 2–3 months
   - In patients with initial blood lymphocyte counts of less than 30×10^9/L (30,000/μL), LDT should not be used as a single parameter to define a treatment indication
   - Factors contributing to lymphocytosis or lymphadenopathy other than CLL (e.g., infections) should be excluded
5. Autoimmune anemia and/or thrombocytopenia that is poorly responsive to corticosteroids or other standard therapy
6. Constitutional symptoms, defined as any one or more of the following disease-related symptoms or signs
   - (a) Unintentional weight loss of 10% or more within the previous 6 months
   - (b) Significant fatigue (i.e., ECOG PS 2, or worse; inability to work or perform usual activities)
   - (c) Fevers higher than 100.5°F or 38.0°C for 2 or more weeks without other evidence of infection
   - (d) Night sweats for more than 1 month without evidence of infection

[a]Hypogammaglobulinemia or monoclonal or oligoclonal paraproteinemia does not by itself constitute a basis for initiating therapy. The absolute lymphocyte count should not be used as the sole indicator for treatment

Several prospective randomized studies from the 1990s failed to show an overall survival (OS) benefit in newly diagnosed patients treated with immediate as compared to delayed interventions [40]. While the recent discovery and validation of novel prognostic markers raise the possibility of risk stratifying appropriate asymptomatic patients for treatment at diagnosis and the development of new therapeutic agents may change the natural history of the disease, studies investigating risk-based early treatment and treatment with newer agents and combinations have not yet demonstrated improvements in OS. As a result, current guidelines recommend that unless in a clinical trial, treatment should not be initiated until patients develop signs of progressive or symptomatic disease. Indications for treatment according to the 2008 updated National Cancer Institute – International Workshop on Chronic Lymphocytic Leukemia Working Group guidelines are summarized in Table 3.6 [25].

The current standard of care for early stage CLL is to provide reassurance and closely monitor patients – "watch and wait." This approach can be challenging for both patients and clinicians. For patients, it can lead to substantial anxiety and is counter to the view in most malignancies that early detection and treatment improve outcomes. For clinicians, it is known that survival of Rai stage 0 CLL patients is substantially shorter than that of age-matched controls, that traditional staging is inadequate for predicting individual patients' courses, and that 70% of patients will ultimately require therapy [41, 42]. Several ongoing trials investigating risk stratified early treatment using novel prognostic markers, including the German phase III CLL7 study and an NCBI phase III intergroup study, may result in improved outcomes among selected patients.

Assessment of Disease Response

Prior to initial therapy, disease assessment should include physical examination for the presence of lymphadenopathy (LAD) and hepatosplenomegaly, complete blood cell count (including reporting the proportion of prolymphocytes if they are present), and bone marrow biopsy. Computed tomography (CT) scans are currently generally not recommended for initial evaluation or follow-up because enlarged lymph nodes detected only on CT do not change Rai or Binet staging [25]. However, limited data suggest that the presence of abdominal LAD in Rai stage 0 patients may predict progression of disease [43]. Further research examining the role of both CT and positron emission tomography (PET) may broaden the indications for the use of these tests.

Assessment of response should include a physical exam as well as evaluation of the peripheral blood and bone marrow. Responses should be considered complete (CR), partial (PR), or progressive disease (PD), and criteria for each response are described in Table 3.7. The term CR with incomplete marrow recovery (CRi) is recommended to describe patients who fulfill all criteria for CR but who maintain persistent anemia, thrombocytopenia, and/or neutropenia that is presumed to be related to drug toxicity [25].

An additional emerging consideration in the assessment of treatment responses is the significance of eradicating minimal residual disease (MRD) in patients who achieve conventional CR. Multicolor flow cytometry and allele-specific polymerase chain reactions (PCR) allow sensitive monitoring for MRD, and growing evidence suggests that achieving MRD negativity leads to longer PFS and, in some patients, the potential for cure. To further understand the significance of MRD negativity, it is recommended that novel clinical trials include MRD assessment using either four-color flow cytometry or PCR with a sensitivity of one CLL cell per 10,000 leukocytes [25].

Therapy

Overview

Once indications for treatment have been met, an increasing variety of therapies are available for initial treatment of CLL. Alkylating agents, primarily chlorambucil, cyclophosphamide (C), and bendamustine (B); nucleoside analogs

Table 3.7   Response definition after treatment for patients with CLL

Parameter	CR[a]	PR[a]	PD[a]
Group A			
Lymphadenopathy[b]	None >1.5 cm	Decrease ≥50%	Increase ≥50%
Hepatomegaly	None	Decrease ≥50%	Increase ≥50%
Splenomegaly	None	Decrease ≥50%	Increase ≥50%
Blood lymphocytes	<4,000/μL	Decrease ≥50% from baseline	Increase ≥50% over baseline
Marrow[c]	Normocellular, <30% lymphocytes, no B-lymphoid nodules. Hypocellular marrow defines incomplete CR	50% Reduction in marrow infiltrate, or B-lymphoid nodules	
Group B			
Platelet count	>100,000/μL	>100,000/μL or increase ≥50% over baseline	Decrease of ≥50% from baseline secondary to CLL
Hemoglobin	>11.0 g/dL	>11 g/dL or increase ≥50% over baseline	Decrease of >2 g/dL from baseline secondary to CLL
Neutrophils[c]	>1,500/μL	>1,500/μL or >50% improvement over baseline	

Group A criteria define the tumor load; group B criteria define the function of the hematopoietic system (or marrow)

[a]CR (complete remission): all of the criteria have to be met, and patients have to lack disease-related constitutional symptoms; PR (partial remission): at least two of the criteria of group A plus one of the criteria of group B have to be met; SD is absence of progressive disease (PD) and failure to achieve at least a PR; PD: at least one of the above criteria of group A or group B has to be met

[b]Sum of the products of multiple lymph nodes (as evaluated by CT scans in clinical trials or by physical examination in general practice)

[c]These parameters are irrelevant for some response categories

including fludarabine (F), pentostatin (P), and cladribine; and the monoclonal antibodies rituximab (R) and alemtuzumab (A) have all been extensively investigated, and modern initial treatment regimens incorporate various combinations of these drugs. Regimen decisions require an assessment of relative risks and benefits and treatment goals for the individual patient. While more intensive regimens may offer higher rates of response, attendant toxicities, particularly immunosuppression, may not be appropriate for all patients. For patients who relapse, time to relapse is the most important prognostic indicator. A variety of strategies are available, and as discussed below, treatment decisions depend on several factors. Figures 3.1 and 3.2 provide algorithms summarizing treatment options and outcomes for both initial therapy and treatment of relapsed disease, respectively.

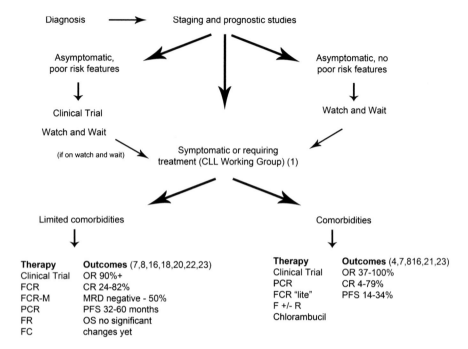

Fig. 3.1 Algorithm for front-line treatment of CLL including outcomes from a series of clinical trials in patients with limited or more extensive comorbidities. *F* fludarabine, *C* cyclophosphamide *R* rituximab, *M* mitoxantrone, *P* pentostatin, *OR* overall response, *CR* complete remission, *MRD* minimal residual disease, *PFS* progression-free survival, *OS* overall survival

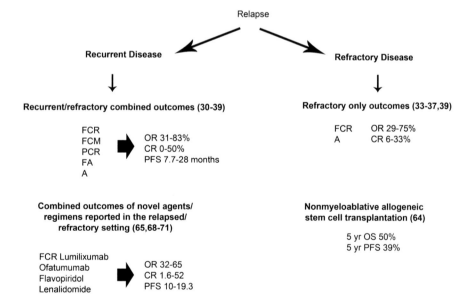

Fig. 3.2 Outcomes for CLL patients receiving therapy for relapsed or refractory disease. *F* fludarabine, *C* cyclophosphamide, *R* rituximab, *M* mitoxantrone, *P* pentostatin, *A* alemtuzumab, *OR* overall response, *CR* complete remission, *MRD* minimal residual disease, *PFS* progression-free survival, *OS* overall survival

Initial Therapy

In 2000, Rai et al. published the pivotal US intergroup study that initiated the modern era of CLL therapy. In a comparison of initial treatment with chlorambucil, the standard of care for decades, versus fludarabine versus combination therapy, fludarabine demonstrated an improved overall response rate (ORR) (63% vs 37%), CR (20% vs 4%), and PFS (25 months vs 14 months) as compared to chlorambucil [44]. The combined therapy arm was stopped early due to increased toxicity without improved outcomes as compared to the single-agent fludarabine arm. Single-agent fludarabine did not demonstrate an OS advantage, though crossover was allowed. These results, which were confirmed in several additional studies comparing nucleoside analogs to alkylator-based therapy, [45, 46] established nucleoside analog–based therapy as the de facto standard of care for first-line treatment among patients suitable for relatively aggressive therapy.

More recent studies have examined the potential to improve outcomes by adding agents to nucleoside analogs. Because nucleoside analogs inhibit the repair of alkylating agent-induced DNA interstrand cross-links, their combination with an alkylating agent is appealing. In next-generation randomized studies, combination of fludarabine and cyclophosphamide (FC) demonstrated superior outcomes to fludarabine alone in terms of ORR (74–95% vs 60–83%), CR (23–17% vs 5%), and PFS (31.6–40 months vs 19.2–20 months) [47–49]. Again, however, no OS improvements were observed, and FC was associated with increased myelosuppression as compared to single-agent fludarabine. Pentostatin combined with cyclophosphamide, as well as sequential fludarabine and then cyclophosphamide, has also been investigated and demonstrated improved results over single-agent therapy [50, 51]. Cladribine in combination with cyclophosphamide did not yield significant improvement over cladribine alone, and enthusiasm for cladribine in CLL treatment has waned [52]. Recently, the addition of mitoxantrone (M) to FC has also demonstrated encouraging results without markedly increased toxicity (64% CR with 26% MRD negativity by flow and PCR) [53].

The development of monoclonal antibodies has provided additional therapeutic strategies. Rituximab, an anti-CD20 chimeric monoclonal antibody, has been integrated into a variety of upfront regimens. As a single agent, rituximab has been less active against CLL than other indolent non-Hodgkin lymphomas. This relative lack of single-agent efficacy has been attributed to the relatively lower CD20 expression on CLL cells as well as the presence of soluble CD20 in the plasma of CLL patients that acts as an antigen sink and shortens the half-life of the drug [54, 55]. While more intensive dose regimens may increase the efficacy of single-agent rituximab, when rituximab is used in conjunction with other agents, it appears to markedly improve outcomes. FR has been investigated in a prospective randomized trial comparing concurrent and sequential dosing strategies [56, 57]. Following induction therapy, patients in both arms with stable disease or better received an additional four weekly doses of rituximab. Concurrent FR was associated with higher OR (90% vs 77%) and CR (47% vs 28%) without improved PFS or OS as compared to sequential therapy, but both strategies yielded improved CR, ORR, and 2-year PFS when compared to a historical cohort treated with single-agent F therapy.

A large phase II study has demonstrated that the addition of rituximab to FC has resulted in increased rates of CR (72%), with 82% and 42% of evaluable patients in CR achieving flow cytometric and PCR-negative remissions, respectively. MRD-negative patients had significantly longer PFS (85–89 months) versus MRD-positive patients (49 months) [58]. To date, no published studies have demonstrated an OS advantage associated with FCR, but preliminary evidence from a phase III randomized international trial comparing FCR to FC does demonstrate improved OS [59]. FCR is associated with a high degree of myelosuppression (52% grade 3–4 neutropenia per course) with persistent cytopenias in 19% of patients and late cytopenias in 28% of patients. Another recent study of 72 patients investigating the addition of mitoxantrone to FCR has demonstrated CR rates of 82% with 46% of patients MRD negative by multicolor flow cytometry, but longer follow-up and larger studies are needed to confirm the efficacy of this regimen, particularly with regard to toxicity [60]. FCR and FCR-M may not be suitable for highly comorbid patients or older patients with limited marrow reserve.

To overcome the toxicity of FCR, investigators have examined alternative dosing strategies. Dose-reduced fludarabine and cyclophosphamide combined with upfront and maintenance rituximab, "FCR-lite," have demonstrated good response rates (79% CR) and significantly reduced grade 3/4 neutropenia (13% of cycles) as compared to standard FCR [61]. Sequential FCR has also been investigated as a strategy to administer dose-dense therapy with decreased toxicity [62]. Though a small study has demonstrated the feasibility of this strategy, its benefits versus standard FCR therapy are uncertain.

Pentostatin, which is associated with possible relatively reduced myelosuppression as compared to fludarabine, has been investigated in combination with cyclophosphamide and rituximab and has been reported to yield high rates of response (63% CR) and to be well tolerated in older patients and patients with poor renal function [63, 64]. Preliminary results of a phase III study conducted in the community setting comparing FCR to the combination of pentostatin, cyclophosphamide, and rituximab have not demonstrated significant differences in outcomes, including infectious complications, between the regimens [65].

Alemtuzumab, which is established as a monotherapy in relapsed disease, is a humanized monoclonal antibody targeting CD52, a receptor that is highly expressed on CLL cells as well as normal B- and T-cells, which has recently gained approval for first-line therapy. Alemtuzumab was approved on the basis of a phase III study demonstrating a favorable ORR (83% vs 55%), CR (24% vs 2%), and PFS (23.3 months vs 14.7 months) compared to chlorambucil [66]. Notably, alemtuzumab has been suggested to have improved efficacy in patients with 17p deletions, and the 11 patients with 17p deletions in this study achieved 63% OR with median PFS of 10.7 months. Given the small numbers of patients with 17p deletions, these numbers were not statistically significantly superior to the 20% ORR and 2.2-month PFS in the chlorambucil arm. Alemtuzumab is significantly immunosuppressive, particularly lymphosuppressive, and is associated with high rates of CMV reactivation. When given intravenously, as in this study, alemtuzumab is also associated with high rates of infusional toxicity. Critics of the study leading to approval of alemtuzumab in the first-line setting argue that given alternative modern regimens, chlorambucil may not have been an appropriate comparative arm for initial efficacy. Several phase II studies examining the efficacy of upfront alemtuzumab combined with other agents, including the addition of alemtuzumab to FCR [67] as well as alemtuzumab combined with rituximab [68], are currently accruing, but insufficient data are available to reach conclusions regarding the efficacy and toxicity of the regimens.

Finally, bendamustine, an alkylating agent with purine-like properties, has also recently been approved for initial therapy based on improved CR (31% vs 2%), ORR (68% vs 31%), and PFS (21.6 months vs 8.3 months) in a phase III trial comparing outcomes to initial treatment with chlorambucil [69]. Bendamustine was associated with significantly more grade 3–4 adverse events and severe infections. As in the case of alemtuzumab, critics of the study note that chlorambucil again may not have been an appropriate comparative arm. Preliminary data, however, suggest that bendamustine combined with rituximab yields high response rates with limited toxicity [70]. In relapsed CLL, depending on the dose and patient population, the ORR ranges from 40% to 93%, and the CR rate ranges from 7% to 30% [71].

Most recently, ofatumumab, a fully humanized anti-CD20 monoclonal antibody, was approved for treatment of relapsed/refractory CLL in 2009 based on encouraging results using single-agent ofatumumab in fludarabine refractory patients [72]. Positive preliminary results of a phase II trial of ofatumumab in combination with fludarabine and cyclophosphamide in previously untreated patients were reported in 2009 [73].

Maintenance Therapy

The potential to improve outcomes with additional therapy combined with reported improved outcomes in MRD-negative patients has resulted in investigation of ongoing or consolidation therapy using monoclonal antibodies. Goals include improving initial incomplete responses or, for patients with CR but persistent MRD, eliminating detectable disease. Consolidation with alemtuzumab following FCR therapy is the most intensively investigated strategy. In studies performed thus far, alemtuzumab consolidation has been associated with increased rates of MRD negativity and improved PFS, but toxicities have been significant, and the overall efficacy of this strategy is not yet clear [74]. Rituximab consolidation for patients with MRD following FR induction has also been demonstrated to increase PFS [75]. At this time, given the risk of additional toxicity, consolidation strategies cannot be recommended outside context of clinical trial.

Initial Treatment Summary

As described above, a wide variety of therapies are available for initial treatment of CLL, and several additional investigational agents are being explored as adjunct therapies in the frontline setting. As possible, patients requiring treatment and those with poor prognostic features at presentation should be enrolled in clinical trials. For suitably fit patients without access to clinical trials, FCR has demonstrated impressive results to date and has been shown to be appropriate first-line therapy, though no prospective randomized trials using this regimen have matured sufficiently to definitively demonstrate OS or PFS benefit. BR, FR, FCR-lite, and pentostatin, cyclophosphamide, and rituximab are reasonable regimens for patients in whom toxicities are a significant concern. For older, poor performance status patients, single-agent chlorambucil remains a reasonable upfront strategy. For patients with 17p deletions, upfront alemtuzumab might be considered, and enrollment in trials of more aggressive therapy, including possible allogeneic HCT, might be particularly appropriate.

Treatment of Relapse

Given current treatment strategies, relapse remains a significant issue. Approximately 50% of patients treated initially with FCR will relapse by 6 years, and long-term PFS curves following FCR treatment show no plateau. While a reassessment of goals of care, comorbidities, and prior therapy at the time of relapse is important in determining second-line treatment regimens, time to relapse may be the most meaningful prognostic factor determining long-term outcomes. Based on current treatment strategies, patients who relapse are commonly considered to have either recurrent or refractory disease. Patients who do not experience at least PR or progress within 6 months of treatment with a fludarabine-based regimen are considered refractory, while patients who progress ≥6 months after previous therapy are considered recurrent.

Treatment algorithms for patients with recurrent disease are similar to those for initial therapy. Patients often respond well to fludarabine-based regimens, even if fludarabine was included in initial treatment. As in the initial treatment setting, FCR appears associated with higher rates of response than FC or fludarabine alone and may result in improved OS. In a large series, fludarabine sensitive relapsed patients achieved a 76% ORR and 31% CR rate following FCR [76]. FC combined with mitoxantrone [77], pentostatin, cyclophosphamide, rituximab [78], and fludarabine combined with alemtuzumab [79] have also been explored in the recurrent setting and have yielded similar ORR to FCR, CR rates ranging from 25% to 50% and PFS from 13 to 25 months.

For patients with refractory disease, the prognosis is typically poor and treatment decisions more challenging. The observation that greater than half of fludarabine refractory patients present initially with poor-risk clinical or genetic features further emphasizes the need for improved upfront strategies for these patients. Therapeutic strategies again range from additional established chemotherapy ± immunotherapy to investigational agents/clinical trials to HCT. Alemtuzumab has been extensively investigated in the fludarabine refractory setting. Optimal dosing schedules have not been determined, but data suggest that the subcutaneous injection may be similarly efficacious and associated with significantly fewer infusional reactions than intrave-nous administration. These studies have demonstrated response rates ranging from 33% to 50% [80–82], with better responses in patients with disease confined to the peripheral blood and bone marrow and no bulky lymphadenopathy.

Retreatment with a fludarabine-based regimen is also an option, and as in the initial and recurrent treatment settings, FCR appears to offer superior, albeit unsat-isfactory, response rates when compared to fludarabine alone or FC combination. Among 37 fludarabine-refractory patients the ORR was 59%, but only 5% achieved a CR [76]. Alemtuzumab combined with FCR (CFAR) [83] or FR [84], as well as oxaliplatin, fludarabine, cytarabine, and rituximab (OFAR) [85], FC-M and dexam-ethasone [86], and FA [87] have been investigated in smaller studies, as have non-fludarabine-based regimens including pentostatin, cyclophosphamide, rituximab [78], alemtuzumab and rituximab [88], rituximab and high-dose glucocorticoids [89–91], and BM-R [92]. Unfortunately, none of these combinations have demon-strated marked improvements in this challenging patient population.

Hematopoietic Cell Transplantation

Hematopoietic cell transplantation remains a more aggressive strategy for poor prognosis or relapsed/refractory patients, and both autologous and allogeneic strate-gies have been investigated. In the early 1990s, several phase II studies of autolo-gous HCT in multiply relapsed patients, many of whom proceeded to transplantation with active refractory disease, achieved disappointing results [93, 94]. Subsequent studies investigated transplant earlier in the disease course. While these studies of patients transplanted in states of MRD with aggressively purged stem cell products demonstrated low rates of transplant-related mortality (TRM), high rates of CR, and prolonged remissions in some patients, a continuous pattern of relapse has been observed [95–99]. In addition, data suggested that autologous HCT did little to sig-nificantly overcome poor prognostic markers [97, 98]. Finally, longer follow-up demonstrated an appreciable risk (~8–9%) of secondary myelodysplasia or acute myeloid leukemia as well as a 19% incidence of other solid tumors [95, 96]. No prospective studies have compared outcomes following standard chemotherapy and autologous HCT in the treatment of CLL, but given the current expected CR rates and remission durations following FCR, as well as the increasing numbers of addi-tional agents available for treatment, little data suggest significant benefit for autol-ogous transplantation, and the procedure has fallen out of favor.

Allogeneic HCT offers potentially curative therapy, but the risks associated with the procedure make it unsuitable for many patients and raise difficult questions about when in the disease course it should be offered. Earlier studies of myeloabla-tive allogeneic HCT in suitable younger patients demonstrated survival curve pla-teaus emerging 1–2 years following transplantation, but registry data demonstrating TRM rates between 38% and 50% tempered enthusiasm for the strategy [100]. The recent introduction of reduced-intensity transplant regimens has increased interest in the allogeneic approach and has extended the potential for transplant to older patients and those with more extensive comorbidities. By altering the conditioning regimen to provide only the immunosuppression necessary to enable engraftment of donor cells, reduced-intensity regimens are markedly less toxic than myeloablative regimens and largely rely on the graft-versus-leukemia effect to cure disease. Various reduced-intensity regimens have been reported, with 2-year survivals in heavily pretreated patients ranging between 50% and 80% [101–105]. Researchers from The Fred Hutchinson Cancer Research Center have recently updated results for 82 patients with advanced fludarabine refractory CLL demonstrating 5-year OS of 50% with 39% disease-free survival and 23% TRM [106]. Notably, in contrast to autologous HCT, allogeneic transplantation appears to overcome negative prognostic factors; patients with 17p deletions as well as ZAP-70 positivity have achieved long-term survival rates comparable to patients without these negative features. Tumor bulk and chemosensitivity at the time of transplantation have emerged as the most important prognostic factors following reduced-intensity transplants for CLL, as patients with chemosensitive disease and LAD <5 cm have improved outcomes.

Given the apparent curative potential of allogeneic HCT, as well as improvements in supportive care and the decreased toxicity of reduced-intensity regimens, the role of allogeneic transplantation in CLL may continue to increase. As possible, suitable candidates with fludarabine-refractory disease should be offered the option of transplantation, and investigational studies of upfront transplant for patients with poor prognostic factors, particularly 17p deletions, are underway.

Novel and Investigational Strategies

Monoclonal Antibodies

Several novel monoclonal antibodies are in development. Lumiliximab is the most mature. Lumiliximab is a chimeric macaque and human monoclonal antibody targeted against CD23, which is highly expressed on CLL cells. Phase I testing demonstrated an excellent toxicity profile but limited activity when administered as monotherapy. When added to FCR in relapsed patients, results compared favorably to outcomes in historic FCR cohorts, and a phase III trial comparing FCR and FCR + lumiliximab has been initiated [107]. SGN-40 and CHIR-12.12, antibodies targeting CD40, an antigen present on CLL cells, are in early stage testing in CLL [108, 109].

Flavopiridol and CDK Inhibitors

Flavopiridol inhibits cyclin-dependant kinases (CDKs) and induces cell-cycle arrest. In spite of impressive in vitro activity against CLL, early clinical trials using continuous infusion yielded suboptimal results. Development of bolus schedules has yielded ORR of 60–63% in fludarabine refractory patients with no statistically different response rates in patients with poor prognostic factors [110]. Flavopiridol may also be minimally immunosuppressive, and therefore has appeal as an agent to be used in combination therapy. Several other CDK inhibitors are in earlier stages of development.

Lenalidomide

Lenalidomide is an immunomodulatory drug whose precise mechanism of antileukemic activity is uncertain. Lenalidomide has demonstrated activity in two phase II trials, yielding ORR of 47% and 32% in relapsed/refractory patients [111, 112]. A distinct tumor flare reaction, characterized by painful lymphadenopathy, with or without fever and bone pain, has been reported following lenalidomide therapy and has raised questions about the efficacy of this approach. Optimized dosing strategies, however, may decrease the incidence and severity of the reaction. Preliminary data suggest that lenalidomide in combination with rituximab may improve responses without additional toxicity [113].

Bcl-2 Inhibitors

Several antiapoptotic Bcl-2 family proteins, including Bcl-2, Bcl-xl, Bcl-w, and Mcl-1, are highly expressed in a significant portion of CLL patients. Recently, a number of small molecules, including obatoclax, AT101, SPC2996, ABT263, and oblimersen, have been developed that are capable of down regulating these antiapoptotic proteins and enhancing programmed cell death. The furthest developed of these Bcl-2 antagonists, oblimersen, is an antisense phosphothioate oligonucleotide that targets the messenger RNA of Bcl-2. In spite of limited activity as a single agent in relapsed/refractory patients, when added to fludarabine and cyclophosphamide, oblimersen increased response rates in patients with recurrent CLL [114].

Miscellaneous Early Stage Drugs

Several additional drugs, which operate through a variety of pathways, are also in preclinical or early stage testing for CLL. CAL-101, a phosphatidylinositol 3-kinase inhibitor, has demonstrated in vitro activity against CLL cells [115]. Cloretazine, an alkylating agent, and CNF2024, a heat shock protein inhibitor, are in phase I testing. Numerous novel and established tyrosine kinase inhibitors, including AZD2171, byrostatin-1, dasatinib, enzastaurin, CCI779, and sunitinib, are in early stage testing, as are the interleukin-2 receptor blockers denileukin diftitox and LMB-2 immunotoxin, and the vascular endothelial growth factor inhibitor bevacizumab [116]. Forodesine and clofarabine are newer nucleoside analogs that are also being evaluated [117, 118].

Vaccine and Adoptive Immunotherapy

T-cell-based therapy is an alternative strategy that holds promise in CLL. The potent graft-versus-CLL effect demonstrated following allogeneic HCT raises hope that immune manipulation may be harnessed to treat the disease. After years of investigation, T-cell-based therapies are beginning to yield results. Strategies include adoptive transfer of T-lymphocytes that have been genetically manipulated to either express tumor specific T-cell receptors or chimeric antigen receptors targeted against surface antigens on CLL cells. Alternatively, development of dendritic cell–based vaccines is also under investigation.

Conclusions

CLL management is evolving rapidly. Novel combinations and dosing schedules of existing drugs have yielded significant improvements in outcomes for patients requiring initial therapy. Fludarabine, alemtuzumab, and bendamustine have, as single agents, demonstrated improved response rates as compared to traditional chlorambucil. Addition of cyclophosphamide or rituximab to fludarabine increases response rates and PFS as compared to single-agent fludarabine. FCR provides longer PFS compared to historical controls receiving FC, and preliminary data suggest that FCR may prolong OS.

Prospective trials examining the efficacy of integrating novel prognostic markers into treatment algorithms may lead to earlier treatment for selected patients, and examination of strategies to achieve MRD negativity may lead to new goals of MRD residual disease testing; however, it is essential to establish the widespread utilization of these tests.

For patients with relapsed and refractory disease, few randomized trials are available to determine a standard of care. Patient heterogeneity across trials makes comparisons difficult. Numerous promising new agents, as well as reduced-intensity HCT, are currently in clinical trial and will likely lead to continued improvement in outcomes in the future.

References

1. Goldin LR, Caporaso NE. Family studies in chronic lymphocytic leukaemia and other lymphoproliferative tumours. Br J Haematol. 2007;139:774–9.
2. Boelens J, Lust S, Vanhoecke B, Offner F. Chronic lymphocytic leukaemia. Anticancer Res. 2009;29:605–15.
3. Jemal A, Siegel R, Xu J, Ward E. Cancer statistics, 2010. CA Cancer J Clin. 2010;60:277–300.
4. Linet MS, Schubauer-Berigan MK, Weisenburger DD, et al. Chronic lymphocytic leukaemia: an overview of aetiology in light of recent developments in classification and pathogenesis. Br J Haematol. 2007;139:672–86.

5. Molica S, Levato D. What is changing in the natural history of chronic lymphocytic leukemia? Haematologica. 2001;86:8–12.
6. Shanafelt TD, Byrd JC, Call TG, Zent CS, Kay NE. Narrative review: initial management of newly diagnosed, early-stage chronic lymphocytic leukemia. Ann Intern Med. 2006;145:435–47.
7. Dores GM, Anderson WF, Curtis RE, et al. Chronic lymphocytic leukaemia and small lymphocytic lymphoma: overview of the descriptive epidemiology. Br J Haematol. 2007;139: 809–19.
8. Finch SC, Hoshino T, Itoga T, Ichimaru M, Ingram Jr RH. Chronic lymphocytic leukemia in Hiroshima and Nagasaki, Japan. Blood. 1969;33:79–86.
9. Gluzman D, Imamura N, Sklyarenko L, Nadgornaya V, Zavelevich M, Machilo V. Patterns of hematological malignancies in Chernobyl clean-up workers (1996–2005). Exp Oncol. 2006;28:60–3.
10. Institute of Medicine of the National Academies. Veterans and agent orange. Washington, DC: National Academies Press; 2003. p. 242–392.
11. Yee KW, O'Brien SM. Chronic lymphocytic leukemia: diagnosis and treatment. Mayo Clin Proc. 2006;81:1105–29.
12. Gomez SL, Quach T, Horn-Ross PL, et al. Hidden breast cancer disparities in Asian women: disaggregating incidence rates by ethnicity and migrant status. Am J Public Health. 2010;100 Suppl 1:S125–31.
13. Mauro FR, Giammartini E, Gentile M, et al. Clinical features and outcome of familial chronic lymphocytic leukemia. Haematologica. 2006;91:1117–20.
14. Yuille MR, Matutes E, Marossy A, Hilditch B, Catovsky D, Houlston RS. Familial chronic lymphocytic leukaemia: a survey and review of published studies. Br J Haematol. 2000;109:794–9.
15. Goldin LR, Pfeiffer RM, Li X, Hemminki K. Familial risk of lymphoproliferative tumors in families of patients with chronic lymphocytic leukemia: results from the Swedish family-cancer database. Blood. 2004;104:1850–4.
16. Slager SL, Kay NE. Familial chronic lymphocytic leukemia: what does it mean to me? Clin Lymphoma Myeloma. 2009;9 Suppl 3:S194–7.
17. Chiorazzi N, Rai KR, Ferrarini M. Chronic lymphocytic leukemia. N Engl J Med. 2005; 352:804–15.
18. Moreno C, Montserrat E. New prognostic markers in chronic lymphocytic leukemia. Blood Rev. 2008;22:211–9.
19. Cheson BD, Bennett JM, Rai KR, et al. Guidelines for clinical protocols for chronic lymphocytic leukemia: recommendations of the National Cancer Institute-Sponsored Working Group. Am J Hematol. 1988;29:152–63.
20. Keating MJ, O'Brien S, Lerner S, et al. Long-term follow-up of patients with chronic lymphocytic leukemia (CLL) receiving fludarabine regimens as initial therapy. Blood. 1998;92:1165–71.
21. Robak E, Robak T. Skin lesions in chronic lymphocytic leukemia. Leuk Lymphoma. 2007;48:855–65.
22. Wierda WG, Lamanna N, Weiss MA. Chronic lymphocytic leukemia. In: Cancer management: a multidisciplinary approach. 11th ed. Lawrence: CMPMedica; 2008. Chapter 34.
23. Dearden C. Disease-specific complications of chronic lymphocytic leukemia. Hematol Am Soc Hematol Educ Progr. 2008:450–6.
24. Diehl LF, Ketchum LH. Autoimmune disease and chronic lymphocytic leukemia: autoimmune hemolytic anemia, pure red cell aplasia, and autoimmune thrombocytopenia. Semin Oncol. 1998;25:80–97.
25. Hallek M, Cheson BD, Catovsky D, et al. Guidelines for the diagnosis and treatment of chronic lymphocytic leukemia: a report from the international workshop on chronic lymphocytic leukemia updating the National Cancer Institute-Working Group 1996 guidelines. Blood. 2008;111:5446–56.
26. Ghia P, Ferreri AM, Caligaris-Cappio F. Chronic lymphocytic leukemia. Crit Rev Oncol Hematol. 2007;64:234–46.

27. Rawstron AC, Bennett FL, O'Connor SJ, et al. Monoclonal B-cell lymphocytosis and chronic lymphocytic leukemia. N Engl J Med. 2008;359:575–83.

28. Rossi D, Sozzi E, Puma A, et al. The prognosis of clinical monoclonal B cell lymphocytosis differs from prognosis of Rai 0 chronic lymphocytic leukaemia and is recapitulated by biological risk factors. Br J Haematol. 2009;146:64–75.

29. Rawstron AC, Hillmen P. Clinical and diagnostic implications of monoclonal B-cell lymphocytosis. Best Pract Res Clin Haematol. 2010;23:61–9.

30. Rai KR, Sawitsky A, Cronkite EP, Chanana AD, Levy RN, Pasternack BS. Clinical staging of chronic lymphocytic leukemia. Blood. 1975;46:219–34.

31. Rai KR. A critical analysis of staging in CLL. In: Gale RP, Rai KR, editors. Chronic lymphocytic leukemia: recent progress and future directions. New York: Liss; 1987. p. 253–64.

32. Binet JL, Auquier A, Dighiero G, et al. A new prognostic classification of chronic lymphocytic leukemia derived from a multivariate survival analysis. Cancer. 1981;48:198–206.

33. Wierda WG, O'Brien S, Wang X, et al. Prognostic nomogram and index for overall survival in previously untreated patients with chronic lymphocytic leukemia. Blood. 2007;109:4679–85.

34. Bergmann MA, Eichhorst BF, Busch R, et al. Prospective evaluation of prognostic parameters in early stage chronic lymphocytic leukemia (CLL): results of the CLL1-protocol of the German CLL Study Group (GCLLSG). Blood (ASH Annu Meeting Abstr). 2007;110:625.

35. Dohner H, Stilgenbauer S, Benner A, et al. Genomic aberrations and survival in chronic lymphocytic leukemia. N Engl J Med. 2000;343:1910–6.

36. Dal-Bo M, Bertoni F, Forconi F, et al. Intrinsic and extrinsic factors influencing the clinical course of B-cell chronic lymphocytic leukemia: prognostic markers with pathogenetic relevance. J Transl Med. 2009;7:76.

37. Hamblin TJ. Prognostic markers in chronic lymphocytic leukaemia. Best Pract Res Clin Haematol. 2007;20:455–68.

38. Kay NE, O'Brien SM, Pettitt AR, Stilgenbauer S. The role of prognostic factors in assessing 'high-risk' subgroups of patients with chronic lymphocytic leukemia. Leukemia. 2007;21:1885–91.

39. Crespo M, Bosch F, Villamor N, et al. ZAP-70 expression as a surrogate for immunoglobulin-variable-region mutations in chronic lymphocytic leukemia. N Engl J Med. 2003;348:1764–75.

40. CLL Trialists' Collaborative Group. Chemotherapeutic options in chronic lymphocytic leukemia: a meta-analysis of the randomized trials. J Natl Cancer Inst. 1999;91:861–8.

41. Shanafelt TD, Rabe KG, Kay NE, et al. Age at diagnosis and the utility of prognostic testing in patients with chronic lymphocytic leukemia. Cancer. 2010;116:4777–87.

42. Shanafelt TD. Predicting clinical outcome in CLL: how and why. Hematol Am Soc Hematol Educ Progr. 2009:421–9.

43. Muntanola A, Bosch F, Arguis P, et al. Abdominal computed tomography predicts progression in patients with Rai stage 0 chronic lymphocytic leukemia. J Clin Oncol. 2007;25:1576–80.

44. Rai KR, Peterson BL, Appelbaum FR, et al. Fludarabine compared with chlorambucil as primary therapy for chronic lymphocytic leukemia. N Engl J Med. 2000;343:1750–7.

45. Johnson S, Smith AG, Loffler H, et al. Multicentre prospective randomised trial of fludarabine versus cyclophosphamide, doxorubicin, and prednisone (CAP) for treatment of advanced-stage chronic lymphocytic leukaemia. The French Cooperative Group on CLL. Lancet. 1996;347:1432–8.

46. Leporrier M, Chevret S, Cazin B, et al. Randomized comparison of fludarabine, CAP, and ChOP in 938 previously untreated stage B and C chronic lymphocytic leukemia patients. Blood. 2001;98:2319–25.

47. Flinn IW, Neuberg DS, Grever MR, et al. Phase III trial of fludarabine plus cyclophosphamide compared with fludarabine for patients with previously untreated chronic lymphocytic leukemia: US Intergroup Trial E2997. J Clin Oncol. 2007;25:793–8.

48. Eichhorst BF, Busch R, Hopfinger G, et al. Fludarabine plus cyclophosphamide versus fludarabine alone in first-line therapy of younger patients with chronic lymphocytic leukemia. Blood. 2006;107:885–91.

49. Catovsky D, Richards S, Matutes E, et al. Assessment of fludarabine plus cyclophosphamide for patients with chronic lymphocytic leukaemia (the LRF CLL4 trial): a randomised controlled trial. Lancet. 2007;370:230–9.

50. Weiss MA, Maslak PG, Jurcic JG, et al. Pentostatin and cyclophosphamide: an effective new regimen in previously treated patients with chronic lymphocytic leukemia. J Clin Oncol. 2003;21:1278–84.

51. Robak T, Blonski JZ, Wawrzyniak E, et al. Activity of cladribine combined with cyclophosphamide in frontline therapy for chronic lymphocytic leukemia with 17p13.1/TP53 deletion: report from the Polish Adult Leukemia Group. Cancer. 2009;115:94–100.

52. Robak T, Blonski JZ, Gora-Tybor J, et al. Cladribine alone and in combination with cyclophosphamide or cyclophosphamide plus mitoxantrone in the treatment of progressive chronic lymphocytic leukemia: report of a prospective, multicenter, randomized trial of the Polish Adult Leukemia Group (PALG CLL2). Blood. 2006;108:473–9.

53. Bosch F, Ferrer A, Villamor N, et al. Fludarabine, cyclophosphamide, and mitoxantrone as initial therapy of chronic lymphocytic leukemia: high response rate and disease eradication. Clin Cancer Res. 2008;14:155–61.

54. McLaughlin P, Grillo-Lopez AJ, Link BK, et al. Rituximab chimeric anti-CD20 monoclonal antibody therapy for relapsed indolent lymphoma: half of patients respond to a four-dose treatment program. J Clin Oncol. 1998;16:2825–33.

55. Manshouri T, Do KA, Wang X, et al. Circulating CD20 is detectable in the plasma of patients with chronic lymphocytic leukemia and is of prognostic significance. Blood. 2003;101:2507–13.

56. Byrd JC, Peterson BL, Morrison VA, et al. Randomized phase 2 study of fludarabine with concurrent versus sequential treatment with rituximab in symptomatic, untreated patients with B-cell chronic lymphocytic leukemia: results from Cancer and Leukemia Group B 9712 (CALGB 9712). Blood. 2003;101:6–14.

57. Byrd JC, Rai K, Peterson BL, et al. Addition of rituximab to fludarabine may prolong progression-free survival and overall survival in patients with previously untreated chronic lymphocytic leukemia: an updated retrospective comparative analysis of CALGB 9712 and CALGB 9011. Blood. 2005;105:49–53.

58. Tam CS, O'Brien S, Wierda W, et al. Long-term results of the fludarabine, cyclophosphamide, and rituximab regimen as initial therapy of chronic lymphocytic leukemia. Blood. 2008;112:975–80.

59. Hallek M, Fingerle-Rowson G, Fink A, et al. First-line treatment with fludarabine, cyclophosphamide, and rituximab improves overall survival in previously untreated patients with advanced chronic lymphocytic leukemia (CLL): results of a randomized phase III trial on behalf of an International Group of Investigators and the German CLL Study Group. Blood (ASH Annu Meeting Abstr). 2009;114:535.

60. Bosch F, Abrisqueta P, Villamor N, et al. Rituximab, fludarabine, cyclophosphamide, and mitoxantrone: a new, highly active chemoimmunotherapy regimen for chronic lymphocytic leukemia. J Clin Oncol. 2009;27:4578–84.

61. Foon KA, Boyiadzis M, Land SR, et al. Chemoimmunotherapy with low-dose fludarabine and cyclophosphamide and high dose rituximab in previously untreated patients with chronic lymphocytic leukemia. J Clin Oncol. 2009;27:498–503.

62. Lamanna N, Jurcic JG, Noy A, et al. Sequential therapy with fludarabine, high-dose cyclophosphamide, and rituximab in previously untreated patients with chronic lymphocytic leukemia produces high-quality responses: molecular remissions predict for durable complete responses. J Clin Oncol. 2009;27:491–7.

63. Kay NE, Geyer SM, Call TG, et al. Combination chemoimmunotherapy with pentostatin, cyclophosphamide, and rituximab shows significant clinical activity with low accompanying toxicity in previously untreated B chronic lymphocytic leukemia. Blood. 2007;109:405–11.

64. Shanafelt TD, Lin T, Geyer SM, et al. Pentostatin, cyclophosphamide, and rituximab regimen in older patients with chronic lymphocytic leukemia. Cancer. 2007;109:2291–8.

65. Reynolds C, Di Bella N, Lyons RM, et al. Phase III trial of fludarabine, cyclophosphamide, and rituximab vs pentostatin, cyclophosphamide, and rituximab in B-cell chronic lymphocytic leukemia. Blood (ASH Annu Meeting Abstr). 2008;112:327.

66. Hillmen P, Skotnicki AB, Robak T, et al. Alemtuzumab compared with chlorambucil as first-line therapy for chronic lymphocytic leukemia. J Clin Oncol. 2007;25:5616–23.

67. Parikh SA, Keating M, O'Brien S, et al. Frontline combined chemoimmunotherapy with fludarabine, cyclophosphamide, alemtuzumab and rituximab in high-risk chronic lymphocytic leukemia. Blood (ASH Annu Meeting Abstr). 2009;114:208.

68. Zent CS, Call TG, Shanafelt DT, et al. Alemtuzumab and rituximab for initial treatment of high risk, early stage chronic lymphocytic leukemia. Blood (ASH Annu Meeting Abstr). 2007;110:2050.

69. Knauf WU, Lissichkov T, Aldaoud A, et al. Phase III randomized study of bendamustine compared with chlorambucil in previously untreated patients with chronic lymphocytic leukemia. J Clin Oncol. 2009;27:4378–84.

70. Fischer K, Cramer P, Stilgenbauer S, et al. Bendamustine combined with rituximab in first-line therapy of advanced CLL: a multicenter phase II trial of the German CLL Study Group (GCLLSG). Blood (ASH Annu Meeting Abstr). 2009;114:205.

71. Cheson BD, Rummel MJ. Bendamustine: rebirth of an old drug. J Clin Oncol. 2009;27:1492–501.

72. Wierda WG, Kipps TJ, Mayer J, et al. Ofatumumab as single-agent CD20 immunotherapy in fludarabine-refractory chronic lymphocytic leukemia. J Clin Oncol. 2010;28:1749–55.

73. Wierda WG, Kipps TJ, Dürig J, et al. Ofatumumab combined with fludarabine and cyclophosphamide shows high activity in patients with previously untreated chronic lymphocytic leukemia: results from a randomized, multicenter, international, two-dose, parallel group, phase II trial. Blood (ASH Annu Meeting Abstr). 2009;114:207.

74. Schweighofer CD, Ritgen M, Eichhorst BF, et al. Consolidation with alemtuzumab improves progression-free survival in patients with chronic lymphocytic leukaemia (CLL) in first remission: long-term follow-up of a randomized phase III trial of the German CLL Study Group (GCLLSG). Br J Haematol. 2009;144:95–8.

75. Del Poeta G, Del Principe MI, Buccisano F, et al. Consolidation and maintenance immunotherapy with rituximab improve clinical outcome in patients with B-cell chronic lymphocytic leukemia. Cancer. 2008;112:119–28.

76. Wierda W, O'Brien S, Wen S, et al. Chemoimmunotherapy with fludarabine, cyclophosphamide, and rituximab for relapsed and refractory chronic lymphocytic leukemia. J Clin Oncol. 2005;23:4070–8.

77. Bosch F, Ferrer A, Lopez-Guillermo A, et al. Fludarabine, cyclophosphamide and mitoxantrone in the treatment of resistant or relapsed chronic lymphocytic leukaemia. Br J Haematol. 2002;119:976–84.

78. Lamanna N, Kalaycio M, Maslak P, et al. Pentostatin, cyclophosphamide, and rituximab is an active, well-tolerated regimen for patients with previously treated chronic lymphocytic leukemia. J Clin Oncol. 2006;24:1575–81.

79. Elter T, Borchmann P, Schulz H, et al. Fludarabine in combination with alemtuzumab is effective and feasible in patients with relapsed or refractory B-cell chronic lymphocytic leukemia: results of a phase II trial. J Clin Oncol. 2005;23:7024–31.

80. Keating MJ, Flinn I, Jain V, et al. Therapeutic role of alemtuzumab (Campath-1H) in patients who have failed fludarabine: results of a large international study. Blood. 2002;99:3554–61.

81. Stilgenbauer S, Zenz T, Winkler D, et al. Subcutaneous alemtuzumab in fludarabine-refractory chronic lymphocytic leukemia: clinical results and prognostic marker analyses from the CLL2H study of the German Chronic Lymphocytic Leukemia Study Group. J Clin Oncol. 2009;27:3994–4001.

82. Moreton P, Kennedy B, Lucas G, et al. Eradication of minimal residual disease in B-cell chronic lymphocytic leukemia after alemtuzumab therapy is associated with prolonged survival. J Clin Oncol. 2005;23:2971–9.

83. Badoux XC, Keating M, O'Brien S, et al. Chemoimmunotherapy with cyclophosphamide, fludarabine, alemtuzumab and rituximab is effective in relapsed patients with chronic lymphocytic leukemia. Blood (ASH Annu Meeting Abstr). 2009;114:3431.

84. Lin TS, Donohue KA, Byrd JC, et al. Consolidation therapy with subcutaneous alemtuzumab after fludarabine and rituximab induction therapy improves the complete response rate in chronic lymphocytic leukemia and eradicates minimal residual disease but is associated with severe infectious toxicity: final analysis of CALGB study 10101. Blood (ASH Annu Meeting Abstr). 2009;114:210.

85. Tsimberidou AM, Wierda WG, Plunkett W, et al. Phase I-II study of oxaliplatin, fludarabine, cytarabine, and rituximab combination therapy in patients with Richter's syndrome or fludarabine-refractory chronic lymphocytic leukemia. J Clin Oncol. 2008;26:196–203.
86. Mauro FR, Foa R, Meloni G, et al. Fludarabine, ara-C, novantrone and dexamethasone (FAND) in previously treated chronic lymphocytic leukemia patients. Haematologica. 2002;87:926–33.
87. Engert A, Gercheva L, Robak T, et al. Improved progression-free survival of alemtuzumab plus fludarabine versus fludarabine alone as second-line treatment of patients with B-cell chronic lymphocytic leukemia: preliminary results from a phase III randomized trial. Blood (ASH Annu Meeting Abstr). 2009;114:537.
88. Faderl S, Ferrajoli A, Wierda W, O'Brien S, Lerner S, Keating MJ. Alemtuzumab by continuous intravenous infusion followed by subcutaneous injection plus rituximab in the treatment of patients with chronic lymphocytic leukemia recurrence. Cancer. 2010;116:2360–5.
89. Castro JE, Sandoval-Sus JD, Bole J, Rassenti L, Kipps TJ. Rituximab in combination with high-dose methylprednisolone for the treatment of fludarabine refractory high-risk chronic lymphocytic leukemia. Leukemia. 2008;22:2048–53.
90. Bowen DA, Call TG, Jenkins GD, et al. Methylprednisolone-rituximab is an effective salvage therapy for patients with relapsed chronic lymphocytic leukemia including those with unfavorable cytogenetic features. Leuk Lymphoma. 2007;48:2412–7.
91. Dungarwalla M, Evans SO, Riley U, Catovsky D, Dearden CE, Matutes E. High dose methylprednisolone and rituximab is an effective therapy in advanced refractory chronic lymphocytic leukemia resistant to fludarabine therapy. Haematologica. 2008;93:475–6.
92. Weide R, Pandorf A, Heymanns J, Koppler H. Bendamustine/mitoxantrone/rituximab (BMR): a very effective, well tolerated outpatient chemoimmunotherapy for relapsed and refractory CD20-positive indolent malignancies. Final results of a pilot study. Leuk Lymphoma. 2004;45:2445–9.
93. Khouri IF, Keating MJ, Vriesendorp HM, et al. Autologous and allogeneic bone marrow transplantation for chronic lymphocytic leukemia: preliminary results. J Clin Oncol. 1994;12:748–58.
94. Pavletic ZS, Bishop MR, Bierman PJ, Armitage JO. Bone marrow transplantation in chronic lymphocytic leukemia and lymphomas. Biomed Pharmacother. 1996;50:118–24.
95. Milligan DW, Fernandes S, Dasgupta R, et al. Results of the MRC pilot study show autografting for younger patients with chronic lymphocytic leukemia is safe and achieves a high percentage of molecular responses. Blood. 2005;105:397–404.
96. Gribben JG, Zahrieh D, Stephans K, et al. Autologous and allogeneic stem cell transplantations for poor-risk chronic lymphocytic leukemia. Blood. 2005;106:4389–96.
97. Ritgen M, Lange A, Stilgenbauer S, et al. Unmutated immunoglobulin variable heavy-chain gene status remains an adverse prognostic factor after autologous stem cell transplantation for chronic lymphocytic leukemia. Blood. 2003;101:2049–53.
98. Dreger P, Stilgenbauer S, Benner A, et al. The prognostic impact of autologous stem cell transplantation in patients with chronic lymphocytic leukemia: a risk-matched analysis based on the VH gene mutational status. Blood. 2004;103:2850–8.
99. Jantunen E, Itala M, Siitonen T, et al. Autologous stem cell transplantation in patients with chronic lymphocytic leukaemia: the Finnish experience. Bone Marrow Transplant. 2006;37:1093–8.
100. Michallet M, Archimbaud E, Bandini G, et al. HLA-identical sibling bone marrow transplantation in younger patients with chronic lymphocytic leukemia. European Group for Blood and Marrow Transplantation and the International Bone Marrow Transplant Registry. Ann Intern Med. 1996;124:311–5.
101. Khouri IF, Lee MS, Saliba RM, et al. Nonablative allogeneic stem cell transplantation for chronic lymphocytic leukemia: impact of rituximab on immunomodulation and survival. Exp Hematol. 2004;32:28–35.
102. Khouri IF, Saliba RM, Admirand J, et al. Graft-versus-leukaemia effect after non-myeloablative haematopoietic transplantation can overcome the unfavourable expression of ZAP-70 in refractory chronic lymphocytic leukaemia. Br J Haematol. 2007;137:355–63.

103. Brown JR, Kim HT, Li S, et al. Predictors of improved progression-free survival after nonmyeloablative allogeneic stem cell transplantation for advanced chronic lymphocytic leukemia. Biol Blood Marrow Transplant. 2006;12:1056–64.
104. Schetelig J, Thiede C, Bornhauser M, et al. Evidence of a graft-versus-leukemia effect in chronic lymphocytic leukemia after reduced-intensity conditioning and allogeneic stem-cell transplantation: the Cooperative German Transplant Study Group. J Clin Oncol. 2003;21: 2747–53.
105. Delgado J, Thomson K, Russell N, et al. Results of alemtuzumab-based reduced-intensity allogeneic transplantation for chronic lymphocytic leukemia: a British Society of Blood and Marrow Transplantation Study. Blood. 2006;107:1724–30.
106. Sorror ML, Storer BE, Sandmaier BM, et al. Five-year follow-up of patients with advanced chronic lymphocytic leukemia treated with allogeneic hematopoietic cell transplantation after nonmyeloablative conditioning. J Clin Oncol. 2008;26:4912–20.
107. Byrd JC, Kipps TJ, Flinn IW, et al. Phase 1/2 study of lumiliximab combined with fludarabine, cyclophosphamide, and rituximab in patients with relapsed or refractory chronic lymphocytic leukemia. Blood. 2010;115:489–95.
108. Furman RR, Forero-Torres A, Shustov A, Drachman JG. A phase I study of dacetuzumab (SGN-40, a humanized anti-CD40 monoclonal antibody) in patients with chronic lymphocytic leukemia. Leuk Lymphoma. 2010;51:228–35.
109. Luqman M, Klabunde S, Lin K, et al. The antileukemia activity of a human anti-CD40 antagonist antibody, HCD122, on human chronic lymphocytic leukemia cells. Blood. 2008;112: 711–20.
110. Lin TS, Ruppert AS, Johnson AJ, et al. Phase II study of flavopiridol in relapsed chronic lymphocytic leukemia demonstrating high response rates in genetically high-risk disease. J Clin Oncol. 2009;27:6012–8.
111. Chanan-Khan A, Miller KC, Musial L, et al. Clinical efficacy of lenalidomide in patients with relapsed or refractory chronic lymphocytic leukemia: results of a phase II study. J Clin Oncol. 2006;24:5343–9.
112. Ferrajoli A, Lee BN, Schlette EJ, et al. Lenalidomide induces complete and partial remissions in patients with relapsed and refractory chronic lymphocytic leukemia. Blood. 2008;111: 5291–7.
113. Ferrajoli A, Badoux XC, O'Brien S, et al. Combination therapy with lenalidomide and rituximab in patients with relapsed chronic lymphocytic leukemia. Blood (ASH Annu Meeting Abstr). 2009;114:206.
114. O'Brien S, Moore J, Ding L, Novick S, Rai K. Addition of oblimersen (Bcl-2 antisense) to fludarabine cyclophosphamide for relapsed/refractory chronic lymphocytic leukemia extends survival in patients who achieve CR/nPR: results from a randomized phase 3 study. Blood (ASH Annu Meeting Abstr). 2007;110:751.
115. Herman SE, Gordon AL, Wagner AJ, et al. The phosphatidylinositol 3-kinase-{delta} inhibitor CAL-101 demonstrates promising pre-clinical activity in chronic lymphocytic leukemia by antagonizing intrinsic and extrinsic cellular survival signals. Blood. 2010;116(12): 2078–88.
116. Pinilla-Ibarz J, McQuary A. Chronic lymphocytic leukemia: putting new treatment options into perspective. Cancer Control. 2010;17:4–15; quiz 16.
117. Balakrishnan K, Verma D, O'Brien S, et al. Phase II and pharmacodynamic study of oral forodesine in patients with advanced and/or fludarabine-treated chronic lymphocytic leukemia. Blood. 2010;116(6):886–92.
118. Gandhi V, Plunkett W, Bonate PL, et al. Clinical and pharmacokinetic study of clofarabine in chronic lymphocytic leukemia: strategy for treatment. Clin Cancer Res. 2006;12:4011–7.

Chapter 4
Chronic Myeloid Leukemia (CML)

Andrew Coveler and Vivian G. Oehler

Abstract Chronic myeloid leukemia (CML) is a relatively rare form of leukemia, comprising ~15% of all leukemia cases. According to the National Cancer Institute's Surveillance Epidemiology and End Result (SEER) Cancer Statistics database, an estimated 2,800 men and 2,070 women will be diagnosed with CML in 2010. Among these patients, 440 men and women are expected to die. Mortality did not change between 1975 and 1984, decreased slightly between 1984 and 1997, but decreased significantly after the introduction of the ABL-targeted tyrosine kinase inhibitor (TKI) imatinib mesylate (IM). The prevalence of CML in the USA could increase to 200,000 or more cases over the next 20 years.

Keywords Chronic myeloid leukemia • Leukemia • CML • Mortality • Tyrosine kinase inhibitor • Imatinib mesylate • Hematopoietic stem cell • Clonal disorder

Introduction

Chronic myeloid leukemia (CML) is a relatively rare form of leukemia, comprising ~15% of all leukemia cases [1]. According to the National Cancer Institute's Surveillance Epidemiology and End Result (SEER) Cancer Statistics database, an

A. Coveler, M.D.
Assistant Professor, Division of Medical Oncology, Department of Medicine, University of Washington School of Medicine, Seattle, WA, USA

Clinical Research Division, Fred Hutchinson Cancer Research Center, Seattle, WA, USA

V.G. Oehler, M.D. (✉)
Assistant Member, Clinical Research Division, Fred Hutchinson Cancer Research Center, Seattle, WA, USA

Division of Hematology, Department of Medicine, University of Washington School of Medicine, Seattle, WA, USA
e-mail: voehler@u.washington.edu

E.H. Estey and F.R. Appelbaum (eds.), *Leukemia and Related Disorders: Integrated Treatment Approaches*, Contemporary Hematology,
DOI 10.1007/978-1-60761-565-1_4, © Springer Science+Business Media, LLC 2012

estimated 2,800 men and 2,070 women will be diagnosed with CML in 2010 [2]. Among these patients, 440 men and women are expected to die. Mortality did not change between 1975 and 1984, decreased slightly between 1984 and 1997, but decreased significantly after the introduction of the ABL-targeted tyrosine kinase inhibitor (TKI) imatinib mesylate (IM) [2]. The prevalence of CML in the USA could increase to 200,000 or more cases over the next 20 years [3]. Thus, managing CML patients is and will become a more common practice for hematologists and oncologists. Drug design, development, and testing are active areas of research in CML, and optimal treatment strategies continue to evolve. Several comprehensive clinical guidelines exist, including those from the European LeukemiaNet (ELN) and National Comprehensive Cancer Network (NCCN), which provide guidance on patient management [1, 4–7]. This chapter will focus on the diagnosis and treatment of CML in all phases and will describe the rationale and strategies for monitoring disease, and for selection of second- and third-line therapies for resistant disease.

CML Diagnosis, Prognosis, and Biology

Diagnosing CML

CML is a clonal disorder arising from a hematopoietic stem cell (HSC) [8]. The reciprocal translocation between chromosomes 9 and 22 juxtaposes the BCR gene from chromosome 22 and the ABL tyrosine kinase gene on chromosome 9 and drives the phenotype of CML, particularly in chronic phase (CP) [9–11]. Targeting the ABL tyrosine kinase, as pioneered by Brian J. Druker, has been enormously successful and has dramatically altered treatment of CML.

CP CML is characterized by an elevation in white blood cells consisting primarily of differentiated myeloid cells (metamyelocytes, myelocytes, bands, and neutrophils), basophilia, and in certain patients increased platelets and splenomegaly. The diagnosis is often made by submitting peripheral blood for either qualitative or quantitative reverse-transcription polymerase chain reaction (QPCR) or interphase fluorescence in situ hybridization (FISH) to identify the BCR-ABL translocation. Three BCR-ABL proteins have been described, p210, p190, and p230, which are named based on their respective molecular weights [12]. The 210 kDa protein is the predominant protein in CML, although rarely the p190 protein can be seen and has been associated with a poorer outcome [13]. The p190 protein is seen in Philadelphia (Ph) chromosome positive acute lymphoblastic leukemia (ALL), and the rare p230 protein is associated with a more indolent chronic myeloproliferative disorder. Numerous breakpoints occur in the ABL gene, as a consequence of mRNA splicing; however, BCR is fused to ABL predominantly at the same location within exon 2 of ABL for all proteins. It is the breakpoint in BCR that determines the size of BCR-ABL. The BCR breakpoints "cluster" in three regions (known as breakpoint cluster regions or BCR).

Although the diagnosis of CML is often made from peripheral blood, a bone marrow exam is an essential part of the initial workup for CML. It will differentiate CP, accelerated phase (AP), or blast crisis (BC) CML, and is needed for prognosis. Identifying features consistent with AP or BC disease at diagnosis is important, because these patients have inferior therapeutic responses. There are several sets of criteria for AP disease as published by Sokal et al. [14], the International Bone Marrow Transplant Registry (IBMTR) [15], MD Anderson Cancer Center [16], and the World Health Organization (WHO) [17]. These criteria are described in detail in the NCCN Clinical Practice guidelines [1, 7]. At our institution, we use the WHO criteria. The WHO criteria for AP CML include blasts in the peripheral blood or bone marrow of 10–19%, basophils ≥20% in the peripheral blood, persistent thrombocytopenia (<100 × 10^9/L) not related to therapy or persistent thrombocytosis (>1,000 × 10^9/L) that is unresponsive to therapy, increasing spleen size and white blood cell count unresponsive to therapy, and evidence of cytogenetic clonal evolution (i.e., the acquisition of other cytogenetic changes in addition to the Ph chromosome). Frequent additional cytogenetic abnormalities, in descending order of frequency, include trisomy 8, an additional Ph chromosome, isochromosome 17, trisomy 19, loss of the Y chromosome, trisomy 21, and monosomy 7 [11, 18]. BC CML is defined as ≥20% blasts. Among BC patients, myeloid BC occurs in ~2/3 of cases and lymphoid BC in ~1/3 of cases.

Prognostic Markers in CP CML

The Sokal Risk Score has been a standard tool to define the risk of disease progression and survival time in CML patients treated with chemotherapy or interferon alpha (IFN) [19]. The Hasford Risk Score is a modified Sokal Risk Score that incorporates basophil and eosinophil counts in addition to the Sokal Risk factors of age, spleen size, peripheral blast percentage, and platelet number. For IFN-treated patients, the Hasford Risk Score appeared to be better at predicting survival time and for TKI-treated patients, the Sokal Risk Score still has some predictive value [20, 21] [22–24]. The phase 3 International Randomized Interferon vs. STI571 (IRIS) trial, which randomized patients to receive either IFN or IM, patients were risk stratified by Sokal Risk Score. At 12 months, complete cytogenetic response (CCyR) rate was 76%, 67%, and 49% in low, intermediate, and high Sokal score patients, respectively. Disease progression at 5 years follow-up among low, intermediate, and high Sokal Risk Score patients was statistically significantly different at 3%, 8%, and 17%, respectively [24]. Recently, a new score for patients treated with first-line TKI therapy, the EUTOS Score, has been proposed based primarily on percent basophils and spleen size. In 2,060 patients, 5-year progression-free survival (PFS) was 90% vs. 82% for low- vs. high-risk patients [25].

In approximately 10–15% of CML cases, variant translocations exist [26–28]. These typically involve 3-way (or more) rearrangements of BCR-ABL with other regions of the genome. However, the prognostic significance of these variants remains unknown [28]. A frequent genetic abnormality seen in CP CML is deletion of the derivative chromosome 9 (or der 9q del). Studies of over 400 patients treated prior to the availability of IM, and who did not undergo allogeneic transplantation, demonstrated that der 9q del was associated with early CML progression and poorer overall survival [29]. Although an early study suggested poorer responses to IM in patients with der 9q del, recent data from over 500 patients suggest that der 9q del does not impact response rate, duration of response, or risk of progression [30, 31]. A recent study of patients receiving second-generation TKIs confirmed that der 9q del did not adversely affect major cytogenetic response (MCyR), CCyR, or overall survival (OS) [32].

Technological advances over the past 10 years have dramatically improved our ability to detect global differences in the expression of genes, proteins, and novel regulators of gene and protein expression, called microRNAs (miRNAs), as well as detect single nucleotide polymorphism (SNP) variations. Recently, genome sequencing efforts have begun. These approaches will continue to identify new therapeutic and prognostic targets in leukemia, and this field remains an exciting one to watch [33–40]. Recently, a genome-wide association study suggested that several loci are associated with an increased susceptibility to CML [41]. Prognostic predictor candidates have been identified for CML. For example, microarray-based gene expression profiling (GEP) has identified distinct expression signatures associated with disease progression and therapy resistance, while SNP profiling has identified SNPs associated with outcomes on TKI therapy [42–48]. However, these candidates have not, as of yet, been applied more broadly to clinical practice.

Biology in Brief

An in-depth review of the molecular biology of CML is beyond the scope of this chapter, and a number of excellent review papers exist [10–12, 49–51]. However, a basic understanding of CML biology is helpful to understand new directions in drug development and clinical trials. Unlike many other cancers, the phenotype of CP CML is uniquely driven by a single genetic alteration, the BCR-ABL translocation. For this reason, CP CML can be targeted with single-agent TKI therapy directed against the ABL tyrosine kinase. The Bcr-Abl fusion protein activates downstream signaling through several pathways including JAK/STAT, PI3 kinase/AKT, MAP kinase, SRC, and RAS, and ultimately activates transcription factors such as the various STATs, MYC, and NFKB. These pathways mediate cell proliferation and protection from apoptosis. Consequently, several of these are targets for drug development (e.g., PI3 kinase inhibitors, mTOR inhibition) [10–12, 49–51]. Dasatinib also targets SRC kinases such as LYN, in addition to ABL, providing a possible mechanism for activity in refractory or relapsed CML [52].

Bcr-Abl also mediates altered adhesion and may promote cell survival in response to TKI therapy through processes such as autophagy [53]. Autophagy is a process by which cells breakdown intracellular material in lysosomes in response to stress.

These functions are also viable drug targets. In CML, leukemia progenitor cells are found in the peripheral blood, spleen, and sometimes at extramedullary sites, suggesting that BCR-ABL alters adhesion and homing to the bone marrow. Impaired integrin responses, as well as BCR-ABL-induced changes in chemokines such as SDF1 and chemokine receptors such as CXCR4, contribute to impaired adhesion and increased migration of CML cells [54–60]. Upregulation of CXCR4, which occurs with effective treatment of CML by IM, promotes migration of CML cells to the bone marrow where they become quiescent and protected from therapy [61]. These observations may suggest a role for CXCR4 inhibition in overcoming TKI resistance [62].

Although still limited, our understanding of events involved in CML progression is growing. The amount of BCR-ABL, as well as the duration of exposure to BCR-ABL, appears to impact CML disease progression. Several groups have described that BCR-ABL mRNA expression increases with CML disease progression [63–66]. It is thought that BCR-ABL expression in CML progression contributes to genetic instability resulting in further genetic lesions (some of which are BCR-ABL independent) [56, 67–73]. Success with single-agent TKI therapy may be short-lived because of these additional genetic events. For example, SET expression increases as CML disease progresses [74]. SET is an inhibitor of the tumor suppressor protein phosphatase 2a (PP2A) and regulates cell proliferation and differentiation, as well as the proteasomal degradation of BCR-ABL [74]. Drugs that activate PP2A are candidates for investigation in advanced and resistant CML [74]. Other events contribute to the block in differentiation seen with progression. The loss of Ikaros is associated with the block in lymphoid differentiation in Ph+ ALL and lymphoid BC [75], whereas the loss of CEBPA or increase in HES1 contributes to the block in myeloid differentiation in myeloid BC [76, 77].

The increased frequency of ABL tyrosine kinase domain (TKD) point mutations in more advanced disease [78, 79], the acquisition of additional chromosomal abnormalities, and the loss of tumor suppressor genes such as TP53, RB1, and CDKN2A [11] are thought to be due to increased DNA damage in the setting of faulty repair and surveillance. Reactive oxygen species (ROS)-dependent DNA damage is increased in BCR-ABL-containing cells as compared to normal cells [68–71]. BCR-ABL expression also results in increased DNA double-strand breaks and checkpoint disruption leading to inappropriate repair [68, 72, 73, 80]. Recent reports suggest that the GC-rich ABL kinase domain is more predisposed to ROS-induced double-strand breaks, which, in the presence of faulty repair, contributes to ABL TKD point mutations [68].

The ability to preferentially target leukemia stem cells (LSCs), but not normal HSC, is a significant focus of current leukemia research. It is thought that CML cannot be eradicated without targeting CML stem cells. TKI therapy does not appear to eradicate CML stem cells [81, 82], thus patients currently stay on therapy lifelong. A better understanding of pathways regulating CML LSC proliferation and survival is required to design drugs that can eradicate these cells but not normal HSCs. WNT signaling, an important pathway regulating normal HSCs and normal development, is upregulated not only in CML stem cells but also in CML progenitor cells through beta-catenin [66, 83]. Recently, a role for another stem cell pathway, Hedgehog, has been implicated in CML [83, 84]. Certain drugs may target LSCs preferentially. In addition to drugs that inhibit smoothened in the Hedgehog pathway, some histone deacytelase inhibitors in combination with IM improve the eradication of LSCs but not normal HSCs [85]. Drugs targeting these pathways are the focus of several ongoing CML phase 1 and phase 2 trials.

The Treatment of CML

Rational for Monitoring and Monitoring Guidelines

CML has transformed from a frequently fatal disease to a disease that is successfully treated in the majority of patients. However, continuous and adequate TKI dosing is essential to achieve treatment goals. The impact of compliance on outcome is not as evident in carefully monitored patients participating in clinical trials. However, in 169 patients recruited from 34 centers in Belgium (the ADAGIO study), the authors reported that only 14.2% of patients were 100% compliant with prescribed IM and that noncompliance was associated with poorer responses [86]. Age, living alone, dose of IM, and being male adversely impacted compliance. Additionally in multivariate modeling, length of time from diagnosis and length of IM treatment also adversely impacted compliance. Factors that positively influenced compliance included increased knowledge about CML disease and treatment, at least a secondary education, and taking other medications chronically [86]. Another recent study reported that for patients with an adherence rate of ≤85% vs. those >85% were statistically significantly more likely to lose CCyR at 2 years (26.8% vs. 1.5%, respectively) [87].

Although most CP CML patients respond to therapy, approximately 20–25% of patients become resistant to IM. Adequate monitoring is important to identify which patients are not responding optimally so that early treatment interventions may occur and progression to AP and BC can be avoided, if possible. Published guidelines, including the NCCN and ELN [1, 4] guidelines, are based on patient characteristics at presentation, such as phase, and expected responses at various time points during therapy as established from various clinical trials [4, 71].

How We Measure Response

Before reviewing individual TKIs, it is important to understand how response to therapy is measured in CML. Reflecting the sensitivity of each test, hematologic responses precede cytogenetic responses, which in turn typically precede major or complete molecular responses. A complete hematologic response (CHR) in the peripheral blood is defined as a WBC $<10 \times 10^9/L$ with no immature granulocytes, less than 5% basophils, and platelets $<450 \times 10^9/L$. In addition, the spleen should not be palpable [88]. Cytogenetic responses are determined by the percentages of cells by G-banding of metaphase preparations that remain Philadelphia chromosome positive and are classified as complete (0%), partial (1–35%), minor (36–65%), minimal (66–94%), or lacking (≥95%) [5]. Major cytogenetic response (MCyR) encompasses both CCyR and partial cytogenetic response. Although interphase FISH using probes directed against BCR-ABL breakpoints is a more sensitive tool for monitoring disease than metaphase cytogenetic preparations [89, 90], almost all clinical trial outcomes are reported using metaphase cytogenetic preparations and not interphase FISH responses.

CML also provides a unique target to monitor at the molecular level. Sensitive PCR assays were developed and tested extensively in the 1990s, first as qualitative PCR (positive vs. negative result) and then as quantitative PCR (QPCR), in the allogeneic transplantation setting. QPCR provides an extremely sensitive measure of *bcr-abl* and depending on the assay can detect as few as 1–10 CML cells in 1,000,000 cells [91–94]. Nested qualitative PCR, which involves two amplification steps using two sets of primers (one "nested" inside the other), is typically more sensitive, and a patient who is negative by a nonnested QPCR assay may be positive by a nested qualitative PCR assay [64, 94–98]. However, QPCR is performed routinely, and qualitative PCR is primarily a research test at this time.

Thus, the tools were already in place to monitor CML disease on TKI therapy. In the IRIS trial that led to FDA approval of IM as frontline CML therapy [23], molecular response was measured every 3 months as a $\log_{10}$ (log) change from the median baseline of a group of 30 patient samples [22]. Although reported as log reductions, these reductions were not changes from a patient-specific baseline, but rather changes from a standardized population. As compared to CML patients after allogeneic transplantation, the vast majority of patients with a CCyR on the IRIS trial were still positive by QPCR testing [22]. Molecular response as well as cytogenetic response impacted PFS. Over time, many patients exhibited a continued decline in *bcr-abl*, and those with the largest log-decrease had the best PFS [99]. The first definition of a major molecular response (MMR), a 3-log or greater reduction in BCR-ABL mRNA levels, stems from this trial [22]. Among 368 patients at a median follow-up of 25 months, PFS was 85% in patients who did not achieve a CCyR, 95% in patients with a CCyR and <3-log reduction in *bcr-abl*, and 100% in patients with a CCyR and ≥3-log reduction in *bcr-abl* [22, 23]. Updates at 5 years follow-up demonstrated that for patients with at least a 3-log reduction in *bcr-abl*, estimated PFS rates remained 100% [24].

The definition of major molecular response has changed over time. It is now primarily defined as a percent *bcr-abl/abl* (or *bcr-abl/bcr*). This approach does not require a baseline PCR value and is easier to use in the community setting. One of the first reports using this method was a study of 280 CP CML patients treated with IM, including 117 treated previously with IFN [100]. A major molecular response was initially defined as less than 0.05%. In this study, the median baseline *bcr-abl/abl* was 39.4%, thus <0.05% was essentially the equivalent of a 3-log or greater reduction. At a median follow-up of 31 months, MMR, as defined in this way, was achieved by 62% of patients, and a complete molecular response (CMR) was achieved by 34% [100]. This difference in CMR incidence between this trial and the IRIS trial (4%) likely reflects assay sensitivity and the length of follow-up. Notably, molecular responses for IM-treated patients on the IRIS trial did deepen over time [99]. In a subset of 29 patients treated on the IRIS trial in Australia and New Zealand, by 81 months, the cumulative probability of MMR was 87%. Among this group, 70% had a >4-log reduction, and 52% had undetectable *bcr-abl* [99]. Achievement of MMR affects durability of CCyR. Among IRIS trial patients evaluable at 7 years, only 3% of patients with MMR at 18 months lost CCyR as compared to 26% who had achieved CCyR but not MMR at 18 months [101]. As the incidence of CMR increases over time on IM and second-generation TKIs, the influence of CMR on outcomes has come under greater scrutiny.

Although molecular monitoring of the peripheral blood is an important method to monitor patients, a few issues remain to be fully addressed. It is important to note that bone marrow and peripheral blood are not interchangeable in the serial evaluation of *bcr-abl* [102]. It has been difficult to translate log reductions into percent reductions that correlate with the patient outcome milestones on the IRIS trial. Additionally, what is considered "standard monitoring" has not been standardized universally. At this time, the use of various control genes, as well as differences in reagents and amounts of RNA analyzed, makes it difficult to compare results between laboratories. These discrepancies led to several publications on standardization of assays [103]. One solution is to provide internationally accepted reference reagents, but until this proposal becomes feasible, an international reporting scale has been proposed [103]. A defined international scale (IS) molecular response is derived after adjustment for laboratory specific conversion factors. The IS approach allows for the continued use of various control genes such as *B2M*, *GUSB*, *ABL*, and *BCR*. However, to date, some private and academic labs do not report IS responses, most likely because it requires extensive validation and comparison to a reference laboratory to arrive at the appropriate conversion factor for each lab. Additionally, this conversion factor does not take into account variations in sensitivity between assays. Several retrospective studies applied the IS approach to *bcr-abl* measurements from the IRIS study and the German CML Study IV [104, 105]. In the latter study for patient receiving 400 mg/day of IM, minimum molecular response levels predictive of EFS were established: 10% after 6 months, 1% after 12 months, and 0.1% at 18 months. These values are used commonly in practice with MMR defined as ≤0.1% IS, and this MMR values is endorsed in the most recent ELN guidelines [5, 88].

Treatment Before IM

Rationally designed TKIs targeting ABL have dramatically altered the treatment of CML. Prior to IM, HSCT was pursued as first-line therapy in CML patients, despite the significant upfront mortality, in patients, particularly young patients, with available donors and adequate performance status (~1/3 of patients). Transplantation is discussed in the section entitled "The Role of Allogeneic Transplantation." IFN with or without the addition of cytarabine (Ara-C) was the main drug therapy prior to IM [106]. Achievement of a CCyR on IFN is associated with good long-term prognosis; however, only ~10–25% of patients achieved a CCyR [107–110]. Interestingly, durable responses continued in a small subset of patients with CCyR who stopped IFN [107, 108, 110]. Biological studies also suggest that IFN may target CML stem cells [111–114]. As a consequence of these clinical and biological observations, there is a continued interest in combining IFN with TKI, despite the significant side effects of IFN.

First-Line Therapy

Imatinib Mesylate

IM belongs to the class of 2-phenyl-amino-pyrimidines and is a potent inhibitor of several tyrosine kinases: ABL, platelet-derived growth factor receptor (PDGFR)α, PDGRFβ, and c-KIT. IM is a highly selective and specific inhibitor that binds to the ATP binding pocket and stabilizes ABL in its inactive conformation, thereby preventing phosphorylation of the kinase and downstream proteins [115]. IM quickly demonstrated impressive responses in phase I and II studies of over 1,000 patients at 30 centers who had failed other therapies. Similar to other therapies for CML, response was significantly dependent on phase. The best outcomes were observed in CP and the worst in BC [116–120]. In subsequent sections, we will focus first on TKI outcomes in CP patients and address outcomes in AP and BC patients separately.

The randomized phase III IRIS study of 1,106 patients compared first-line IM at 400 mg by mouth daily vs. IFN and low-dose Ara-C for newly diagnosed CP CML. Not only was IM much better tolerated, but at 18 months, the estimated MCyR incidence rate was 87.1% in IM-treated patients as compared with 34.7% in the IFN- and Ara-C-treated patients [23]. Even more impressively, the estimated CCyR incidence rate was 76.2% in IM-treated patients as compared to 14.5% in IFN- and Ara-C-treated patients [23]. Over time, it has been increasingly difficult to compare IM to IFN plus Ara-C directly as the study allowed for crossover between the 2 arms and 359 patients (or 65%) crossed over to the IM arm. The main reason for crossover was intolerance to IFN (26%) [24, 120]. Eight-year follow-up of 553 patients randomized to first-line IM indicates that 304 (55%) remain on IM therapy [122]. IM was stopped due to unsatisfactory therapeutic response (16%), death (3%), HSCT (3%), and other or unknown reason (17%). Estimated OS was 85%, freedom from progression to AP or BC was 92%, and event-free survival (EFS) was 81%. The annual event rate is defined as either a loss of CHR, loss of MCyR, progression to AP or BC, or death during treatment [122]. The annual estimated event rates were 3.3% in year 1, 7.5% in year 2, 4.8% in year 3, 1.5% in year 4, 0.8% in year 5, and 0.4% in year 6 [121]. One death from disease progression occurred in year 8, the first in 2 years. Focusing on progression only in years 4–8, the annual rates of progression were 0.9%, 0.5%, 0%, 0%, and 0.4%, respectively [122].

Cytogenetic response is associated with outcome, and only patients achieving a CCyR demonstrate durable responses. The IRIS trial has reported cumulative CCyR incidences, which refer to the percent of patients achieving a particular response (or the best response), not the percent of patients maintaining that response. The cumulative best CCyR rate on IM was 82% (456 patients), and among patients who achieved a CCyR on IM and remained on study treatment, 63% (349 patients) remain in documented CCyR [121]. Time to cytogenetic response after treatment initiation also matters. Analyses suggest that 3 months is too early to determine if a patient will achieve a CCyR on IM as 50% of patients with >95% Ph chromosomes present still achieve a CCyR. However, by 6 months, only ~15% of patients with more than 95% Ph chromosomes present will achieve a CCyR. By 12 months, only patients with at least an MCyR are likely to achieve a CCyR [4, 6, 88]. The ELN guidelines, initially published in 2006, have proposed cytogenetic milestones for response and have defined failure and suboptimal responses on IM based on these observations [6].

Can IM Be Stopped?

The ability of patients to achieve a CMR has prompted interest in IM cessation, although a number of studies have shown that CML stem and progenitor cells remain detectable in IM-treated patients in CCyR, as well as in prolonged CCyR [123, 124]. A study in France examined 69 patients who were QPCR negative for at least 2 years prior to enrolling on the STIM (Stop IM) study. With a median follow-up of 21 months, the probability of remaining in CMR at 12 months was 41%. There was no statistically significant difference in maintaining a CMR between patients who had been treated with IM alone vs. those who had received IM after IFN. Among the 41 patients with molecular relapse, 27 occurred within the first 6 months of IM cessation; all patients could be rescued with reinstitution of IM. Factors associated with persistent CMR off IM included Sokal Risk Score (low), sex (male) and duration of IM prior to its cessation (50 months or longer) [125]. At this time stopping IM should only be considered in the setting of a clinical trial.

Dasatinib and Nilotinib as First-Line Therapy in CP CML

Nilotinib and dasatinib are now approved as first-line therapy for CP CML. Phase 2 studies of both drugs as second-line therapy demonstrated rapid cytogenetic and molecular responses [126–129]. However, two phase 3 trials suggested that PFS was better on second-generation TKIs, leading to expedited FDA approval of dasatinib and nilotinib [130, 131]. Although the number of patients progressing on IM was quite small, this reported difference has led to a rapid increase in the use of second-generation TKIs as first-line therapy.

The phase 3 randomized ENESTnd trial compared nilotinib to IM in 846 newly diagnosed CP CML patients at 217 centers [130]. Patients were randomized 1:1:1 to nilotinib at 300 mg twice per day (282 patients), nilotinib at 400 mg twice per day (281 patients), or IM at 400 mg once per day (283 patients). Patients were stratified by Sokal Risk Score so that all groups contained the same number of patients in the low, intermediate, and high Sokal Risk Score categories. The primary endpoint was MMR at 12 months; the secondary endpoint was CCyR at 12 months. Other endpoints included time to and duration of MMR and CCyR, EFS, PFS, and OS. At 12 months, CCyR rates were statistically significantly different between both nilotinib arms and IM. CCyR was no different between 300 and 400 mg twice per day (80% and 78%, respectively), but was statistically significantly lower in the IM arm (65%). At 12 months, MMR rates were also statistically significantly higher in the nilotinib arms as compared to the IM arm: 44% and 43% for nilotinib at 400 or 300 mg twice per day, respectively, vs. 22% for the IM arm. MMR rates for the nilotinib arms were also higher at 3, 6, and 9 months. One caveat to the MMR data is that the rate of MMR on nilotinib and IM is lower than has been reported in other studies. A key observation leading to FDA approval was the statistically significant difference in PFS: 11 patients in the IM arm progressed to AP or BC (3.9%) vs. 2 and 1 (total 3 patients) in the 300 and 400 mg twice per day nilotinib arms (0.7% and 0.4%, respectively). It should be noted, however, that no patient with MMR, irrespective of treatment, progressed, although 3 of 11 IM-treated patients with CCyR progressed [130].

Newly diagnosed CP CML patients (519 patients) were randomized to dasatinib at 100 mg daily or to IM at 400 mg daily in the multinational DASISION trial [131]. The primary endpoint was CCyR at 12 months. Secondary endpoints included MMR at any time, duration of MMR and CCyR, and EFS and PFS. The rate of MMR by 12 months was statistically significantly higher in dasatinib vs. IM-treated patients (46% vs. 28%, respectively). Confirmed CCyR by 12 months was also higher in dasatinib-treated patients at 77% vs. 66% in IM-treated patients. Similar to the ENESTnd trial, cytogenetic and molecular responses occurred more quickly. Progression to AP or BC occurred in 5 dasatinib patients (1.9%) and in 9 IM patients (3.5%), but this observed trend did not reach the statistical significance threshold. For the DASISION trial, similar to the ENESTnd trial, no patients with MMR progressed [131].

If the statistically significant observations and trend toward improved PFS for nilotinib and dasatinib, respectively, continue and impact OS, then these drugs may prove to be "better" first-line therapy for some patients. Clearly, responses on nilotinib and dasatinib are faster, but 82% of patients ultimately achieved a CCyR on IM on the IRIS trial [24, 121]. The answer to which therapy to choose may depend, in part, upon whether waiting for a CCyR in IM-treated patients is detrimental. The optimal milestones utilized in the ELN and NCCN guidelines suggest CCyR should occur within 12–18 months [1, 4, 5, 132]. Thereafter, the likelihood of achieving a CCyR is lower, and the likelihood of progressing on therapy is higher. Data from the recently published ENESTnd and DASISION trials also suggest that early CCyR and MMR translate into better PFS [130, 131]. This observation may ultimately translate into better OS.

However, we may end up "overtreating" a significant proportion of patients in order to benefit a few. IM has a proven efficacy and safety record with no significant long-term sequelae observed [24, 133], and careful monitoring can successfully identify patients at risk for treatment failure. Dasatinib and nilotinib have unique side effects that may (or may not) be significant in the long run when utilized outside of the carefully selected clinical trial population. These include QT prolongation, pancreatitis, glucose elevations, and pleural effusion [130, 131]. Using second-generation TKIs as first-line therapy may also limit second-line therapy choices. The significance of this issue is unknown, and patients who fail first-line second-generation TKIs may have CML that is more difficult to treat. But time and experience with these drugs should put these issues into perspective. For now, a decision on which drug to use as first-line in CP may depend upon risk features such as Sokal or Hasford Risk Scores, patient medical history, side effect profile of each drug, patient's history of compliance, patient family history, and patient preference. The observation that high Sokal or Hasford Risk Score patients had higher MMR rates at 12 months on second-generation TKIs [130, 131] could be used to stratify patients at diagnosis. Additionally, the identification of other molecular diagnostic predictors could facilitate decision-making to first- vs. second (vs. third)-generation TKIs. However, when IM becomes available in generic form, cost will likely be the major factor in treatment decision-making, unless dasatinib and nilotinib show a significant survival benefit.

Resistance to Therapy Mechanisms of Resistance

Resistance to TKI therapy is often characterized as primary or secondary (i.e., acquired) resistance. What causes primary resistance, for the most part, still remains elusive, but reported mechanisms include altered drug transport, BCR-ABL independent mechanisms (where BCR-ABL remains inhibited, but disease is not significantly altered, or disease progression occurs), clonal evolution, and the retention of a reservoir of quiescent CML stem cells. The last mechanism may explain why most patients cannot stop TKI therapy. Point mutations in the ABL tyrosine kinase domain (TKD) are seen more rarely in primary resistance but are the most common mechanism of acquired TKI resistance. Assays to detect ABL TKD mutations are available clinically.

Plasma Levels and Drug Transport

In primary resistance decreased drug bioavailability either through poor absorption or increased hepatic metabolism; increased IM cellular efflux through ABC drug transporters such as MDR1 or ABCG2 [134, 135] and decreased IM influx through the SLC family transporter hOCT1 [136, 137] likely play a significant role.

A study of day 29 trough plasma levels for IM and its metabolite CGP74588 in 351 patients enrolled on the IRIS study suggested that trough levels were significantly higher on day 29 in patients who ultimately achieved CCyR [138]. Trough IM plasma levels after at least 12 months of IM therapy were also associated with cytogenetic and molecular responses [139]. These data suggest that a trough plasma level threshold of 1,000 ng/mL may be a determinant in achieving a CCyR. However, it remains unclear whether or not plasma levels are a reliable method to evaluate resistance. Discontinuation or nonadherence to IM likely influenced these early clinical observations. As may be expected, the discontinuation rate was highest in the group with the lowest plasma trough levels [138].

Drug transport into (influx) and out of (efflux) CML cells plays a role in IM resistance. Notably, IM plasma trough levels do not measure the amount of drug *within* cells. Early studies of CML primary patient cells exposed to IM demonstrated upregulation of the expression of the efflux transporter MDR1 and downregulation of the expression of the influx transporter hOCT1 (SLC22A1 or OCT-1) implying that the balance of these two transporters plays a role in IM resistance [134, 140]. Drug transporters such as MDR1, ABCG2, and OCT-1 are thought to play a role in CML stem cell resistance to IM [135, 136, 141]. MDR1 inhibition, however, does not sensitize CML cells to IM [142]. Modulating drug transporters, however, is difficult for many reasons, including that MDR1 is not solely responsible for drug resistance [82].

OCT-1 is a primary mediator of IM influx and has received attention as a possible predictor of IM response. There have been conflicting data on whether OCT-1 mRNA expression at diagnosis predicts response to IM [143]. Radiolabeled assays that measure "activity" (or intracellular uptake and retention) of drug suggest that OCT-1 mediates uptake of IM but not of nilotinib, and that "activity" correlates with better molecular response to IM [136]. The ability of "activity" to predict molecular response, however, is abrogated by higher doses of IM [137].

BCR-ABL Amplification and Independence

Amplification of the BCR-ABL gene was the first IM resistance mechanism described [144]. However, subsequent studies have shown that it is an infrequent cause of resistance [145]. BCR-ABL independent resistance has been most extensively described in the context of SRC kinases [146]. LYN kinase overexpression mediates IM resistance primarily in advanced CML, but also in some CP cases in the absence of ABL TKD mutations [147–149]. LYN kinase activation contributes to persistent bcr-abl independent tyrosine phosphorylation [148, 149]. At this time, the prevalence of increased expression or activity of LYN in mutation-negative TKI-resistant CML is unknown, but for resistance mediated by increased LYN, dasatinib, which also targets SRC kinase [150], is a reasonable choice. LYN overexpression may also be associated with resistance to nilotinib [151]. However, excellent responses to nilotinib in mutation-negative CP patients suggest that upregulated LYN may occur infrequently. Lastly, at this time, no clinical assays exist to determine LYN kinase expression or activity in resistant patients [152].

Clonal Evolution

Clonal evolution (CE) in patients treated with TKIs has been reported in both Ph+ and Ph− cells. As discussed earlier, CE in Ph+ cells is a feature of CML disease progression. In an early study of 498 patients with CP or AP CML, Ph+ CE was observed in 70 CP and 51 AP patients [153]. Ph+ CE was not associated with significant differences in MCyR or CCyR rates; however, Ph+ CE was associated with poorer OS. A subsequent study of 141 patients found that Ph+ CE was associated with a higher risk of relapse (50%) as compared to patients without Ph+ CE (9%) [154].

Approximately 3–9% of patients achieving a CCyR show evidence of CE in Ph− cells [155–158]. Ph− CE has also been described in IFN-treated patients [159, 160]. The most common secondary chromosomal abnormality in Ph− CE, similar to Ph+ CE, is trisomy 8, but cytogenetic lesions associated with myelodysplasia (−5 and −7 deletions and complex cytogenetics) have also been described [161, 162]. Unlike Ph+ CE, Ph− CE does not impact outcomes except in the rare cases of MDS-associated abnormalities, typically accompanied by cytopenias. In these cases, progression to MDS and in some cases AML can occur [161, 162]. In a study of 515 (primarily) CP patients previously treated with IFN before IM, 30 patients (5%) had confirmed Ph− CE most commonly involving chromosomes Y, 8, and 7. Ph− CE had no impact on PFS and OS in patients achieving an MCyR, suggesting that IM response is more important than CE [163]. Two patients developed MDS (median follow-up 51 months). In a subsequent study of 258 de novo CML patients receiving IM (median follow-up 37 months), 9% developed Ph− CE in at least one metaphase [164]. This study confirmed that −Y and trisomy 8 are the most common abnormalities. Notably, −Y also occurs with aging in men. The incidence of Ph− CE decreased to 3% if only patients with the abnormalities present in at least two or more metaphases were considered. In most Ph-negative patients, CE was transient and disappeared in 18 of 21 patients. In a subanalysis of patients with at least 36 months of follow-up, the development of Ph− CE was associated with worse PFS but no difference in OS; estimated 4-year PFS was 63% in CE vs. 88% in no CE ($p = 0.05$) [165]. One patient developed AML in association with −7. Ph− CE has also been observed in dasatinib-treated patients after IM failure. In conclusion, the detection of CE may warrant closer follow-up, but no change in treatment strategy is indicated unless evidence of dysplasia is noted.

ABL Tyrosine Kinase Domain Point Mutations

ABL tyrosine kinase domain (TKD) point mutations are the main mechanism of resistance occurring after an initial response to therapy [166–170]. The appearance of ABL TKD point mutations raises several issues: are all mutations equal in terms of resistance, and how do we treat point-mutated CML? Currently, direct nucleotide sequencing, in which the *bcr-abl* transcript is amplified and the product sequenced to detect the point mutation, is the main method of ABL TKD mutation detection. This is a fairly insensitive technique, and the mutation must represent ~15–25% of the BCR-ABL clone in order to be detected [168]. Other more sensitive point mutation detection methods are not readily available outside of research institutions [171–173]. It remains unclear whether detection of very low amounts of point-mutated ABL using highly sensitive assays is clinically helpful [171]. A very informative review on this topic was recently published [174].

More than 100 point mutations have been described after IM exposure, leading to amino acid changes in the activation loop, ATP phosphate-binding loop (or p-loop), and the hinge region along the C- and N-terminal lobes of the kinase [174]. In vitro studies suggest other mutations may exist in the N-terminal cap and the SRC homology domains 2 and 3 (SH2 and SH3); however, the clinical relevance of these mutations is unknown [175]. Ultimately, these mutations result in impaired IM binding and decreased inhibition of downstream ABL signaling. IM binds to and stabilizes the inactive Abl conformation where there is distortion of the ATP binding loop [115]. Mutations at the direct contact sites or sites that prevent Abl from adopting the confirmation needed for IM binding result in resistance. Nilotinib was designed to provide a "better fit" than IM and thus is resistant to far fewer mutations [176, 177]. However, ABL proteins harboring T315I and p-loop mutations (e.g., L248V, G250E, Q252H, Y253F/H, and E255K/V) remain resistant to nilotinib. In contrast, dasatinib binds to the active confirmation (and perhaps the inactive confirmation) of ABL. Thus, mutations that confer resistance to dasatinib impede direct binding (e.g. T315I) [178, 179].

The prevalence of mutations increases as CML progresses [168–170]. Early CP patients have the lowest rate of mutation development, followed by "late" CP (CML for >1 year before starting IM), AP, and BC patients. The GIMEMA Working Party on CML examined 256 IM-treated CML patients and found ABL TKD point mutations in 26% of CP cases (but only 4% in a subset of early CP cases), 44% of AP cases, 73% of myeloid BC cases, and 81% of lymphoid BC cases [180]. Not only is the prevalence of mutations higher in advanced disease, but there also appears to be a variation in mutation type by disease phase. The pan-resistant T315I occurs as much as three times more frequently in advanced phase CML as compared to CP CML patients [174]. Furthermore, the frequency of multiple mutations is also lower in CP patients as compared with other phases: 17% in CP vs. 30% in AP vs. 36% in myeloid BC vs. 27% of lymphoid BC and Ph+ ALL [174].

Early studies suggested that substitutions at seven amino acid residues accounted for a large proportion of mutations in IM-treated patients [180]. In the GIMEMA Working Party study, discussed above, 7 amino acid residues (10 point mutations) were the most common and comprised 85% of the mutations detected [180]. Furthermore, the p-loop and T315I mutations comprised 55% of the point mutations detected. In IM-treated patients, p-loop mutations and the T315I mutation are associated with poorer outcomes or more rapid evolution to advanced phase disease as compared to other mutations or no mutations [169, 180, 181]. Two more recent studies that have collated mutations, one of more than 800 mutations and the other of more than 500 mutations, support these original observations [174, 182, 183]. These studies found that the T315, Y253, E255, M351, G250, F359, and H396 were the most frequent and accounted for 66% of mutations and 60% of mutations in each study, respectively. With regard to dasatinib resistance associated mutations (besides T315I), mutations involving amino acid residues 317 and 299 were rare. The frequency for F317L was 5.7%. For nilotinib, T315I, F359V, E255K, Y253H, E255V, and F359C/I are the most frequent mutations associated with resistance [174, 177, 184].

When should ABL sequencing be pursued? It should be considered when appropriate clinical milestones, as discussed later, are not achieved or are lost. Additionally, several groups have reported and confirmed that small changes in the burden of molecular disease, measured by *bcr-abl* QPCR, may indicate the development of point mutations. It should be noted this observation only applies to serial monitoring done in the same laboratory using IS standardization. It has been reported that a >2-fold rise in BCR-ABL mRNA is associated with the emergence of ABL TKD mutations [79]. In 214 patients, 61% of patients with a >2-fold increase in *bcr-abl* had detectable mutations compared to <1% of patients with stable or decreasing *bcr-abl* [79]. This earlier observation has been confirmed by a more recent study where a 2.6-fold increase was considered the optimal cut-off for point mutation detection in the laboratory used for this study [185]. This observation reinforces the need for an aggressive monitoring strategy for patients on TKI therapy and suggests that waiting for a tenfold or more increase in *bcr-abl* may cause a delay in point mutation detection under current guidelines. However, given current differences in laboratory monitoring of *bcr-abl* using QPCR, an optimal cut-off may vary between laboratories which makes these recommendations more difficult to implement uniformly in the community.

Monitoring Response

The excellent outcomes achieved with TKI therapy in CML mandate careful monitoring to ensure these outcomes are obtained. The NCCN and ELN provide excellent guidelines for monitoring CML patients in all phases based on the clinical trials data accrued over the past decade [1, 4, 6, 88]. The initial ELN guidelines were published in 2006 and validated in 2008 [88]. These guidelines will likely be altered to accommodate observations using dasatinib and nilotinib as first-line therapy. The ELN guidelines provide response definitions; timing of expected responses; and definitions of optimal response, suboptimal response, and failure. Based on data from the IRIS trial, patients who fail to achieve these responses within the specified time are unlikely to achieve these responses and consequently have decreased PFS and OS compared to patients meeting these milestones [88]. To summarize briefly, the expected optimal responses on IM are to achieve: a CHR by 3 months, major cytogenetic response (includes partial and CCyR) by 6 months, CCyR by 12 months, and an MMR by 18 months. Failure is defined as no CHR by 6 months, no MCyR by 12 months, and no CCyR by 18 months [88]. Treatment milestones are shown in Table 4.1 and recommendations for disease monitoring in Table 4.2. These guidelines highlight the importance of bone marrow exams and routine metaphase

Table 4.1 Expected treatment outcomes

Time from diagnosis	Treatment milestones	Milestone definition	Suboptimal	Failure
3 months	Complete hematologic response (CHR)[a]	Normal CBC and differential, no evidence of extramedullary disease	< CHR	No response
6 months	Major cytogenetic response (MCyR)[b]	1–35% Ph-positive metaphases[c] or 0% Ph-positive metaphases[c]	< MCyR	< CHR
12 months	Complete cytogenetic response (CCyR)	0% Ph-positive metaphases[c]	< CCyR	< MCyR
18 months	Major molecular response (MMR)	≥3-log reduction of BCR-ABL mRNA or ≤0.1% BCR-ABL IS	< MMR	< CCyR
	Complete molecular response (CMR)	No evidence of BCR-ABL by RT-PCR		

Adapted from the 2011 NCCN guidelines and ELN guidelines [1, 5–7]

[a] A complete hematologic response requires a leukocyte count of $<10 \times 10^9$/L, platelet count of $<450 \times 10^9$/L, and a normal differential with no early forms, no splenomegaly

[b] Additional cytogenetic responses definitions: a major cytogenetic response comprises complete and partial cytogenetic responses

[c] Based on at least 20 metaphases

Table 4.2 Recommendations for monitoring disease

At time of:	Complete blood count and white cell differential	Metaphase cytogenetics (bone marrow)	Quantitative RT-PCR (peripheral blood)
Diagnosis	Every 1–2 weeks until blood counts are stable	Prior to therapy	Prior to therapy
CHR	Every 3 months	Every 3–6 months[a]	Every 3 months
CCyR	Every 3 months	*In evolution*[b]	Every 3 months
MMR	Every 3 months	*In evolution*[b]	Every 3–6[c] months
CMR	Every 3 months	*In evolution*[b]	Every 3–6[c] months

Adapted from the 2011 NCCN guidelines and ELN guidelines [1, 5–7]

CHR complete hematologic response, *MMR* major molecular response, *CCyR* complete cytogenetic response, *CMR* complete molecular response

[a] The NCCN guidelines suggest bone marrow aspirates at 6, 12, and 18 months. A bone marrow exam with cytogenetics at 12 months not required if CCyR at 6 months, or at 18 months if CCyR at 6 and/or 12 months

[b] Recommendations for the frequency of bone marrow aspirates in patients with CCyR continue to evolve. For patients with stable CCyR, previous recommendations suggested ~ every 18 months due to concerns regarding Ph-negative clonal evolution (CE). However, in the absence of Ph-negative CE in patients with stable CCyR and MMR, it is likely that the period between marrows will continue to lengthen

[c] For patients with stable MMR or CMR, it is reasonable to consider monitoring at 6-month intervals

cytogenetic examination at diagnosis and for monitoring response until a CCyR is achieved. PFS and OS on the IRIS trial were defined primarily by cytogenetic response [23, 24]. Although universally standardized molecular monitoring of the peripheral blood by QPCR, together with FISH, may someday supplant the need for bone marrow metaphase cytogenetics, this is not currently the case. However, once a stable CCyR is achieved, molecular monitoring of the peripheral blood is sufficient in reliable clinical laboratories [1, 4, 6, 88]. A bone marrow exam is indicated for loss of response, but indications for follow-up bone marrows in patients with durable CCyRs continue to evolve. One indication is unexpected cytopenias, which may be an indicator of disease progression or more rarely MDS or AML (arising from Ph– clonal evolution). Cytopenias in the first 3–6 months are not unexpected and are thus not of similar concern.

An evaluation of the ELN guidelines was reported in 2008; 224 consecutive patients between June 2000 and May 2007 with CP CML receiving IM as first-line therapy were evaluated to determine the predictive value of these guidelines [88]. None of the patients classified as a failure at 3 or 12 months reversed their failure status [88]. At the 6-month milestone, 4 of 37 patients classified as failure subsequently satisfied criteria for response. However, of these 4 patients, one failed at 18 months and 2 lost their CCyR. Comparing patients who met failure criteria at any time during the first 12 months to those who never met failure criteria, OS and PFS at 5 years were statistically significantly different at 80.6% vs. 96.1% and 63.8% vs. 90.8%, respectively. Of note, suboptimal responses at 18 months were not statistically significantly predictive of PFS or OS at 5 years. Patients who achieved a CCyR but failed to achieve an MMR at 12 or 18 months were more likely to lose their cytogenetic response. Specifically, among patients who did not achieve an MMR at 12 months, 23.6% lost their CCyR as compared to 2.6% among those who achieved an MMR ($p=0.04$). At 18 months, 24.6% of patients who did not achieve an MMR lost their CCyR as compared to 0% among those who achieved this milestone ($p=0.006$) [88]. Milestones are shown in Table 4.1, and an algorithm adapted from these guidelines is shown in Fig. 4.1.

Monitoring and early detection is based on the premise that altering therapeutic strategy is more effective in the setting of more limited resistance. In an analysis of 293 patients receiving dasatinib for IM failure, patients receiving dasatinib for loss of MCyR rather than loss of both MCyR and loss of a CHR were more likely to achieve a CCyR (72% vs. 42%) and also had improved 24-month EFS (89% vs. 29%) [186]. More recent retrospective reviews suggest that patients with suboptimal responses as defined by ELN guidelines may have outcomes that are more similar to patients defined as ELN failures [88, 132]. Suboptimal responders at 6 months were less likely to achieve a CCyR than optimal responders (30% vs. 97%), and EFS and transformation-free survival (TFS) were similar for suboptimal responders and failures at this time point. However, suboptimal responses were less worrisome at 12 and 18 months. At 12 months, TFS was the same for suboptimal responders and optimal responders, but EFS was worse in the former group. By 18 months, there was no difference between the two groups. Notably, the 18-month guidelines are primarily driven by molecular response. Thus, these data suggest that meeting hematologic and cytogenetic milestones early may be more important than the time required achieving molecular milestones.

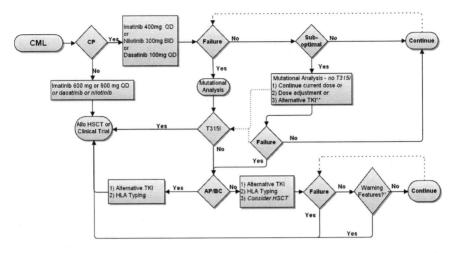

Fig. 4.1 A suggested monitoring strategy. *Patients who achieve a partial or complete cytogenetic response at 6 months or a CCyR by 12 months on second-line therapy have significantly improved survival [284]. Patients without a cytogenetic response at 3 or 6 months should receive alternative therapy [7]. **Choice may depend on milestone. No change may be appropriate for a patient with CCyR and declining *bcr-abl* but no MMR at 18 months, whereas the absence of CCyR at 12 months may warrant switching to an alternative TKI (based on mutation profile). Additionally, the presence of a resistance-conferring mutation warrants a change in treatment strategy

Second (and Third)-Line Therapy

Increased IM and Building on IM in CP CML

With the availability of highly active second-generation TKIs, IM dose escalation has become primarily a thing of the past. Several studies have reported that CCyR, MMR, and CMR rates are higher on increased IM doses of 600 or 800 mg [187–189]. Two studies have compared frontline IM at 400–800 mg/day prospectively: the European LeukemiaNet Study and Novartis-sponsored Tyrosine Kinase Inhibitor Optimization and Selectivity (TOPS) study [190, 191]. A major difference between the two studies is that the ELN study focused on high Sokal Risk Score patients, who, as demonstrated in the IRIS trial, had poorer outcomes as compared to low and intermediate Sokal Risk Score patients. The ELN study randomly assigned 216 patients to receive IM at 800 or 400 mg; median follow-up was 26 months [190]. At 1 year, the CCyR rate in these high-risk patients was 64% vs. 58% in the high-dose vs. the standard-dose arm (p = .435). No differences were observed in CCyR at 3 and 6 months either, and there was no statistically significant difference in molecular responses at 3, 6, and 12 months. The TOPS study stratified patients by Sokal score and randomized patients in a 2:1 design to IM at 800 mg/day or IM at 400 mg/day [191]. The primary outcome was MMR. Only at 3 and 6 months was there a statistically significant difference in MMR rates; thereafter no difference was observed. These data suggest that dose intensity impacted time to MMR, but did not increase the numbers of patients achieving an MMR. Additionally, there were no differences in MMR between low and intermediate Sokal Risk Score patients stratified by dose. Furthermore, the incidence of cytopenias and dose interruptions was significantly higher in patients receiving IM at 800 mg. Lastly, and perhaps most importantly, there were no statistically significant differences between the two arms with regard to EFS, PFS, and OS [191]. In conclusion, at this time, these data support the continued use of IM at 400 mg/day as first-line therapy.

Mutation data should be used to guide the feasibility of dose escalation if it is considered. All patients with evidence of ABL TKD point mutations should be switched to a second-generation TKI based on the mutation detected and the known mutation profile of dasatinib or nilotinib. As discussed, dasatinib and nilotinib yield more rapid cytogenetic and molecular responses and, are associated with improved PFS. These observations coupled with the increased side effects of IM at 800 mg daily suggest a limited role for dose escalation in the future, but it could be considered in patients unable to tolerate second-generation TKIs.

IFN has remained of interest in the clinical community for two reasons: the fact that a small subset of patients maintains a CCyR off IFN and the possibility that IFN may target a CML stem cell [107–114]. Attempting to preferentially target leukemia stem cells, which does not occur with TKI therapy, is an active area of research. Although data presented in abstract form for the German CML Study IV suggested no improvement in outcomes with the addition of IFN [192], the recently published French SPIRIT trial suggested a benefit, although discontinuation rates for IFN were high [193]. Patients were randomized to 1 of 4 arms: IM at 400 mg/day, IM at 600 mg/day, IM + cytarabine at 20 mg/m^2 for 14 days/month, and IM + pegylated IFN alpha 2a at 90mcg/week. At 12 months, the IM + pegylated IFN arm showed a statistically significant improvement in molecular response: 57% achieved MMR (<0.1) on this combination vs. 38% in the IM at 400 mg daily arm. Additionally, a superior molecular response, as defined as <0.01%, was also statistically significantly higher in the IFN arm vs. IM at 400 mg daily arm, 30% vs. 14%, respectively. A major caveat is that 45% of patients stopped pegylated IFN due to side effects within the first year as compared to 7% who stopped IM at 400 mg daily [193].

Dasatinib and Nilotinib in CP CML Patients Intolerant or Resistant to Imatinib

Nilotinib (Tasigna) is a selective ABL TKI that also targets PDGFR, KIT, and EPHB4 [194]. It is approximately 30-fold more potent than IM and has activity similar to IM against KIT and PDGFRB [176]. Nilotinib treats most IM mutants, but does not treat T315I-, E255K-, and E255V-mutated ABL and has intermediate sensitivity to several other point mutations located in the p-loop. Dasatinib (Sprycel) is less selective but is an even more potent inhibitor of ABL, ~300 times more potent. Dasatinib, unlike IM and nilotinib, can bind to both the inactive and active conformation of the ABL tyrosine kinase [150, 178]. It also significantly inhibits the SRC family of tyrosine kinases including FGR, FYN, HCK, LCK, LYN, and YES. LYN, as noted above, has been implicated in progression to lymphoid BC and IM resistance. Dasatinib also has some activity against KIT and PDGFR and the ephrin family of tyrosine kinases [195]. It lacks activity against T315I-mutated ABL and, uniquely, to ABL mutated at codons 317 and 299 [196]. The last two mutations are sensitive to IM. Bosutinib is effective as second-line therapy but is not available outside of clinical trial in the USA [197].

Dasatinib

Dasatinib has FDA approval to treat patients resistant or intolerant of IM in all phases of CML, as well as Ph+ ALL [194]. Phase 2 clinical trial data from 4 trials of 445 patients who received primarily 70 mg twice per day suggested that a significant proportion of IM resistant and intolerant patients responded to dasatinib. An unexpectedly high, although transient, response was also seen in lymphoid BC and Ph+ ALL, and is thought to be due to targeting of SRC kinases [194].

An open-label phase 2 trial of 150 CP CML patients resistant to IM randomized patients in a 2:1 design to 140 mg of dasatinib per day ($n=101$) or imatinib at 800 mg/day ($n=49$) [126]. At a median follow-up of 15 months, all responses were statistically significantly better in the dasatinib arm than in the high-dose IM arm, suggesting that switching to dasatinib is a more successful strategy than dose escalation in IM resistant patients. CHR was seen in 93% vs. 82%, MCyR was seen in 52% vs. 33%, and CCyR was 40% vs. 16% in dasatinib-treated vs. IM dose-escalated patients, respectively. MMR was also higher at 16% vs. 4%. Notably, there was a statistically significant decrease in risk of treatment failure as well as an improvement in PFS in dasatinib-treated patients (hazard ratio (HR)=0.16 and HR=0.14), respectively. As compared to IM, grade 3 to 4 cytopenias and pleural effusions (17% vs. 0%) were more common on dasatinib [126]. A retrospective analysis of 88 CP patients enrolled on the START-C and START-R trials reported superior responses in IM intolerant as compared to IM resistant patients; CCyR was 44%, and MMR was 33% in IM resistant patients as compared to CCyR of 78% and MMR of 63% in IM intolerant patients after 24 months follow-up [198, 199]. Achieving a CCyR or MMR by 12 months significantly impacted PFS, but did not affect OS at 24 months. These data provided strong evidence that IM resistant and intolerant CP patients can achieve excellent and durable responses on second-line dasatinib.

Current dosing recommendations for dasatinib are derived from an open-label phase 3 trial in which randomized 670 patients were randomized in a 1:1:1:1 design to 4 different dasatinib doses or dosing schedules: 100 mg/day, 50 mg twice per day, 140 mg/day, and 70 mg twice per day [200]. There were no statistically significant differences in cytogenetic responses or PFS between the arms, but the 100 mg/day dosing resulted in lowest side effect profile. Among 167 CP CML patients, MCyR rates were 53% in IM resistant patients and 74% in IM intolerant patients. CCyR rates were 34% in IM resistant patients and 63% in IM intolerant patients. Disease progression was seen in 8–11% of patients across the 4 treatment arms.

With regard to adverse events (AEs), significantly fewer patients experienced pleural effusions on dasatinib at 100 vs. 70 mg twice per day (7% vs. 16%). With regard to hematologic AEs, there were no differences between the two groups except for grade 3 or 4 thrombocytopenia, which was seen in 22% of patients on 100 mg/day as compared to 37% of patients on 70 mg twice per day arm [200]. This study established the recommended dasatinib dose of 100 mg/day in CP CML patients.

Predictors of long-term cytogenetic response on dasatinib were recently reported [201]. Multivariate analysis revealed that younger age, lower percentage of Ph+ cells, prior MCyR on IM, IM intolerance rather than resistance as the cause for IM failure, and shorter time from diagnosis to dasatinib use correlated with achievement of MCyR and CCyR.

Nilotinib

Nilotinib has FDA approval to treat CP and AP CML patients, resistant or intolerant of IM at doses of 400 mg BID [128]. An initial report of 280 IM resistant and intolerant CP CML patients receiving nilotinib at 400 mg by mouth twice per day demonstrated MCyR in 48% at 6 months [202]. Median time to achievement of an MCyR was 2.8 months; estimated survival at 12 months was 95% [202]. In recent updates of this study at 24 months, CHR, MCyR, and CCyR were 94%, 59%, and 44%, respectively [203]. Among patients achieving CCyR, 56% achieved MMR. Notably, CCyR was durable in 84% of patients at 24 months. Estimated PFS and OS at 24 months were 64% and 87%, respectively. These data are similar to those reported for dasatinib and suggest that resistant and intolerant CP patients can achieve excellent and durable responses on second-line nilotinib. Variables that predict response and long-term outcomes on nilotinib have been identified: BCR-ABL molecular response at 3 months (BCR-ABL <10% IS) predicted MCyR and MMR at 24 months [204] [similar to IM response at 3 months on the IRIS trial [22]] irrespective of baseline mutation status. MCyR by 12 months, no high IC_{50} point mutations, hemoglobin >120 g/L, and baseline basophilia <4% predicted for superior PFS [205].

Choosing Between Dasatinib and Nilotinib

When selecting second-line TKI therapy, mutation profile is often the key determinant. Other factors to consider include treatment tolerance, medical history, and comorbid conditions, as well as patient choice. Mounting clinical evidence suggests that the presence of a mutation at the time second-line therapy is initiated is associated not only with recurrence of the same mutation but also with the development of new mutations on therapy [206]. In a study of 95 patients receiving second- or third-line therapy with dasatinib or nilotinib, 83% of patients relapsed due to newly acquired mutations [207].

Currently, in vitro data from mutation resistance screening of transformed cell lines and clinical data from phase 2 and 3 clinical trials can inform the choice between dasatinib and nilotinib. It should be noted that there are differences between what is predicted in vitro and what is observed in patients clinically. These differences may stem, in part, from the differing transforming ability of each of the different mutated kinases in vitro as compared to in vivo [208]. These differences have been addressed in a recent review on how to select optimal second-line TKI therapy [174]. The authors ranked mutations based on frequency and provide evidence to support resistance from several sources: class A = no clinical evidence to support resistance, B = in vitro data suggesting intermediate insensitivity/resistance with some clinical data (but insufficient clinical data to impact clinical decisions), C = compelling clinical evidence to recommend an alternative TKI, and D = no role in therapy (i.e., T315). This review provides one of the most comprehensive surveys of point mutations.

Clinical and in vitro data suggest that T315I, F317L/I/C/V, V299L, and T315A mutations confer resistance to dasatinib [196, 207, 209–212]. Except for the T315I mutation, these mutations are rare and are sensitive to nilotinib or imatinib. In contrast, certain p-loop mutations, in particular the E255K and Y253F/H and E255V [177, 184, 213], which are associated with intermediate or high dasatinib resistance in vitro, are not as clearly associated with clinical resistance.

Although data for dasatinib and nilotinib suggest that the presence of ABL TKD point mutations prior to second-line therapy adversely affected responses [206, 207], larger retrospective studies combining studies suggest this may not be the case. In a study of 1,043 patients receiving dasatinib as second-line therapy, no significant differences were detected; CCyR rates were 40% and 41%, respectively, in patients with no mutation vs. any mutation [212]. There was also no impact on PFS or OS at 24 months. PFS was 80% in patients without mutations vs. 70% in patients with a baseline mutation; OS was 92% and 88%, respectively. However, no patient with T315I- or F317L-mutated ABL achieved a CCyR. For the Y253H, E255K, and E255V mutations, (p-loop mutations), CCyR was achieved in 61% (14 patients), 38% [6], and 36% [4] of patients, respectively. For the Q252H, CCyR was observed in 1 patient (17%), and MCyR was observed in another. Another retrospective report of 670 patients receiving dasatinib after IM failure, reported that 53% of patients with baseline mutations retained those mutations, 19% of patients with no baseline mutations developed new mutations, and 47% of patients with baseline mutations developed new mutations [214]. In conclusion, these data suggest that T315I, F317L/I/C/V, V299L, and T315A mutations cause clinically relevant resistance to dasatinib. For the p-loop mutations, which are resistant to nilotinib, clinical efficacy is seen for the most part on dasatinib.

Similar to dasatinib-treated patients, recent reports suggest that outcomes stratified by mutation status (present vs. absent) are similar in patients receiving second-line nilotinib therapy, except for mutations with IC_{50} >150 nM [206]. Among 281 patients, 114 (41%) had point mutations, and the incidence of baseline point mutations was higher in IM resistant as compared to IM intolerant patients (55% vs. 10%) [206]. Thirty percent of patients with baseline mutations developed new mutations as compared to 11% without baseline mutations. Among patients with no baseline mutation, 60% achieved an MCyR, 40% achieved a CCyR, and 29% achieved an MMR at 12 months. The rates for patients with baseline mutations with

$IC_{50} \leq 150$ nM were not significantly different at 58%, 40%, and 29%, respectively. Among 26 patients with high IC_{50} point mutations (Y253H, E255K, E255V, F359C, F259V), treated with nilotinib only 5 (19%) achieved MCyR and none achieved CCyR. Among this group, 18 of 26 (69%) progressed during nilotinib treatment. Notably, clinical responses, including CCyR, were observed in patients with other p-loop mutations including L248V, G250E, and Q252H. In conclusion, Y253H, E255K/V, and F359V/C mutations appear to be clinically resistant to nilotinib, and dasatinib is a better choice [202, 206, 215]. Rare mutations such as the F317I/V/C and T315A, which are less sensitive or resistant to dasatinib, can be treated with nilotinib (or IM). The T315I mutation requires treatment with new agents on clinical trial as discussed later or allogeneic HSCT. Lastly, it should be noted that unlike response to second-line therapy, responses to third-line TKI therapy with either nilotinib or dasatinib (or bosutinib) are limited and short-lived. In a report of 48 patients, 34 were treated with dasatinib after IM/nilotinib, and 14 were treated with nilotinib after IM/dasatinib [216]. Among 25 CP patients, responses included 5 MMR, 3 CCyR, 2 PCyR, 3 minor CyR, 6 CHR, and 6 had no response. The median CCyR duration was 16 months with only 3 patients (all treated in CP) having a CCyR sustained for more than 12 months. Median failure-free survival was 20 months for these CP patients [216].

Treating Advanced CML

Unfortunately, as CML progresses to AP or BC response to TKI therapy, similar to all other therapies, becomes poorer. A likely explanation, as discussed above, is that other genetic events drive the disease. The median time from diagnosis of CP CML to progression to BC in untreated patients is ~3 to 5 years [217], but the range of timing is quite broad, encompassing a range of 0.5–15 years [218]. The vast majority of patients are diagnosed in CP, but ~15% of patients present in AP or BC. Some patients who present with AP CML respond to TKI therapy [219–222]. In BC disease, TKI therapy with or without chemotherapy can lead to second CP before allogeneic HSCT is pursued. The current convention is to treat de novo advanced phase CML with higher doses of IM starting at 600 mg daily [223]. However, most patients with AP or BC disease are patients whose disease has progressed on frontline IM therapy and often harbor resistance mutations [117].

Accelerated Phase

Phase 2 study results of 181 AP CML patients previously treated with IFN or other therapies demonstrated that IM at 400 or 600 mg resulted in sustained hematologic responses in 69% of patients with 34% achieving a CHR. MCyR was reported in 24% of patients and CCyR in 17%. Estimated PFS and OS at 12 months were 59%

and 74%, respectively [117]. These early data suggested that 600 mg was a more effective dose than 400 mg in AP CML. The GIMEMA Working Party study of 111 AP patients treated with IM at 600 mg/daily confirmed this observation. CHR occurred in 71% of patients and most patients, 96%, returned to CP [219]. MCyR and CCyR occurred in 30% and 21% of patients, respectively. The median time to CHR was 2 months and to CCyR was 6 months. Notably, among the patients who did achieve a CCyR, this response was durable in 65% (median observation time of 73 months) [219]. The estimated OS for patients who presented in AP was 37 months but was significantly improved in patients who obtained CCyR.

In the era of IM, many patients who develop AP disease do so in the setting of IM failure or intolerance. Consequently, we have more limited data on dasatinib or nilotinib as first-line therapy in patients with AP CML. Even though more potent TKIs may ultimately prove to be better in treating CP disease, because CML progression can be associated with Bcr-Abl independence, it less likely (and unlikely for BC disease) that second- and third-generation TKIs alone will be sufficient to treat advanced disease. Thus, these patients, whenever possible, should be treated on clinical trials or proceed to HSCT.

Dasatinib has received FDA approval for the treatment of AP CML intolerant or resistant to IM [194]. The START-A trial evaluated dasatinib 70 mg twice daily with potential dose escalation to 100 mg twice daily for inadequate responses in AP CML resistant (161 patients) or intolerant of IM (13 patients) [220]. Forty-five percent achieved a CHR, 39% MCyR, and 32% CCyR. The 12-month PFS was 66%, and the OS was 82%. Nonhematologic adverse events were mostly mild with diarrhea being the most common in 52% of patients; grade 3 or 4 diarrhea was observed in only 8%. Gastrointestinal bleeding was observed in 6%. Pleural effusions of any grade occurred in 27% of patients, but grade 3–4 pleural effusions occurred in only 5%. The median time to the development of grade 2–4 pleural effusions was 124 days (range, 15–500 days). Cytopenias were common and may predict for worse outcomes. Grade 3 or 4 neutropenia and thrombocytopenia was observed in 76% and 82% of patients, respectively. Cytopenias were frequent and managed with transient dose interruptions or reductions. Dose reductions and interruptions were required by 65% and 85% of patients, respectively. Dose escalation to greater than 140 mg a day occurred in 35% of the patients and 52% discontinued therapy with the most common reason being progressive disease [220]. The phase 3 CA180-035 study compared dasatinib at 140 mg once daily (158 patients) to dasatinib 70 mg twice daily (159 patients) in AP patients [221]. Overall, there was no statistically significant difference in response stratified by dose; however, once daily dosing demonstrated an improved safety profile. This observation has led to the recommended dosing for advanced disease at 140 mg once daily. For patients receiving 140 mg daily, the incidence of MCyR was 66%, CCyR was 39%, and estimated PFS and OS rates at 24 months were 51% and 63%, respectively [221].

Nilotinib has also received FDA approval for AP CML intolerant or resistant to imatinib [128]. In a single-arm open-label phase 2 study of 119 AP CML patients treated with nilotinib at 400 mg by mouth twice per day with a median duration of treatment of 202 days, hematologic responses occurred in 47% [222].

MCyR occurred in 29% and CCyR in 16% of patients. Median time to MCyR was 2 months, and the median duration of response was 15.4 months (range, 0.6–17.9 months). Estimated OS at 12 months was 79%. The most common reported nonhematologic side effects were rash (22%), pruritus (20%), constipation (11%), and headache, fatigue, and nausea (10% each). Grade 3 or 4 thrombocytopenia and neutropenia occurred in 35% and 21%, respectively. Nilotinib is associated with transaminitis, elevated bilirubin, lipase, and amylase. The first was seen rarely (~2% of patients), increased bilirubin was seen in 9%, lipase elevations in 18%, and amylase elevations in 2% of these patients [222].

Similar to CP CML, responses to third-line TKI therapy in advanced CML are limited and of short duration [216]. In a study of 48 CML patients in all phases, among 10 AP patients, 1 achieved MMR, 1 CCyR, 2 PCyR, 1 minor cytogenetic response, 4 CHR, and 1 had no response. Among 13 BC patients, 1 achieved an MMR, 2 CCyR, 1 PCyR, 1 minor CyR, 2 returned to CP, and 6 had no response. Median failure-free survivals were 5 and 3 months, respectively, for AP and BC CML patients [216].

These poorer responses to first-, second-, and third-line therapy merit consideration of allogeneic HSCT at the time of diagnosis for patients who present with AP disease. Reserving HSCT until patients demonstrate suboptimal responses or failure on first-line therapy may be reasonable given the upfront mortality risk associated with allogeneic transplantation. Waiting, however, requires close monitoring per established guidelines with a plan to proceed to allogeneic HSCT if optimal monitoring milestones are not met. It also necessitates prior identification of potential donors for patients who are transplant candidates so that transplant can proceed in a timely manner in the case of therapy failure. Proceeding to allogeneic transplantation is appropriate for all patients who are transplant candidates who fail TKI therapy with progression of disease.

Blast Crisis

Historically, BC CML is extremely difficult to treat and does not respond well to either acute myeloid leukemia (AML) induction regimens for myeloid BC (MBC) or acute lymphoblastic leukemia (ALL) regimens for lymphoid BC (LBC) [224]. TKIs are active in BC CML; however, responses are typically of short duration [52, 119, 225, 226]. Thus, the goal of therapy for BC CML patients is to return disease to second CP or better and proceed to allogeneic HSCT for patients who are candidates for this procedure. For myeloid BC CML, aggressive regimens as initial strategy may not be warranted, and the choice to treat patients more aggressively with TKI plus induction chemotherapy will depend upon age, performance status, and subsequent plan for therapy (i.e., plans to proceed to HSCT). The duration of response to single-agent TKI is shorter in LBC as compared to MBC. Median OS is 11.8 months in MBC as compared to 5.3 months in LBC [227, 228]. Thus, TKI therapy alone for LBC is typically not sufficient.

Phase 2 study results of 229 BC patients treated at 400–600 mg orally daily of IM demonstrated that 52% of patients achieved sustained hematologic responses and 8% achieved CHR [119]. MCyR was achieved in 16%, and CCyR was achieved in 7% of patients. The median survival time was 6.9 months with estimated survival rates of 43% at 9 months, 32% at 12 months, and 20% at 18 months [119]. Other studies have confirmed these observations: a large single institution study (which combined 3 studies) reported on 75 patients and a GIMEMA Working Party phase 2 study reported on 92 patients [116, 229]. In the first study, overall CHR for BC CML was ~20%; it was 23% for myeloid BC and 10% for lymphoid BC. Cytogenetic responses were seen in approximately 10% of patients, and 1-year survival was ~25% [116]. As compared to historical control patients who received cytarabine, IM was less toxic and yielded better responses. Dose also appeared to be important as BC patients treated with IM at 600 vs. 400 mg had higher cytogenetic response rates, 18% vs. 6%, respectively [224]. The second study reported on longer-term outcomes, as long as 6-year follow-up for some patients [229]. Survival rates for the 72 myeloid and 20 lymphoid BC patients were 53% at 6 months, 29% at 12 months, 23% at 18 months, and 11% at 36 months. Two baseline characteristics prior to therapy correlated with improved outcomes: performance status <2 and blast count <50%. Additionally, although only 10 patients achieved this milestone, median survival was longer in patients who achieved MCyR as compared to those who did not, 20.5 months vs. 6 months, respectively [230].

Dasatinib at 140 mg daily is approved for the treatment of BC CML that is resistant or intolerant of IM. The START-B and START-L phase 2 open-label trials examined 157 BC CML patients: 109 myeloid (START-B) and 48 lymphoid BC (START-L) BC CML patients [226]. A major hematologic response was obtained in 34% MBC and 35% LBC patients, and an MCyR was observed in 33% and 52% of MBC and LBC patients, respectively. The higher response to dasatinib in LBC patients is thought to be due to targeting of SRC kinases by this drug. However, despite the fact that patients do achieve MCyRs, these responses are short-lived. OS is poor with a median PFS of only 6.7 and 3 months for MBC and LBC, respectively [226]. Nilotinib is not approved for the treatment of BC CML, but in the rare case of dasatinib resistance-associated point mutations that are sensitive to nilotinib, approval for this drug can be requested.

Given the poor outcomes in BC CML, attempts to treat BC patients with a more aggressive initial strategy are most appropriate in the setting of clinical trials. Outside of the clinical trials, the choice of which induction regimen to use in combination with TKI may be considered based on historical data [227, 228, 230, 231]. Because the duration of response to TKI therapy is so short for LBC patients (~3–4 months), these patients are more commonly treated with TKI plus ALL regimens (e.g., HyperCVAD) [227]. For MBC, either TKI alone or TKI plus AML induction chemotherapy may be considered [227, 228]. TKI therapy alone may be successful in the rare patient who presents with de novo MBC CML. If HSCT is not feasible, the addition of chemotherapy is more likely to result in side effects rather than benefit. However, for patients with good PS and who are transplant candidates, the addition of induction therapy to second-line TKI, although more toxic, may result in more rapid responses. It is because the duration of response in BC is so short that it remains critical, whenever possible, to anticipate the transition to more advanced disease through close monitoring and to proceed to HSCT as quickly as possible in patients who are candidates for this therapy.

The Role of Allogeneic Transplantation

CML was one of the first major success stories in transplantation [232] and was the leading indication for an allogeneic HSCT worldwide at the end of the last millennium [233]. HSCT is associated with a greater than 85% survival at select centers if performed in CP, but only 40% in AP and <20% in BC [234–236]. With the introduction of TKIs, the trend of increasing CML transplants has now been reversed. It is now the fourth and seventh most common indication for HSCT worldwide and in North America, respectively [237]. The factors that influence outcomes for CML transplants are reviewed in detail in several excellent reviews dedicated to the topic of HSCT in CML [238, 239]. These reviews discuss the impact of conditioning, donor source, graft source, and the indications for the use of TKIs during and after HSCT. This section will briefly review HSCT, indications to proceed to HSCT, and the use of TKIs after HSCT.

Indications for HSCT include presentation in AP or BC, failure or intolerance of second-line TKI therapy, and T315I mutations. With third-generation TKIs that appear to target T315I-mutated CML being tested on clinical trials, the last indication may change [240]. Secondary to the high lifetime cost of IM and appropriate monitoring, HSCT in developing countries may be pursued earlier in young patients with available donors. Although some patients in AP may have durable responses to first-line TKI therapy, it is a minority [219]. Thus, patients in AP and those who present in BC are candidates for HSCT at diagnosis, as are all patients with evidence of disease progression at the time of resistance [116]. Similar to IM [241, 242], preliminary data for dasatinib and nilotinib demonstrate no increase in transplant-related toxicity to date due to treatment with TKIs prior to HSCT [243]. In fact, certain studies suggest that patients responding to IM, in particular CP patients, may have improved survival after transplantation [242, 244] and decreased incidence of chronic graft-versus-host disease [241, 245]. Thus, for patients diagnosed in AP or BC, initial treatment with IM is recommended as long as the treating physician and patient understand that responses are generally short. These patients should be evaluated for HSCT at diagnosis and proceed to HSCT when suitable donors are available.

It is estimated that 15–30% of CP patients who start IM therapy develop resistance or intolerance [23, 121]; among these patients, ~50% will respond to second-line therapy [200, 202]. Thus, CP patients and siblings should be typed when resistance is detected. HSCT is often pursued at the time of suboptimal response or failure of second-line therapy. Despite the hypothetical concern that a delay in HSCT would adversely affect outcomes, most studies suggest that treatment with

TKI in CP patients prior to HSCT does not result in worse outcomes [164, 241, 242]. However, it is crucial to monitor patients closely for optimal response on second-line therapy as half will fail and because HSCT outcomes are worse for more advanced disease. Thus, intervention before progression is crucial. For patients with T315I mutations, HSCT or treatment on clinical trial with agents that treat T315I-mutated CML is appropriate as second-line therapy.

The most influential factors predicting outcomes in allogeneic HSCT patients are disease phase, transplant donor type, donor/recipient sex combination, age, and interval from diagnosis to transplantation. These variables comprise the EBMT score [246, 247]. HSCT conditioning can be myeloablative or nonmyeloablative, also known as reduced intensity conditioning (RIC), with bone marrow (BM) or peripheral blood stem cells (PBSC) as the graft source [238, 239]. At most large transplant centers, HSCT is done on a variety of protocols, but historically, conditioning has utilized chemotherapy agents such as cyclophosphamide or busulfan or cyclophosphamide in combination with total body irradiation (TBI) for myeloablative transplants [234, 236, 248]. Given that many patients with CML are over age 60, myeloablative transplantation is often not feasible. RIC is associated with a decrease in transplant-related mortality (TRM), but an increased rate of relapse [249–251]. PBSC recipients typically engraft more rapidly, and have increased graft-versus-leukemia (GvL), but also greater graft-versus-host disease (GvHD) [233, 252–254]. Consequently, PBSC may be a better choice for patients conditioned with RIC regimens. Recently, cord blood has become an increasingly useful approach for patients without available donors. Limiting issues at this time include high nonrelapse mortality [255].

TKIs play an important role as prevention and treatment of relapse after transplantation. Most patients after HSCT, as compared to patients treated with TKI alone, are negative at the molecular level for *bcr-abl* [93, 94]. The risk of relapse at 5 years is 15% for those transplanted in CP, 30% for those in AP, and >60% for those transplanted in BC [233]. TKI therapy after HSCT is often considered for patients at high risk of relapse, such as patients transplanted with AP or BC disease or patients undergoing RIC transplantation. It may be an option to decrease or delay the need for immunologic maneuvers in these patients [256]. For patients treated with IM after HSCT, almost all patients could start IM on schedule (~ day 35) and remain on IM. Approximately 15% of patients needed temporary dose reduction or cessation due to intolerance, which was primarily GI toxicity rather than hematologic toxicity [256]. TKI use decreases relapse risk in higher risk patients and can result in durable cytogenetic and molecular remissions [256–258]. Because data remain limited from controlled series, the use of IM or other TKIs after HSCT is best done in the setting of a clinical trial.

Donor lymphocyte infusions (DLI) are another strategy to treat molecular, cytogenetic, and hematologic relapse and are a mainstay of treatment for patients who relapse after HSCT, either alone or in combination with TKI [259, 260]. In a study of 37 patients with CML who relapsed after HSCT from 1994 to 2004, treatment was initiated with DLI and/or IM [260]. The majority of 11 patients (91%) receiving DLI and IM achieved a molecular remission within 3 months, which was substantially faster than those who received only TKI or DLI therapy. Notably, patients who received DLI+IM (7 patients) remained in a molecular remission, whereas IM only treated patients (4 patients) relapsed, necessitating reinstitution of IM. Lastly, DLI plus TKI therapy has been shown to have superior OS and DFS when compared DLI [260]. These retrospective data suggest that when IM is used alone to treat relapse, it needs to be continued indefinitely, which may not be the case if it used in combination with DLI.

Managing Side Effects and Long-Term Complications

Given the excellent responses to TKI therapy and the availability of clinical trial outcomes data, guidelines to monitor CML patients have been published by NCCN and ELN. However, the ability to take one or two pills daily lifelong is not an easy task. Erratic use of treatment increases the risk for mutations and the development of resistant disease. Side effect and toxicity management of TKI therapy is thus of paramount importance at both initiation of therapy and throughout therapy. Appropriate and aggressive management of side effects in combination with dose reductions or short-term cessation can help limit the development of resistance. An excellent review of this topic for patients treated with IM, dasatinib, and nilotinib was recently published [133]. Toxicities are generally determined by the phase of disease and the dose and/or schedule of administration. Common Terminology Criteria for Adverse Events (CTCAE) (version 3.0 or 4.0), which are used on clinical trials to grade side effects, provide a useful tool to categorize side effects by organ system. Table 4.3 summarizes the frequency of adverse events (AEs) on first-line trials for IM, nilotinib, and dasatinib.

Hematologic Toxicities

The most clinically significant toxicities are hematologic. Regardless of the degree of neutropenia associated with initial TKI therapy, neutropenic fever and other infectious complications are much less common with TKI therapy as compared to chemotherapy. This difference is believed to be secondary to the lack of common chemotherapy side effects such as mucositis that break down the barrier to infection [134]. IM at 400 mg/day initiated for CP CML yields grade 3 or 4 neutropenia in only 14% of patients in the first year of treatment. However, grade 3 or 4 neutropenia is seen in 58% and 64% of patients in the first year when treatment is initiated in AP and BC, respectively [24, 133, 261]. The percentage of patients, in subsequent years, who continue to have high grade cytopenias declines with time in all phases. A phase II study evaluating IM in AP demonstrated the hematologic toxicities were similar in both the 400 and 600 mg dose groups indicating the higher grade toxicities are more likely secondary to the phase of disease than dose [117].

Management of hematologic toxicities is delineated in the FDA labeling and various guidelines such as the NCCN Practice Guidelines [1, 7]. In brief, for an ANC <1,000 or platelet count <50,000, hold drug until ANC >1,500 or platelet count >75,000 and resume at starting dose of 400 mg. If recurrence of ANC <1,000 or platelet count <50,000, again hold and resume at a reduced dose of 300 mg. These guidelines are not absolute recommendations [1, 7]. For example, cytopenias are almost universal in BC patients, but the drug should not necessarily be held. Under certain circumstances, although response may appear to be limited, the removal of TKI may result in a rapid increase in blast counts. Thus, patients should be monitored closely when drug is held in this particular circumstance. The ultimate goal of therapy is continuous therapy. Thus, continuing treatment with close monitoring, even if values fall below what is stated in the recommendations, may be reasonable as cytopenias will typically resolve as the burden of CML disease falls. It is also important to resume full-dose therapy, whenever possible, as full dose may be tolerated despite the initial need for dose reduction and is much more likely to result in optimal therapeutic outcomes.

Dasatinib and nilotinib are associated with a greater incidence of myelosuppression which may be secondary to inherent medication differences, but are more likely related to the patient population in which these medications were initially studied [127, 202, 222]. Many patients treated with dasatinib and nilotinib are IM failures and, similar to patients with AP and BC disease, have greater frequency of cytopenias. Dose optimization studies for dasatinib suggest 100 mg daily for CP disease and 140 mg daily for advanced or resistant disease are yielded similar efficacy with fewer side effects [131, 200, 220, 226]. For nilotinib first-line therapy with 300 mg twice per day is sufficient, whereas 400 mg twice per day is recommended for advanced or resistant disease [130, 202, 222].

Nonhematologic Toxicities

Nonhematologic toxicity is common, although most side effects are mild, i.e., grade 1 or 2 (Table 4.3) [24, 127, 202, 262–264]. Nausea is common, most often not severe, and can frequently be managed by taking the medication with a meal or large class of water for IM and dasatinib. For appropriate absorption, nilotinib must be taken on an empty stomach, i.e., fasting for 1 h prior or 2 h after a meal [263].

Fluid retention or edema is a common and usually a mild toxicity of IM [24]. It resembles congestive heart failure but is not caused by a decrease in cardiac function. That said, it can be managed in similar fashion with diuretics as needed. Periorbital edema may be better treated with topical steroids rather than diuretics [133, 265]. Similar to hematologic toxicities, nonhematologic toxicities are more common in patients with advanced CML. Dasatinib-induced fluid-related events such as pericardial effusions, pulmonary edema, cardiac dysfunction, and pulmonary hypertension are seen infrequently and at 100 mg daily dosing almost not at all [127, 200, 220]. Pleural effusions remain a clinically significant finding, but have

Table 4.3 Summary of common toxicities on tyrosine kinase inhibitor therapy

	Imatinib [23]		Dasatinib [131]		Nilotinib [130]	
	400 mg QD ($n=551$)		100 mg QD ($n=258$)		300 mg bid ($n=279$)	
Grade	All (%)	3/4 (%)	All (%)	3/4 (%)	All (%)	3/4 (%)
Nonhematologic						
Rash	34	2	11	0	31	<1
Headache	31	<1	12	0	14	1
Nausea	44	<1	8	0	11	<1
Alopecia	4	0			8	0
Pruritus	7	<1			15	<1
Myalgia	21	1.5	6	0	10	<1
Fatigue	35	1	8	<1	11	0
Vomiting	17	1.5	5	0	5	0
Diarrhea	33	2	17	<1	8	1
Musculoskeletal pain	37	3	11	0		
Muscle spasm	38	1			7	0
Peripheral edema	55	1	14	1	5	0
Eyelid edema					1	0
Periorbital edema					<1	0
Pleural effusion			10	0		
Hematologic						
Neutropenia	61	14	65	21	43	12
Thrombocytopenia	57	8	70	19	48	10
Anemia	45	3	90	10	38	3
Labs						
Increased total bilirubin					53	4
Increased alkaline phosphatase					21	0
Decreased phosphate					32	5
Increased glucose					36	6
Increased lipase					24	6
Increased amylase					15	<1
Increased creatinine					5	0
Increased ALT					66	4
Increased AST					40	1
Increased AST or ALT	43	5				

Adapted from the IRIS, DASISION, and ENESTnd trials [23, 130, 131]

been reduced to less than 10% at the current recommended 100 mg daily dosing [200, 266]. Diuretic therapy and other supportive care measures are appropriate initial management options for fluid retention [267]. Dose interruption may be needed based on grade, and a short course of steroids, for example, prednisone 20 mg/day for 3 days, is sometimes helpful. In the setting of significant pleural effusion, a lower dose such as 80 mg daily may be possible in lieu of switching to another TKI.

Cutaneous reactions are typically mild to moderate and a frequent complication of IM, dasatinib, and nilotinib therapy [24, 127, 202]. Appropriate initial therapies include observation, antihistamines, and various topical agents [133, 268]. Salves, coal tar preparations, and topical steroids are also useful in the management of skin toxicity. A brief course of systemic steroids is often effective for more diffuse involvement [133, 268].

Laboratory abnormalities that require monitoring include transaminitis and hyperbilirubinemia. Grade 2 or greater abnormalities in liver function tests are an indication for dose interruption and when resolved resumption at a lower dose is indicated [262–264]. Escalation of dose should be considered if the lower dose is well tolerated without a recurrence of abnormalities. Nilotinib is more frequently associated with elevated serum lipase, amylase, bilirubin, and/or transaminases, in addition to glucose [130, 202]. Grade 3 or 4 elevations require interruption of nilotinib, imaging studies as indicated, and resumption when grade 1 or less at once daily dosing. In the absence of recurrent symptoms, dose escalation may be attempted. However, if grade 3 or 4 symptoms recur, alternative TKI therapy may be indicated.

ECG monitoring is also required prior to initiation and 7 days after initiation of therapy, and periodically thereafter, with nilotinib secondary to the risk for QT prolongation [133, 269]. This is particularly important in the setting of other medications associated with QT prolongation. Although recent studies of nilotinib as first-line therapy suggest QT prolongation is rare [130], the more extensive use of this drug outside of the carefully selected and monitored patients on clinical trial merits careful follow-up until we have more experience with this issue. Monitoring during therapy should be pursued when doses are held or changed. Additionally, electrolytes should be monitored, and potassium and magnesium levels should be maintained within normal limits.

Recent studies suggest that there is minimal cross-intolerance between IM and these newer agents [270]. Supportive care is important to maintain quality of life and to ensure patients continue the medication.

The Future: New Directions in Therapy

IM is a highly effective therapy, but ~20% of patients will develop resistance to therapy over time. Dasatinib and nilotinib are effective first- and second-line therapies. Bosutinib (SKI-606) is a second-generation TKI. In phase 1/2 trials, bosutinib was well tolerated and demonstrated promising results in IM intolerant and resistant patients. An open-label phase 3 trial of bosutinib vs. IM as first-line therapy is underway and should be reported shortly [271, 272]. However, no first- or second-generation TKIs treat T315I-mutated CML (~10–15% of mutations) or effectively target LSCs, and the observation that patients who fail two TKIs do not maintain durable responses on third-line TKIs suggest alternative strategies are needed when allogeneic transplantation is not feasible [81, 82, 174, 216].

There are several approaches to treating resistant CML. One approach is to build a TKI that is not resistant to point-mutated CML. New third-generation TKIs are under investigation, which target T315I-mutated ABL. A second approach is "non-kinase" therapy such as omacetaxine, arsenic, and histone deacetylase inhibitors (HDACi) that have activity in a variety of leukemias including CML [85, 272, 274]. A third approach is to target other pathways, in addition to ABL, that may be important in the CML disease phenotype (e.g., aurora kinase inhibitors) [275], or to target pathways that are important in malignant stem cells (e.g., WNT, Notch, or Hedgehog signaling) [66, 83, 84]. The approach of targeting LSCs is difficult because normal and malignant stem cells share common signaling pathways. However, recent reports suggest that certain histone HDAC inhibitors and Hedgehog pathway inhibitors, in combination with TKIs, may eliminate malignant CML stem and progenitor cells, but not normal hematopoietic stem cells [83–85, 276]. Phase 1 clinical trials are underway.

Drugs under investigation that may treat T315I-mutated ABL include DCC-2036, a "switch pocket" inhibitor that stabilizes the ABL kinase in an active form and effectively treated T315I-mutated CML in a murine model [277]. Aurora kinase A, B, and C are serine/threonine kinases that are involved in chromosomal segregation, spindle formation, and progression through mitosis [278]. Drugs targeting aurora kinases are in phase 1 and 2 clinical trials for a number of solid as well as hematologic malignancies. Some of these compounds have significant toxicities, and a recent trial of the pan aurora kinase inhibitor MK-0457 was halted due to cardiac toxicity [272]. On the research front another class of TKI inhibitor that appears promising is the non-ATP-competitive inhibitors that regulate kinase activity allosterically [279]. All other ABL-targeted TKIs discussed so far are ATP-competitive inhibitors. Theoretically, these allosteric inhibitors should treat all mutated CML.

Homoharringtonine (HHT), a natural alkaloid, is a therapy that predates the era of IM. It showed activity in the treatment of CML refractory to IFN or in combination with IFN as frontline therapy [280, 281]. Because it does not target ABL, interest in this compound (now also available as the semisynthetic compound omacetaxine mepesuccinate) in the treatment of T315I-mutated CML or multiple TKI resistant CML has resurfaced [273]. Ongoing trials of omacetaxine in CML have demonstrated hematologic and cytogenetic responses in patients with T315I mutations [273].

Ponatinib (AP24535, ARIAD Pharmaceuticals) is a potent inhibitor of ABL and, in particular, T315I-mutated ABL. It also inhibits VEGFR, FGFR, and PDGFR. In vitro and murine studies of ponatinib demonstrated significant inhibition of all dasatinib and nilotinib resistance associated mutations and suggest that ponatinib may inhibit all clinically relevant mutations [282]. A phase I study to determine the maximum tolerated and recommended dose of oral ponatinib in patients with refractory or advanced CML and other refractory hematologic malignancies was completed and reported in abstract form in 2010 [240, 283]. Most patients were resistant to at least three prior TKIs (65%), and almost all (95%) had been treated with at least two. Among 38 evaluable CP CML patients, CHR was achieved in 95% and 100% with the T315I mutation. MCyR was achieved in 66% of all patients and 100% of patients with T315I mutations, and a CCyR was achieved in 53% and 89%, respectively. For 17 evaluable patients in advanced phases, a major hematologic response was seen in 35% of patients, MCyR in 24%, and CCyR in 12% [284]. Given the general safety and efficacy profile, a phase 2 study (PACE) was initiated in September of 2010.

Conclusion

In conclusion, excellent therapeutic options exist for the treatment of CML. Most CP patients will achieve durable cytogenetic and molecular responses on first-line TKI therapy. Compliance with therapy and careful monitoring are essential for successful outcome.

References

1. O'Brien S, Berman E, Borghaei H, et al. NCCN clinical practice guidelines in oncology: chronic myelogenous leukemia. J Natl Compr Canc Netw. 2009;7(9):984–1023.
2. Altekruse SF, Kosary CL, Krapcho M, et al. SEER Cancer Statistics Review, 1975–2007. National Cancer Institute. 2010. Accessed 07/20/2010. http://seer.cancer.gov/csr/1975_2008/.
3. Jabbour E, Cortes J, Kantarjian H. Optimal first-line treatment of chronic myeloid leukemia. How to use imatinib and what role for newer drugs. Oncology (Williston Park). 2007;21(6):653–62; discussion 663–4, 667–8.
4. Baccarani M, Cortes J, Pane F, et al. Chronic myeloid leukemia: an update of concepts and management recommendations of European LeukemiaNet. J Clin Oncol. 2009;27(35):6041–51. doi:10.1200/JCO.2009.25.0779.
5. Baccarani M, Castagnetti F, Gugliotta G, Palandri F, Soverini S. Response definitions and European Leukemianet Management recommendations. Best Pract Res Clin Haematol. 2009;22(3):331–41. doi:10.1016/j.beha.2009.10.001.
6. Baccarani M, Saglio G, Goldman J, et al. Evolving concepts in the management of chronic myeloid leukemia: recommendations from an expert panel on behalf of the European LeukemiaNet. Blood. 2006;108(6):1809–20. doi:10.1182/blood-2006-02-005686.
7. O'Brien S, Berman E, Moore JO, et al. NCCN Task Force report: tyrosine kinase inhibitor therapy selection in the management of patients with chronic myelogenous leukemia. J Natl Compr Canc Netw. 2011;9 Suppl 2:S1–25.
8. Fialkow PJ, Gartler SM, Yoshida A. Clonal origin of chronic myelocytic leukemia in man. Proc Natl Acad Sci USA. 1967;58(4):1468–71.
9. Knudson AG. Two genetic hits (more or less) to cancer. Nat Rev Cancer. 2001;1(2):157–62. doi:10.1038/35101031.
10. Deininger MW, Goldman JM, Melo JV. The molecular biology of chronic myeloid leukemia. Blood. 2000;96(10):3343–56.
11. Melo JV, Barnes DJ. Chronic myeloid leukaemia as a model of disease evolution in human cancer. Nat Rev Cancer. 2007;7(6):441–53. doi:10.1038/nrc2147.
12. Quintas-Cardama A, Cortes J. Molecular biology of bcr-abl1-positive chronic myeloid leukemia. Blood. 2009;113(8):1619–30. doi:10.1182/blood-2008-03-144790.
13. Verma D, Kantarjian HM, Jones D, et al. Chronic myeloid leukemia (CML) with P190 BCR-ABL: analysis of characteristics, outcomes, and prognostic significance. Blood. 2009;114(11): 2232–5. doi:10.1182/blood-2009-02-204693.

14. Sokal JE, Baccarani M, Russo D, Tura S. Staging and prognosis in chronic myelogenous leukemia. Semin Hematol. 1988;25(1):49–61.
15. Savage DG, Szydlo RM, Chase A, Apperley JF, Goldman JM. Bone marrow transplantation for chronic myeloid leukaemia: the effects of differing criteria for defining chronic phase on probabilities of survival and relapse. Br J Haematol. 1997;99(1):30–5.
16. Kantarjian HM, Deisseroth A, Kurzrock R, Estrov Z, Talpaz M. Chronic myelogenous leukemia: a concise update. Blood. 1993;82(3):691–703.
17. Swerdlow SH, Campo E, Harris NL, et al. WHO classification of tumours of haematopoietic and lymphoid tissues. 4th ed., Vol 2. Lyon: IARC Press; 2008.
18. Johansson B, Fioretos T, Mitelman F. Cytogenetic and molecular genetic evolution of chronic myeloid leukemia. Acta Haematol. 2002;107(2):76–94.
19. Sokal JE, Cox EB, Baccarani M, et al. Prognostic discrimination in "good-risk" chronic granulocytic leukemia. Blood. 1984;63(4):789–99.
20. Hasford J, Ansari H, Pfirrmann M, Hehlmann R. Analysis and validation of prognostic factors for CML. German CML Study Group. Bone Marrow Transplant. 1996;17 Suppl 3:S49–54.
21. Hasford J, Pfirrmann M, Shepherd P, et al. The impact of the combination of baseline risk group and cytogenetic response on the survival of patients with chronic myeloid leukemia treated with interferon alpha. Haematologica. 2005;90(3):335–40.
22. Hughes TP, Kaeda J, Branford S, et al. Frequency of major molecular responses to imatinib or interferon alfa plus cytarabine in newly diagnosed chronic myeloid leukemia. N Engl J Med. 2003;349(15):1423–32. doi:10.1056/NEJMoa030513.
23. O'Brien SG, Guilhot F, Larson RA, et al. Imatinib compared with interferon and low-dose cytarabine for newly diagnosed chronic-phase chronic myeloid leukemia. N Engl J Med. 2003;348(11):994–1004. doi:10.1056/NEJMoa022457.
24. Druker BJ, Guilhot F, O'Brien SG, et al. Five-year follow-up of patients receiving imatinib for chronic myeloid leukemia. N Engl J Med. 2006;355(23):2408–17. doi:10.1056/NEJMoa062867.
25. Hasford J, Baccarani M, Hoffmann V, et al. Predicting complete cytogenetic response and subsequent progression-free survival in 2060 patients with CML on imatinib treatment: the EUTOS score. Blood. 2011;118(3):686–92. doi:10.1182/blood-2010-12-319038. www.refworks.com.
26. Sandberg AA. Chromosomes and causation of human cancer and leukemia: XL. The Ph1 and other translocations in CML. Cancer. 1980;46(10):2221–6.
27. Heim S, Billstrom R, Kristoffersson U, Mandahl N, Strombeck B, Mitelman F. Variant Ph translocations in chronic myeloid leukemia. Cancer Genet Cytogenet. 1985;18(3):215–27.
28. Fisher AM, Strike P, Scott C, Moorman AV. Breakpoints of variant 9;22 translocations in chronic myeloid leukemia locate preferentially in the CG-richest regions of the genome. Genes Chromosomes Cancer. 2005;43(4):383–9. doi:10.1002/gcc.20196.
29. Huntly BJ, Bench A, Green AR. Double jeopardy from a single translocation: deletions of the derivative chromosome 9 in chronic myeloid leukemia. Blood. 2003;102(4):1160–8. doi:10.1182/blood-2003-01-0123.
30. Kim DH, Popradi G, Sriharsha L, et al. No significance of derivative chromosome 9 deletion on the clearance kinetics of BCR/ABL fusion transcripts, cytogenetic or molecular response, loss of response, or treatment failure to imatinib mesylate therapy for chronic myeloid leukemia. Cancer. 2008;113(4):772–81. doi:10.1002/cncr.23607.
31. Quintas-Cardama A, Kantarjian H, Talpaz M, et al. Imatinib mesylate therapy may overcome the poor prognostic significance of deletions of derivative chromosome 9 in patients with chronic myelogenous leukemia. Blood. 2005;105(6):2281–6. doi:10.1182/blood-2004-06-2208.
32. Quintás-Cardama A, Kantarjian H, Shan J, et al. Prognostic impact of deletions of derivative chromosome 9 in patients with chronic myelogenous leukemia treated with nilotinib or dasatinib. Cancer. 2011;117(22):5085–93. doi:10.1002/cncr.26147.
33. Kirstetter P, Schuster MB, Bereshchenko O, et al. Modeling of C/EBPalpha mutant acute myeloid leukemia reveals a common expression signature of committed myeloid leukemia-initiating cells. Cancer Cell. 2008;13(4):299–310. doi:10.1016/j.ccr.2008.02.008.
34. Marcucci G, Radmacher MD, Maharry K, et al. MicroRNA expression in cytogenetically normal acute myeloid leukemia. N Engl J Med. 2008;358(18):1919–28. doi:10.1056/NEJMoa074256.

35. Figueroa ME, Lugthart S, Li Y, et al. DNA methylation signatures identify biologically distinct subtypes in acute myeloid leukemia. Cancer Cell. 2010;17(1):13–27. doi:10.1016/j.ccr.2009.11.020.

36. Delhommeau F, Dupont S, DellaValle V, et al. Mutation in TET2 in myeloid cancers. N Engl J Med. 2009;360(22):2289–301. doi:10.1056/NEJMoa0810069.

37. Abdel-Wahab O, Mullally A, Hedvat C, et al. Genetic characterization of TET1, TET2, and TET3 alterations in myeloid malignancies. Blood. 2009;114(1):144–7. doi:10.1182/blood-2009-03-210039.

38. Tiu RV, Gondek LP, O'Keefe CL, et al. Prognostic impact of SNP array karyotyping in myelodysplastic syndromes and related myeloid malignancies. Blood. 2011;117(17):4552–60. doi:10.1182/blood-2010-07-295857.

39. Mardis ER, Ding L, Dooling DJ, et al. Recurring mutations found by sequencing an acute myeloid leukemia genome. N Engl J Med. 2009;361(11):1058–66. doi:10.1056/NEJMoa0903840.

40. Ley TJ, Ding L, Walter MJ, et al. DNMT3A mutations in acute myeloid leukemia. N Engl J Med. 2010;363(25):2424–33. doi:10.1056/NEJMoa1005143.

41. Kim DH, Lee ST, Won HH, et al. A genome-wide association study identifies novel loci associated with susceptibility to chronic myeloid leukemia. Blood. 2011;117(25):6906–11. doi:10.1182/blood-2011-01-329797.

42. Bruns I, Czibere A, Fischer JC, et al. The hematopoietic stem cell in chronic phase CML is characterized by a transcriptional profile resembling normal myeloid progenitor cells and reflecting loss of quiescence. Leukemia. 2009;23(5):892–9. doi:10.1038/leu.2008.392.

43. Graham SM, Vass JK, Holyoake TL, Graham GJ. Transcriptional analysis of quiescent and proliferating CD34+ human hemopoietic cells from normal and chronic myeloid leukemia sources. Stem Cells. 2007;25(12):3111–20. doi:10.1634/stemcells.2007-0250.

44. Zheng C, Li L, Haak M, et al. Gene expression profiling of CD34+ cells identifies a molecular signature of chronic myeloid leukemia blast crisis. Leukemia. 2006;20(6):1028–34. doi:10.1038/sj.leu.2404227.

45. Yong AS, Szydlo RM, Goldman JM, Apperley JF, Melo JV. Molecular profiling of CD34+ cells identifies low expression of CD7, along with high expression of proteinase 3 or elastase, as predictors of longer survival in patients with CML. Blood. 2006;107(1):205–12. doi:10.1182/blood-2005-05-2155.

46. Radich JP, Dai H, Mao M, et al. Gene expression changes associated with progression and response in chronic myeloid leukemia. Proc Natl Acad Sci USA. 2006;103(8):2794–9. doi:10.1073/pnas.0510423103.

47. Oehler VG, Guthrie KA, Cummings CL, et al. The preferentially expressed antigen in melanoma (PRAME) inhibits myeloid differentiation in normal hematopoietic and leukemic progenitor cells. Blood. 2009;114(15):3299–308. doi:10.1182/blood-2008-07-170282.

48. McWeeney SK, Pemberton LC, Loriaux MM, et al. A gene expression signature of CD34+ cells to predict major cytogenetic response in chronic-phase chronic myeloid leukemia patients treated with imatinib. Blood. 2010;115(2):315–25. doi:10.1182/blood-2009-03-210732.

49. Goldman JM, Melo JV. BCR-ABL in chronic myelogenous leukemia – how does it work? Acta Haematol. 2008;119(4):212–7. doi:10.1159/000140633.

50. Van Etten RA. Mechanisms of transformation by the BCR-ABL oncogene: new perspectives in the post-imatinib era. Leuk Res. 2004;28 Suppl 1:S21–8. doi:10.1016/j.leukres.2003.10.005.

51. Ren R. Mechanisms of BCR-ABL in the pathogenesis of chronic myelogenous leukaemia. Nat Rev Cancer. 2005;5(3):172–83. doi:10.1038/nrc1567.

52. Cortes J, Rousselot P, Kim DW, et al. Dasatinib induces complete hematologic and cytogenetic responses in patients with imatinib-resistant or -intolerant chronic myeloid leukemia in blast crisis. Blood. 2007;109(8):3207–13. doi:10.1182/blood-2006-09-046888.

53. Fleming A, Noda T, Yoshimori T, Rubinsztein DC. Chemical modulators of autophagy as biological probes and potential therapeutics. Nat Chem Biol. 2011;7(1):9–17. doi:10.1038/nchembio.500.

54. Gordon MY, Dowding CR, Riley GP, Goldman JM, Greaves MF. Altered adhesive interactions with marrow stroma of haematopoietic progenitor cells in chronic myeloid leukaemia. Nature. 1987;328(6128):342–4. doi:10.1038/328342a0.

55. Verfaillie CM, McCarthy JB, McGlave PB. Mechanisms underlying abnormal trafficking of malignant progenitors in chronic myelogenous leukemia. Decreased adhesion to stroma and fibronectin but increased adhesion to the basement membrane components laminin and collagen type IV. J Clin Invest. 1992;90(4):1232–41. doi:10.1172/JCI115985.

56. Salgia R, Li JL, Ewaniuk DS, et al. BCR/ABL induces multiple abnormalities of cytoskeletal function. J Clin Invest. 1997;100(1):46–57. doi:10.1172/JCI119520.

57. Salgia R, Quackenbush E, Lin J, et al. The BCR/ABL oncogene alters the chemotactic response to stromal-derived factor-1alpha. Blood. 1999;94(12):4233–46.

58. Bhatia R, McCarthy JB, Verfaillie CM. Interferon-alpha restores normal beta 1 integrin-mediated inhibition of hematopoietic progenitor proliferation by the marrow microenvironment in chronic myelogenous leukemia. Blood. 1996;87(9):3883–91.

59. Geay JF, Buet D, Zhang Y, et al. p210BCR-ABL inhibits SDF-1 chemotactic response via alteration of CXCR4 signaling and down-regulation of CXCR4 expression. Cancer Res. 2005;65(7):2676–83. doi:10.1158/0008-5472.CAN-04-2152.

60. Peled A, Hardan I, Trakhtenbrot L, et al. Immature leukemic CD34+CXCR4+ cells from CML patients have lower integrin-dependent migration and adhesion in response to the chemokine SDF-1. Stem Cells. 2002;20(3):259–66. doi:10.1634/stemcells.20-3-259.

61. Jin L, Tabe Y, Konoplev S, et al. CXCR4 up-regulation by imatinib induces chronic myelogenous leukemia (CML) cell migration to bone marrow stroma and promotes survival of quiescent CML cells. Mol Cancer Ther. 2008;7(1):48–58. doi:10.1158/1535-7163.MCT-07-0042.

62. Zeng Z, Shi YX, Samudio IJ, et al. Targeting the leukemia microenvironment by CXCR4 inhibition overcomes resistance to kinase inhibitors and chemotherapy in AML. Blood. 2009;113(24):6215–24. doi:10.1182/blood-2008-05-158311.

63. Gaiger A, Henn T, Horth E, et al. Increase of bcr-abl chimeric mRNA expression in tumor cells of patients with chronic myeloid leukemia precedes disease progression. Blood. 1995;86(6):2371–8.

64. Elmaagacli AH, Beelen DW, Opalka B, Seeber S, Schaefer UW. The amount of BCR-ABL fusion transcripts detected by the real-time quantitative polymerase chain reaction method in patients with Philadelphia chromosome positive chronic myeloid leukemia correlates with the disease stage. Ann Hematol. 2000;79(8):424–31.

65. Barnes DJ, Schultheis B, Adedeji S, Melo JV. Dose-dependent effects of Bcr-Abl in cell line models of different stages of chronic myeloid leukemia. Oncogene. 2005;24(42):6432–40. doi:10.1038/sj.onc.1208796.

66. Jamieson CH, Ailles LE, Dylla SJ, et al. Granulocyte-macrophage progenitors as candidate leukemic stem cells in blast-crisis CML. N Engl J Med. 2004;351(7):657–67. doi:10.1056/NEJMoa040258.

67. Melo JV, Chuah C. Resistance to imatinib mesylate in chronic myeloid leukaemia. Cancer Lett. 2007;249(2):121–32. doi:10.1016/j.canlet.2006.07.010.

68. Penserga ET, Skorski T. Fusion tyrosine kinases: a result and cause of genomic instability. Oncogene. 2007;26(1):11–20. doi:10.1038/sj.onc.1209756.

69. Huang P, Feng L, Oldham EA, Keating MJ, Plunkett W. Superoxide dismutase as a target for the selective killing of cancer cells. Nature. 2000;407(6802):390–5. doi:10.1038/35030140.

70. Sattler M, Verma S, Shrikhande G, et al. The BCR/ABL tyrosine kinase induces production of reactive oxygen species in hematopoietic cells. J Biol Chem. 2000;275(32):24273–8. doi:10.1074/jbc.M002094200.

71. Skorski T. BCR/ABL, DNA damage and DNA repair: implications for new treatment concepts. Leuk Lymphoma. 2008;49(4):610–4. doi:10.1080/03093640701859089.

72. Koptyra M, Cramer K, Slupianek A, Richardson C, Skorski T. BCR/ABL promotes accumulation of chromosomal aberrations induced by oxidative and genotoxic stress. Leukemia. 2008;22(10):1969–72. doi:10.1038/leu.2008.78.

73. Stoklosa T, Poplawski T, Koptyra M, et al. BCR/ABL inhibits mismatch repair to protect from apoptosis and induce point mutations. Cancer Res. 2008;68(8):2576–80. doi:10.1158/0008-5472.CAN-07-6858.

74. Neviani P, Santhanam R, Trotta R, et al. The tumor suppressor PP2A is functionally inactivated in blast crisis CML through the inhibitory activity of the BCR/ABL-regulated SET protein. Cancer Cell. 2005;8(5):355–68. doi:10.1016/j.ccr.2005.10.015.

75. Mullighan CG, Miller CB, Radtke I, et al. BCR-ABL1 lymphoblastic leukaemia is characterized by the deletion of Ikaros. Nature. 2008;453(7191):110–4. doi:10.1038/nature06866.

76. Keeshan K, Santilli G, Corradini F, Perrotti D, Calabretta B. Transcription activation function of C/EBPalpha is required for induction of granulocytic differentiation. Blood. 2003;102(4): 1267–75. doi:10.1182/blood-2003-02-0477.

77. Nakahara F, Sakata-Yanagimoto M, Komeno Y, et al. Hes1 immortalizes committed progenitors and plays a role in blast crisis transition in chronic myelogenous leukemia. Blood. 2010;115(14):2872–81. doi:10.1182/blood-2009-05-222836.

78. Branford S, Rudzki Z, Harper A, et al. Imatinib produces significantly superior molecular responses compared to interferon alfa plus cytarabine in patients with newly diagnosed chronic myeloid leukemia in chronic phase. Leukemia. 2003;17(12):2401–9. doi:10.1038/sj.leu.2403158.

79. Branford S, Rudzki Z, Parkinson I, et al. Real-time quantitative PCR analysis can be used as a primary screen to identify patients with CML treated with imatinib who have BCR-ABL kinase domain mutations. Blood. 2004;104(9):2926–32. doi:10.1182/blood-2004-03-1134.

80. Canitrot Y, Falinski R, Louat T, et al. p210 BCR/ABL kinase regulates nucleotide excision repair (NER) and resistance to UV radiation. Blood. 2003;102(7):2632–7. doi:10.1182/blood-2002-10-3207.

81. Graham SM, Jorgensen HG, Allan E, et al. Primitive, quiescent, Philadelphia-positive stem cells from patients with chronic myeloid leukemia are insensitive to STI571 in vitro. Blood. 2002;99(1):319–25.

82. Copland M, Hamilton A, Elrick LJ, et al. Dasatinib (BMS-354825) targets an earlier progenitor population than imatinib in primary CML but does not eliminate the quiescent fraction. Blood. 2006;107(11):4532–9. doi:10.1182/blood-2005-07-2947.

83. Zhao C, Chen A, Jamieson CH, et al. Hedgehog signalling is essential for maintenance of cancer stem cells in myeloid leukaemia. Nature. 2009;458(7239):776–9. doi:10.1038/nature07737.

84. Dierks C, Beigi R, Guo GR, et al. Expansion of Bcr-Abl-positive leukemic stem cells is dependent on Hedgehog pathway activation. Cancer Cell. 2008;14(3):238–49. doi:10.1016/j.ccr.2008.08.003.

85. Zhang B, Strauss AC, Chu S, et al. Effective targeting of quiescent chronic myelogenous leukemia stem cells by histone deacetylase inhibitors in combination with imatinib mesylate. Cancer Cell. 2010;17(5):427–42. doi:10.1016/j.ccr.2010.03.011.

86. Noens L, van Lierde MA, De Bock R, et al. Prevalence, determinants, and outcomes of non-adherence to imatinib therapy in patients with chronic myeloid leukemia: the ADAGIO study. Blood. 2009;113(22):5401–11. doi:10.1182/blood-2008-12-196543.

87. Ibrahim AR, Eliasson L, Apperley JF, et al. Poor adherence is the main reason for loss of CCyR and imatinib failure for chronic myeloid leukemia patients on long-term therapy. Blood. 2011;117(14):3733–6. doi:10.1182/blood-2010-10-309807.

88. Marin D, Milojkovic D, Olavarria E, et al. European LeukemiaNet criteria for failure or suboptimal response reliably identify patients with CML in early chronic phase treated with imatinib whose eventual outcome is poor. Blood. 2008;112(12):4437–44. doi:10.1182/blood-2008-06-162388.

89. Wang YL, Bagg A, Pear W, Nowell PC, Hess JL. Chronic myelogenous leukemia: laboratory diagnosis and monitoring. Genes Chromosomes Cancer. 2001;32(2):97–111.

90. Landstrom AP, Tefferi A. Fluorescent in situ hybridization in the diagnosis, prognosis, and treatment monitoring of chronic myeloid leukemia. Leuk Lymphoma. 2006;47(3):397–402. doi:10.1080/10428190500353133.

91. Roth MS, Antin JH, Ash R, et al. Prognostic significance of Philadelphia chromosome-positive cells detected by the polymerase chain reaction after allogeneic bone marrow transplant for chronic myelogenous leukemia. Blood. 1992;79(1):276–82.

92. Hughes TP, Morgan GJ, Martiat P, Goldman JM. Detection of residual leukemia after bone marrow transplant for chronic myeloid leukemia: role of polymerase chain reaction in predicting relapse. Blood. 1991;77(4):874–8.

93. Radich JP, Gehly G, Gooley T, et al. Polymerase chain reaction detection of the BCR-ABL fusion transcript after allogeneic marrow transplantation for chronic myeloid leukemia: results and implications in 346 patients. Blood. 1995;85(9):2632–8.

94. Radich JP, Gooley T, Bryant E, et al. The significance of bcr-abl molecular detection in chronic myeloid leukemia patients "late," 18 months or more after transplantation. Blood. 2001;98(6):1701–7.

95. Olavarria E, Kanfer E, Szydlo R, et al. Early detection of BCR-ABL transcripts by quantitative reverse transcriptase-polymerase chain reaction predicts outcome after allogeneic stem cell transplantation for chronic myeloid leukemia. Blood. 2001;97(6):1560–5.

96. Branford S, Hughes TP, Rudzki Z. Monitoring chronic myeloid leukaemia therapy by real-time quantitative PCR in blood is a reliable alternative to bone marrow cytogenetics. Br J Haematol. 1999;107(3):587–99.

97. Lin F, van Rhee F, Goldman JM, Cross NC. Kinetics of increasing BCR-ABL transcript numbers in chronic myeloid leukemia patients who relapse after bone marrow transplantation. Blood. 1996;87(10):4473–8.

98. Mensink E, van de Locht A, Schattenberg A, et al. Quantitation of minimal residual disease in Philadelphia chromosome positive chronic myeloid leukaemia patients using real-time quantitative RT-PCR. Br J Haematol. 1998;102(3):768–74.

99. Branford S, Seymour JF, Grigg A, et al. BCR-ABL messenger RNA levels continue to decline in patients with chronic phase chronic myeloid leukemia treated with imatinib for more than 5 years and approximately half of all first-line treated patients have stable undetectable BCR-ABL using strict sensitivity criteria. Clin Cancer Res. 2007;13(23):7080–5. doi:10.1158/1078-0432.CCR-07-0844.

100. Cortes J, Talpaz M, O'Brien S, et al. Molecular responses in patients with chronic myelogenous leukemia in chronic phase treated with imatinib mesylate. Clin Cancer Res. 2005;11(9):3425–32. doi:10.1158/1078-0432.CCR-04-2139.

101. Hughes TP, Hochhaus A, Branford S, et al. Long-term prognostic significance of early molecular response to imatinib in newly diagnosed chronic myeloid leukemia: an analysis from the International Randomized Study of Interferon and STI571 (IRIS). Blood. 2010;116(19):3758–65. doi:10.1182/blood-2010-03-273979.

102. Stock W, Yu D, Karrison T, et al. Quantitative real-time RT-PCR monitoring of BCR-ABL in chronic myelogenous leukemia shows lack of agreement in blood and bone marrow samples. Int J Oncol. 2006;28(5):1099–103.

103. Branford S, Fletcher L, Cross NCP, Müller MC, Hochhaus A, Kim DW. Desirable performance characteristics for BCR-ABL measurement on an international reporting scale to allow consistent interpretation of individual patient response and comparison of response rates between clinical trials. Blood. 2008;112:3330–8.

104. Hughes TP, Hochhaus A, Branford S, et al. Reduction of BCR-ABL transcript levels at 6, 12, and 18 months (mo) correlates with long-term outcomes on imatinib (IM) at 72 Mo: an analysis from the international randomized study of interferon versus STI571 (IRIS) in patients (pts) with chronic phase chronic myeloid leukemia (CML-CP). ASH Annu Meeting Abstr. 2008;112(11):334. http://abstracts.hematologylibrary.org/cgi/content/abstract/ashmtg;112/11/334.

105. Muller MC, Hanfstein B, Erben P, et al. Molecular response to first line imatinib therapy is predictive for long term event free survival in patients with chronic phase chronic myelogenous leukemia – an interim analysis of the randomized German CML study IV. ASH Annu Meeting Abstr. 2008;112(11):333. http://abstracts.hematologylibrary.org/cgi/content/abstract/ashmtg;112/11/333.

106. Guilhot F, Chastang C, Michallet M, et al. Interferon alfa-2b combined with cytarabine versus interferon alone in chronic myelogenous leukemia. French Chronic Myeloid Leukemia Study Group. N Engl J Med. 1997;337(4):223–9.

107. Kantarjian HM, Smith TL, O'Brien S, Beran M, Pierce S, Talpaz M. Prolonged survival in chronic myelogenous leukemia after cytogenetic response to interferon-alpha therapy. The Leukemia Service. Ann Intern Med. 1995;122(4):254–61.

108. Kantarjian HM, O'Brien S, Cortes JE, et al. Complete cytogenetic and molecular responses to interferon-alpha-based therapy for chronic myelogenous leukemia are associated with excellent long-term prognosis. Cancer. 2003;97(4):1033–41. doi:10.1002/cncr.11223.

109. Bonifazi F, de Vivo A, Rosti G, et al. Chronic myeloid leukemia and interferon-alpha: a study of complete cytogenetic responders. Blood. 2001;98(10):3074–81.

110. Mahon FX, Delbrel X, Cony-Makhoul P, et al. Follow-up of complete cytogenetic remission in patients with chronic myeloid leukemia after cessation of interferon alfa. J Clin Oncol. 2002;20(1):214–20.

111. Essers MA, Offner S, Blanco-Bose WE, et al. IFNalpha activates dormant haematopoietic stem cells in vivo. Nature. 2009;458(7240):904–8. doi:10.1038/nature07815.

112. Sato T, Onai N, Yoshihara H, Arai F, Suda T, Ohteki T. Interferon regulatory factor-2 protects quiescent hematopoietic stem cells from type I interferon-dependent exhaustion. Nat Med. 2009;15(6):696–700. doi:10.1038/nm.1973.

113. Dowding C, Gordon M, Guo AP, et al. Potential mechanisms of action of interferon-alpha in CML. Leuk Lymphoma. 1993;11 Suppl 1:185–91.

114. Guilhot F, Roy L, Saulnier PJ, Guilhot J. Interferon in chronic myeloid leukaemia: past and future. Best Pract Res Clin Haematol. 2009;22(3):315–29. doi:10.1016/j.beha.2009.10.005.

115. Schindler T, Bornmann W, Pellicena P, Miller WT, Clarkson B, Kuriyan J. Structural mechanism for STI-571 inhibition of abelson tyrosine kinase. Science. 2000;289(5486):1938–42.

116. Kantarjian HM, Cortes J, O'Brien S, et al. Imatinib mesylate (STI571) therapy for Philadelphia chromosome-positive chronic myelogenous leukemia in blast phase. Blood. 2002;99(10):3547–53.

117. Talpaz M, Silver RT, Druker BJ, et al. Imatinib induces durable hematologic and cytogenetic responses in patients with accelerated phase chronic myeloid leukemia: results of a phase 2 study. Blood. 2002;99(6):1928–37.

118. Kantarjian HM, Talpaz M, O'Brien S, et al. Imatinib mesylate for Philadelphia chromosome-positive, chronic-phase myeloid leukemia after failure of interferon-alpha: follow-up results. Clin Cancer Res. 2002;8(7):2177–87.

119. Sawyers CL, Hochhaus A, Feldman E, et al. Imatinib induces hematologic and cytogenetic responses in patients with chronic myelogenous leukemia in myeloid blast crisis: results of a phase II study. Blood. 2002;99(10):3530–9.

120. Cortes J, Giles F, O'Brien S, et al. Result of high-dose imatinib mesylate in patients with Philadelphia chromosome-positive chronic myeloid leukemia after failure of interferon-alpha. Blood. 2003;102(1):83–6. doi:10.1182/blood-2003-01-0025.

121. Hochhaus A, O'Brien SG, Guilhot F, et al. Six-year follow-up of patients receiving imatinib for the first-line treatment of chronic myeloid leukemia. Leukemia. 2009;23(6):1054–61. doi:10.1038/leu.2009.38 .

122. Deininger M, O'Brien SG, Guilhot F, et al. International randomized study of interferon Vs STI571 (IRIS) 8-year follow up: sustained survival and Low risk for progression or events in patients with newly diagnosed chronic myeloid leukemia in chronic phase (CML-CP) treated with imatinib. Blood (ASH Annu Meeting Abstr). 2009;114(22):1126. http://abstracts.hematologylibrary.org/cgi/content/abstract/ashmtg;114/22/1126.

123. Bhatia R, Holtz M, Niu N, et al. Persistence of malignant hematopoietic progenitors in chronic myelogenous leukemia patients in complete cytogenetic remission following imatinib mesylate treatment. Blood. 2003;101(12):4701–7. doi:10.1182/blood-2002-09-2780.

124. Bocchia M, Ippoliti M, Gozzetti A, et al. CD34+/Ph+cells are still detectable in chronic myeloid leukemia patients with sustained and prolonged complete cytogenetic remission during treatment with imatinib mesylate. Leukemia. 2008;22(2):426–8. doi:10.1038/sj.leu.2404893.

125. Mahon FX, Rea D, Guilhot J, et al. Discontinuation of imatinib in patients with chronic myeloid leukaemia who have maintained complete molecular remission for at least 2 years:

the prospective, multicentre Stop Imatinib (STIM) trial. Lancet Oncol. 2010;11(11):1029–35. doi:10.1016/S1470-2045(10), 70233-3.

126. Kantarjian H, Pasquini R, Hamerschlak N, et al. Dasatinib or high-dose imatinib for chronic-phase chronic myeloid leukemia after failure of first-line imatinib: a randomized phase 2 trial. Blood. 2007;109(12):5143–50. doi:10.1182/blood-2006-11-056028.

127. Hochhaus A, Kantarjian HM, Baccarani M, et al. Dasatinib induces notable hematologic and cytogenetic responses in chronic-phase chronic myeloid leukemia after failure of imatinib therapy. Blood. 2007;109(6):2303–9. doi:10.1182/blood-2006-09-047266.

128. Hazarika M, Jiang X, Liu Q, et al. Tasigna for chronic and accelerated phase Philadelphia chromosome – positive chronic myelogenous leukemia resistant to or intolerant of imatinib. Clin Cancer Res. 2008;14(17):5325–31. doi:10.1158/1078-0432.CCR-08-0308.

129. Cortes JE, Jones D, O'Brien S, et al. Nilotinib as front-line treatment for patients with chronic myeloid leukemia in early chronic phase. J Clin Oncol. 2010;28(3):392–7. doi:10.1200/JCO.2009.25.4896.

130. Saglio G, Kim DW, Issaragrisil S, et al. Nilotinib versus imatinib for newly diagnosed chronic myeloid leukemia. N Engl J Med. 2010;362(24):2251–9. doi:10.1056/NEJMoa0912614.

131. Kantarjian H, Shah NP, Hochhaus A, et al. Dasatinib versus imatinib in newly diagnosed chronic-phase chronic myeloid leukemia. N Engl J Med. 2010;362(24):2260–70. doi:10.1056/NEJMoa1002315.

132. Alvarado Y, Kantarjian H, O'Brien S, et al. Significance of suboptimal response to imatinib, as defined by the European LeukemiaNet, in the long-term outcome of patients with early chronic myeloid leukemia in chronic phase. Cancer. 2009;115(16):3709–18. doi:10.1002/cncr.24418.

133. Mauro MJ, Deininger MW. Management of drug toxicities in chronic myeloid leukaemia. Best Pract Res Clin Haematol. 2009;22(3):409–29. doi:10.1016/j.beha.2009.06.001.

134. Thomas J, Wang L, Clark RE, Pirmohamed M. Active transport of imatinib into and out of cells: implications for drug resistance. Blood. 2004;104(12):3739–45. doi:10.1182/blood-2003-12-4276.

135. Jordanides NE, Jorgensen HG, Holyoake TL, Mountford JC. Functional ABCG2 is overexpressed on primary CML CD34+ cells and is inhibited by imatinib mesylate. Blood. 2006;108(4):1370–3. doi:10.1182/blood-2006-02-003145.

136. White DL, Saunders VA, Dang P, et al. OCT-1-mediated influx is a key determinant of the intracellular uptake of imatinib but not nilotinib (AMN107): reduced OCT-1 activity is the cause of low in vitro sensitivity to imatinib. Blood. 2006;108(2):697–704. doi:10.1182/blood-2005-11-4687.

137. White DL, Saunders VA, Dang P, et al. Most CML patients who have a suboptimal response to imatinib have low OCT-1 activity: higher doses of imatinib may overcome the negative impact of low OCT-1 activity. Blood. 2007;110(12):4064–72. doi:10.1182/blood-2007-06-093617.

138. Larson RA, Druker BJ, Guilhot F, et al. Imatinib pharmacokinetics and its correlation with response and safety in chronic-phase chronic myeloid leukemia: a subanalysis of the IRIS study. Blood. 2008;111(8):4022–8. doi:10.1182/blood-2007-10-116475.

139. Picard S, Titier K, Etienne G, et al. Trough imatinib plasma levels are associated with both cytogenetic and molecular responses to standard-dose imatinib in chronic myeloid leukemia. Blood. 2007;109(8):3496–9. doi:10.1182/blood-2006-07-036012.

140. Mahon FX, Belloc F, Lagarde V, et al. MDR1 gene overexpression confers resistance to imatinib mesylate in leukemia cell line models. Blood. 2003;101(6):2368–73. doi:10.1182/blood. V101.6.2368.

141. Jiang X, Zhao Y, Smith C, et al. Chronic myeloid leukemia stem cells possess multiple unique features of resistance to BCR-ABL targeted therapies. Leukemia. 2007;21(5):926–35. doi:10.1038/sj.leu.2404609.

142. Hatziieremia S, Jordanides NE, Holyoake TL, Mountford JC, Jorgensen HG. Inhibition of MDR1 does not sensitize primitive chronic myeloid leukemia CD34+ cells to imatinib. Exp Hematol. 2009;37(6):692–700. doi:10.1016/j.exphem.2009.02.006.

143. Wang L, Giannoudis A, Lane S, Williamson P, Pirmohamed M, Clark RE. Expression of the uptake drug transporter hOCT1 is an important clinical determinant of the response

to imatinib in chronic myeloid leukemia. Clin Pharmacol Ther. 2008;83(2):258–64. doi:10.1038/sj.clpt.6100268.

144. Gorre ME, Mohammed M, Ellwood K, et al. Clinical resistance to STI-571 cancer therapy caused by BCR-ABL gene mutation or amplification. Science. 2001;293(5531):876–80. doi:10.1126/science.1062538.

145. Hochhaus A, Kreil S, Corbin AS, et al. Molecular and chromosomal mechanisms of resistance to imatinib (STI571) therapy. Leukemia. 2002;16(11):2190–6. doi:10.1038/sj.leu.2402741.

146. Hu Y, Liu Y, Pelletier S, et al. Requirement of Src kinases Lyn, Hck and Fgr for BCR-ABL1-induced B-lymphoblastic leukemia but not chronic myeloid leukemia. Nat Genet. 2004;36(5):453–61. doi:10.1038/ng1343.

147. Donato NJ, Wu JY, Stapley J, et al. BCR-ABL independence and LYN kinase overexpression in chronic myelogenous leukemia cells selected for resistance to STI571. Blood. 2003;101(2):690–8. doi:10.1182/blood.V101.2.690.

148. Wu J, Meng F, Lu H, et al. Lyn regulates BCR-ABL and Gab2 tyrosine phosphorylation and c-Cbl protein stability in imatinib-resistant chronic myelogenous leukemia cells. Blood. 2008;111(7):3821–9. doi:10.1182/blood-2007-08-109330.

149. Wu J, Meng F, Kong LY, et al. Association between imatinib-resistant BCR-ABL mutation-negative leukemia and persistent activation of LYN kinase. J Natl Cancer Inst. 2008;100(13):926–39. doi:10.1093/jnci/djn188.

150. Lombardo LJ, Lee FY, Chen P, et al. Discovery of N-(2-chloro-6-methyl- phenyl)-2-(6-(4-(2-hydroxyethyl)-piperazin-1-yl)-2-methylpyrimidin-4-ylamino)thiazole-5-carboxamide (BMS-354825), a dual Src/Abl kinase inhibitor with potent antitumor activity in preclinical assays. J Med Chem. 2004;47(27):6658–61. doi:10.1021/jm049486a.

151. Mahon FX, Hayette S, Lagarde V, et al. Evidence that resistance to nilotinib may be due to BCR-ABL, Pgp, or Src kinase overexpression. Cancer Res. 2008;68(23):9809–16. doi:10.1158/0008-5472.CAN-08-1008.

152. O'Hare T, Eide CA, Deininger MW. Persistent LYN signaling in imatinib-resistant, BCR-ABL-independent chronic myelogenous leukemia. J Natl Cancer Inst. 2008;100(13):908–9. doi:10.1093/jnci/djn204.

153. Cortes JE, Talpaz M, Giles F, et al. Prognostic significance of cytogenetic clonal evolution in patients with chronic myelogenous leukemia on imatinib mesylate therapy. Blood. 2003;101(10):3794–800. doi:10.1182/blood-2002-09-2790.

154. O'Dwyer ME, Mauro MJ, Blasdel C, et al. Clonal evolution and lack of cytogenetic response are adverse prognostic factors for hematologic relapse of chronic phase CML patients treated with imatinib mesylate. Blood. 2004;103(2):451–5. doi:10.1182/blood-2003-02-0371.

155. Andersen MK, Pedersen-Bjergaard J, Kjeldsen L, Dufva IH, Brondum-Nielsen K. Clonal Ph-negative hematopoiesis in CML after therapy with imatinib mesylate is frequently characterized by trisomy 8. Leukemia. 2002;16(7):1390–3. doi:10.1038/sj.leu.2402634.

156. Bumm T, Muller C, Al-Ali HK, et al. Emergence of clonal cytogenetic abnormalities in Ph-cells in some CML patients in cytogenetic remission to imatinib but restoration of polyclonal hematopoiesis in the majority. Blood. 2003;101(5):1941–9. doi:10.1182/blood-2002-07-2053.

157. O'Dwyer ME, Gatter KM, Loriaux M, et al. Demonstration of Philadelphia chromosome negative abnormal clones in patients with chronic myelogenous leukemia during major cytogenetic responses induced by imatinib mesylate. Leukemia. 2003;17(3):481–7. doi:10.1038/sj.leu.2402848.

158. Lahaye T, Riehm B, Berger U, et al. Response and resistance in 300 patients with BCR-ABL-positive leukemias treated with imatinib in a single center: a 4.5-year follow-up. Cancer. 2005;103(8):1659–69. doi:10.1002/cncr.20922.

159. Hagemeijer A, Smit EM, Lowenberg B, Abels J. Chronic myeloid leukemia with permanent disappearance of the Ph1 chromosome and development of new clonal subpopulations. Blood. 1979;53(1):1–14.

160. Fayad L, Kantarjian H, O'Brien S, et al. Emergence of new clonal abnormalities following interferon-alpha induced complete cytogenetic response in patients with chronic myeloid leukemia: report of three cases. Leukemia. 1997;11(5):767–71.

161. Chee YL, Vickers MA, Stevenson D, Holyoake TL, Culligan DJ. Fatal myelodysplastic syndrome developing during therapy with imatinib mesylate and characterised by the emergence of complex Philadelphia negative clones. Leukemia. 2003;17(3):634–5. doi:10.1038/sj. leu.2402842.

162. Kovitz C, Kantarjian H, Garcia-Manero G, Abruzzo LV, Cortes J. Myelodysplastic syndromes and acute leukemia developing after imatinib mesylate therapy for chronic myeloid leukemia. Blood. 2006;108(8):2811–3. doi:10.1182/blood-2006-04-017400.

163. Deininger MW, Cortes J, Paquette R, et al. The prognosis for patients with chronic myeloid leukemia who have clonal cytogenetic abnormalities in Philadelphia chromosome-negative cells. Cancer. 2007;110(7):1509–19. doi:10.1002/cncr.22936.

164. Jabbour E, Kantarjian HM, Abruzzo LV, et al. Chromosomal abnormalities in Philadelphia chromosome negative metaphases appearing during imatinib mesylate therapy in patients with newly diagnosed chronic myeloid leukemia in chronic phase. Blood. 2007;110(8):2991–5. doi:10.1182/blood-2007-01-070045.

165. Fabarius A, Haferlach C, Muller MC, et al. Dynamics of cytogenetic aberrations in Philadelphia chromosome positive and negative hematopoiesis during dasatinib therapy of chronic myeloid leukemia patients after imatinib failure. Haematologica. 2007; 92(6):834–7.

166. Shah NP, Nicoll JM, Nagar B, et al. Multiple BCR-ABL kinase domain mutations confer polyclonal resistance to the tyrosine kinase inhibitor imatinib (STI571) in chronic phase and blast crisis chronic myeloid leukemia. Cancer Cell. 2002;2(2):117–25.

167. Azam M, Latek RR, Daley GQ. Mechanisms of autoinhibition and STI-571/imatinib resistance revealed by mutagenesis of BCR-ABL. Cell. 2003;112(6):831–43.

168. Branford S, Rudzki Z, Walsh S, et al. High frequency of point mutations clustered within the adenosine triphosphate-binding region of BCR/ABL in patients with chronic myeloid leukemia or Ph-positive acute lymphoblastic leukemia who develop imatinib (STI571) resistance. Blood. 2002;99(9):3472–5.

169. Branford S, Rudzki Z, Walsh S, et al. Detection of BCR-ABL mutations in patients with CML treated with imatinib is virtually always accompanied by clinical resistance, and mutations in the ATP phosphate-binding loop (P-loop) are associated with a poor prognosis. Blood. 2003;102(1):276–83. doi:10.1182/blood-2002-09-2896.

170. Corm S, Nicollini F, Borie D, et al. Mutation status of imatinib mesylate-resistants CML patients and clinical outcomes: a French multicenter retrospective study for the fiLMC Group. ASH Annu Meeting Abstr. 2004;104(11):275. http://abstracts.hematologylibrary.org/cgi/content/abstract/ashmtg;104/11/275.

171. Willis SG, Lange T, Demehri S, et al. High-sensitivity detection of BCR-ABL kinase domain mutations in imatinib-naive patients: correlation with clonal cytogenetic evolution but not response to therapy. Blood. 2005;106(6):2128–37. doi:10.1182/blood-2005-03-1036.

172. Gruber FX, Ernst T, Kiselev Y, Hochhaus A, Mikkola I. Detection of drug-resistant clones in chronic myelogenous leukemia patients during dasatinib and nilotinib treatment. Clin Chem. 2010;56(3):469–73. doi:10.1373/clinchem.2009.133843.

173. Nardi V, Raz T, Cao X, et al. Quantitative monitoring by polymerase colony assay of known mutations resistant to ABL kinase inhibitors. Oncogene. 2008;27(6):775–82. doi:10.1038/sj.onc.1210698.

174. Branford S, Melo JV, Hughes TP. Selecting optimal second-line tyrosine kinase inhibitor therapy for chronic myeloid leukemia patients after imatinib failure: does the BCR-ABL mutation status really matter? Blood. 2009;114(27):5426–35. doi:10.1182/blood-2009-08-215939.

175. Sherbenou DW, Hantschel O, Kaupe I, et al. BCR-ABL SH3-SH2 domain mutations in chronic myeloid leukemia patients on imatinib. Blood. 2010;116(17):3278–85. doi:10.1182/blood-2008-10-183665.

176. Weisberg E, Manley PW, Breitenstein W, et al. Characterization of AMN107, a selective inhibitor of native and mutant Bcr-Abl. Cancer Cell. 2005;7(2):129–41. doi:10.1016/j.ccr.2005.01.007.

177. O'Hare T, Eide CA, Deininger MW. Bcr-Abl kinase domain mutations, drug resistance, and the road to a cure for chronic myeloid leukemia. Blood. 2007;110(7):2242–9. doi:10.1182/blood-2007-03-066936.

178. Tokarski JS, Newitt JA, Chang CY, et al. The structure of Dasatinib (BMS-354825) bound to activated ABL kinase domain elucidates its inhibitory activity against imatinib-resistant ABL mutants. Cancer Res. 2006;66(11):5790–7. doi:10.1158/0008-5472.CAN-05-4187.

179. Manley PW, Cowan-Jacob SW, Fendrich G, et al. Bcr-Abl binding modes of dasatinib, imatinib and nilotinib: an NMR study. ASH Annu Meeting Abstr. 2006;108(11):747. http://abstracts.hematologylibrary.org/cgi/content/abstract/ashmtg;108/11/747.

180. Soverini S, Martinelli G, Rosti G, et al. ABL mutations in late chronic phase chronic myeloid leukemia patients with up-front cytogenetic resistance to imatinib are associated with a greater likelihood of progression to blast crisis and shorter survival: a study by the GIMEMA Working Party on Chronic Myeloid Leukemia. J Clin Oncol. 2005;23(18):4100–9. doi:10.1200/JCO.2005.05.531.

181. Nicolini FE, Corm S, Le QH, et al. Mutation status and clinical outcome of 89 imatinib mesylate-resistant chronic myelogenous leukemia patients: a retrospective analysis from the French intergroup of CML (Fi(phi)-LMC GROUP). Leukemia. 2006;20(6):1061–6. doi:10.1038/sj.leu.2404236.

182. Apperley JF. Part I: mechanisms of resistance to imatinib in chronic myeloid leukaemia. Lancet Oncol. 2007;8(11):1018–29. doi:10.1016/S1470-2045(07)70342-X.

183. Apperley JF. Part II: management of resistance to imatinib in chronic myeloid leukaemia. Lancet Oncol. 2007;8(12):1116–28. doi:10.1016/S1470-2045(07), 70379-0.

184. Redaelli S, Piazza R, Rostagno R, et al. Activity of bosutinib, dasatinib, and nilotinib against 18 imatinib-resistant BCR/ABL mutants. J Clin Oncol. 2009;27(3):469–71. doi:10.1200/JCO.2008.19.8853.

185. Press RD, Willis SG, Laudadio J, Mauro MJ, Deininger MW. Determining the rise in BCR-ABL RNA that optimally predicts a kinase domain mutation in patients with chronic myeloid leukemia on imatinib. Blood. 2009;114(13):2598–605. doi:10.1182/blood-2008-08-173674.

186. Quintas-Cardama A, Cortes JE, O'Brien S, et al. Dasatinib early intervention after cytogenetic or hematologic resistance to imatinib in patients with chronic myeloid leukemia. Cancer. 2009;115(13):2912–21. doi:10.1002/cncr.24325.

187. Kantarjian H, Talpaz M, O'Brien S, et al. High-dose imatinib mesylate therapy in newly diagnosed Philadelphia chromosome-positive chronic phase chronic myeloid leukemia. Blood. 2004;103(8):2873–8. doi:10.1182/blood-2003-11-3800.

188. Hughes TP, Branford S, White DL, et al. Impact of early dose intensity on cytogenetic and molecular responses in chronic-phase CML patients receiving 600 mg/day of imatinib as initial therapy. Blood. 2008;112(10):3965–73. doi:10.1182/blood-2008-06-161737.

189. Cortes JE, Kantarjian HM, Goldberg SL, et al. High-dose imatinib in newly diagnosed chronic-phase chronic myeloid leukemia: high rates of rapid cytogenetic and molecular responses. J Clin Oncol. 2009;27(28):4754–9. doi:10.1200/JCO.2008.20.3869.

190. Baccarani M, Rosti G, Castagnetti F, et al. Comparison of imatinib 400 mg and 800 mg daily in the front-line treatment of high-risk, Philadelphia-positive chronic myeloid leukemia: a European LeukemiaNet Study. Blood. 2009;113(19):4497–504. doi:10.1182/blood-2008-12-191254.

191. Cortes JE, Baccarani M, Guilhot F, et al. Phase III, randomized, open-label study of daily imatinib mesylate 400 mg versus 800 mg in patients with newly diagnosed, previously untreated chronic myeloid leukemia in chronic phase using molecular end points: tyrosine kinase inhibitor optimization and selectivity study. J Clin Oncol. 2010;28(3):424–30. doi:10.1200/JCO.2009.25.3724.

192. Hehlmann R, Jung-Munkwitz S, Lauseker M, et al. Randomized comparison of imatinib 800 Mg Vs. Imatinib 400 Mg +/– IFN in newly diagnosed BCR/ABL positive chronic phase CML: analysis of molecular remission at 12 months; the German CML-study IV. ASH Annu Meeting Abstr. 2009;114(22):339. http://abstracts.hematologylibrary.org/cgi/content/abstract/ashmtg;114/22/339.

193. Preudhomme C, Guilhot J, Nicolini FE, et al. Imatinib plus peginterferon alfa-2a in chronic myeloid leukemia. N Engl J Med. 2010;363(26):2511–21. doi:10.1056/NEJMoa1004095.
194. Brave M, Goodman V, Kaminskas E, et al. Sprycel for chronic myeloid leukemia and Philadelphia chromosome-positive acute lymphoblastic leukemia resistant to or intolerant of imatinib mesylate. Clin Cancer Res. 2008;14(2):352–9. doi:10.1158/1078-0432.CCR-07-4175.
195. Hantschel O, Rix U, Superti-Furga G. Target spectrum of the BCR-ABL inhibitors imatinib, nilotinib and dasatinib. Leuk Lymphoma. 2008;49(4):615–9. doi:10.1080/10428190801896103.
196. Soverini S, Colarossi S, Gnani A, et al. Resistance to dasatinib in Philadelphia-positive leukemia patients and the presence or the selection of mutations at residues 315 and 317 in the BCR-ABL kinase domain. Haematologica. 2007;92(3):401–4.
197. Quintas-Cardama A, Cortes JE. The next generation of therapies for chronic myeloid leukemia. Clin Lymphoma Myeloma. 2009;9 Suppl 4:S395–403. doi:10.3816/CLM.2009.s.040.
198. Baccarani M, Rosti G, Saglio G, et al. Dasatinib time to and durability of major and complete cytogenetic response (MCyR and CCyR) in patients with chronic myeloid leukemia in chronic phase (CML-CP). ASH Annu Meeting Abstr. 2008;112(11):450. http://abstracts.hematologylibrary.org/cgi/content/abstract/ashmtg;112/11/450.
199. Hochhaus A, Muller MC, Radich J, et al. Dasatinib-associated major molecular responses are rapidly achieved in patients with chronic myeloid leukemia in chronic phase (CML-CP) following resistance, suboptimal response, or intolerance on imatinib. ASH Annu Meeting Abstr. 2008;112(11):1095. http://abstracts.hematologylibrary.org/cgi/content/abstract/ashmtg;112/11/1095.
200. Shah NP, Kantarjian HM, Kim DW, et al. Intermittent target inhibition with dasatinib 100 mg once daily preserves efficacy and improves tolerability in imatinib-resistant and -intolerant chronic-phase chronic myeloid leukemia. J Clin Oncol. 2008;26(19):3204–12. doi:10.1200/JCO.2007.14.9260.
201. Jabbour E, Bahceci E, Zhu C, Lambert A, Cortes J. Predictors of long-term cytogenetic response following dasatinib therapy of patients with chronic-phase chronic myeloid leukemia (CML-CP). ASH Annu Meeting Abstr. 2009;114(22):3296. http://abstracts.hematologylibrary.org/cgi/content/abstract/ashmtg;114/22/3296.
202. Kantarjian HM, Giles F, Gattermann N, et al. Nilotinib (formerly AMN107), a highly selective BCR-ABL tyrosine kinase inhibitor, is effective in patients with Philadelphia chromosome-positive chronic myelogenous leukemia in chronic phase following imatinib resistance and intolerance. Blood. 2007;110(10):3540–6. doi:10.1182/blood-2007-03-080689.
203. Kantarjian HM, Giles FJ, Bhalla KN, et al. Nilotinib is effective in patients with chronic myeloid leukemia in chronic phase after imatinib resistance or intolerance: 24-month follow-up results. Blood. 2011;117(4):1141–5. doi:10.1182/blood-2010-03-277152.
204. Branford S, Kim D, Soverini S, et al. Molecular response at 3 months on nilotinib therapy predicts response and long-term outcomes in patients with imatinib-resistant or -intolerant chronic myeloid leukemia in chronic phase (CML-CP). ASH Annu Meeting Abstr. 2009;114(22):3292. http://abstracts.hematologylibrary.org/cgi/content/abstract/ashmtg;114/22/3292.
205. Kantarjian HM, Jabbour E, Giles FJ, et al. Prognostic factors for progression-free survival in patients with imatinib-resistant or -intolerant chronic myeloid leukemia in chronic phase (CML-CP) treated with nilotinib based on 24 month data. ASH Annu Meeting Abstr. 2009;114(22):3298. http://abstracts.hematologylibrary.org/cgi/content/abstract/ashmtg;114/22/3298.
206. Hughes T, Saglio G, Branford S, et al. Impact of baseline BCR-ABL mutations on response to nilotinib in patients with chronic myeloid leukemia in chronic phase. J Clin Oncol. 2009;27(25):4204–10. doi:10.1200/JCO.2009.21.8230.
207. Soverini S, Gnani A, Colarossi S, et al. Philadelphia-positive patients who already harbor imatinib-resistant Bcr-Abl kinase domain mutations have a higher likelihood of developing additional mutations associated with resistance to second- or third-line tyrosine kinase inhibitors. Blood. 2009;114(10):2168–71. doi:10.1182/blood-2009-01-197186.

208. Griswold IJ, MacPartlin M, Bumm T, et al. Kinase domain mutants of Bcr-Abl exhibit altered transformation potency, kinase activity, and substrate utilization, irrespective of sensitivity to imatinib. Mol Cell Biol. 2006;26(16):6082–93. doi:10.1128/MCB.02202-05.

209. Shah NP, Skaggs BJ, Branford S, et al. Sequential ABL kinase inhibitor therapy selects for compound drug-resistant BCR-ABL mutations with altered oncogenic potency. J Clin Invest. 2007;117(9):2562–9. doi:10.1172/JCI30890.

210. Cortes J, Jabbour E, Kantarjian H, et al. Dynamics of BCR-ABL kinase domain mutations in chronic myeloid leukemia after sequential treatment with multiple tyrosine kinase inhibitors. Blood. 2007;110(12):4005–11. doi:10.1182/blood-2007-03-080838.

211. Jabbour E, Kantarjian HM, Jones D, et al. Characteristics and outcome of chronic myeloid leukemia patients with F317L BCR-ABL kinase domain mutation after therapy with tyrosine kinase inhibitors. Blood. 2008;112(13):4839–42. doi:10.1182/blood-2008-04-149948.

212. Muller MC, Cortes JE, Kim DW, et al. Dasatinib treatment of chronic-phase chronic myeloid leukemia: analysis of responses according to preexisting BCR-ABL mutations. Blood. 2009;114(24):4944–53. doi:10.1182/blood-2009-04-214221.

213. Jabbour E, Cortes JE, Kantarjian H. Second-line therapy and beyond resistance for the treatment of patients with chronic myeloid leukemia post imatinib failure. Clin Lymphoma Myeloma. 2009;9 Suppl 3:S272–9. doi:10.3816/CLM.2009.s.023.

214. Shah N, Bahceci E, Lambert A, Ploughman L, Radich J. Resistance, outcome and the development of mutations with dasatinib in patients with chronic-phase chronic myeloid leukemia (CML-CP). ASH Annu Meeting Abstr. 2009;114(22):1122. http://abstracts.hematologylibrary.org/cgi/content/abstract/ashmtg;114/22/1122.

215. Ray A, Cowan-Jacob SW, Manley PW, Mestan J, Griffin JD. Identification of BCR-ABL point mutations conferring resistance to the Abl kinase inhibitor AMN107 (nilotinib) by a random mutagenesis study. Blood. 2007;109(11):5011–5. doi:10.1182/blood-2006-01-015347.

216. Garg RJ, Kantarjian H, O'Brien S, et al. The use of nilotinib or dasatinib after failure to 2 prior tyrosine kinase inhibitors: long-term follow-up. Blood. 2009;114(20):4361–8. doi:10.1182/blood-2009-05-221531.

217. Sawyers CL. Chronic myeloid leukemia. N Engl J Med. 1999;340(17):1330–40.

218. Faderl S, Talpaz M, Estrov Z, Kantarjian HM. Chronic myelogenous leukemia: biology and therapy. Ann Intern Med. 1999;131(3):207–19.

219. Palandri F, Castagnetti F, Alimena G, et al. The long-term durability of cytogenetic responses in patients with accelerated phase chronic myeloid leukemia treated with imatinib 600 mg: the GIMEMA CML Working Party experience after a 7-year follow-up. Haematologica. 2009;94(2):205–12. doi:10.3324/haematol.13529.

220. Apperley JF, Cortes JE, Kim DW, et al. Dasatinib in the treatment of chronic myeloid leukemia in accelerated phase after imatinib failure: the START a trial. J Clin Oncol. 2009;27(21):3472–9. doi:10.1200/JCO.2007.14.3339.

221. Kantarjian H, Cortes J, Kim DW, et al. Phase 3 study of dasatinib 140 mg once daily versus 70 mg twice daily in patients with chronic myeloid leukemia in accelerated phase resistant or intolerant to imatinib: 15-month median follow-up. Blood. 2009;113(25):6322–9. doi:10.1182/blood-2008-11-186817.

222. le Coutre P, Ottmann OG, Giles F, et al. Nilotinib (formerly AMN107), a highly selective BCR-ABL tyrosine kinase inhibitor, is active in patients with imatinib-resistant or -intolerant accelerated-phase chronic myelogenous leukemia. Blood. 2008;111(4):1834–9. doi:10.1182/blood-2007-04-083196.

223. Goldman JM. Initial treatment for patients with CML. Hematology. 2009;2009(1):453–60. doi:10.1182/asheducation-2009.1.453. http://asheducationbook.hematologylibrary.org/cgi/content/abstract/bloodbook;2009/1/453.

224. Silver RT. The blast phase of chronic myeloid leukaemia. Best Pract Res Clin Haematol. 2009;22(3):387–94. doi:10.1016/j.beha.2009.07.006.

225. Fava C, Kantarjian HM, Jabbour E, et al. Failure to achieve a complete hematologic response at the time of a major cytogenetic response with second-generation tyrosine kinase inhibitors

is associated with a poor prognosis among patients with chronic myeloid leukemia in accelerated or blast phase. Blood. 2009;113(21):5058–63. doi:10.1182/blood-2008-10-184960.

226. Cortes J, Kim DW, Raffoux E, et al. Efficacy and safety of dasatinib in imatinib-resistant or -intolerant patients with chronic myeloid leukemia in blast phase. Leukemia. 2008;22(12):2176–83. doi:10.1038/leu.2008.221.

227. Shah NP. Advanced CML: therapeutic options for patients in accelerated and blast phases. J Natl Compr Canc Netw. 2008;6 Suppl 2:S31–6.

228. Giles FJ, DeAngelo DJ, Baccarani M, et al. Optimizing outcomes for patients with advanced disease in chronic myelogenous leukemia. Semin Oncol. 2008;35(1 Suppl 1):S1–17; quiz S18-20. 10.1053/j.seminoncol.2007.12.002.

229. Palandri F, Castagnetti F, Testoni N, et al. Chronic myeloid leukemia in blast crisis treated with imatinib 600 mg: outcome of the patients alive after a 6-year follow-up. Haematologica. 2008;93(12):1792–6. doi:10.3324/haematol.13068.

230. Ottmann OG, Wassmann B. Treatment of Philadelphia chromosome-positive acute lymphoblastic leukemia. Hematology Am Soc Hematol Educ Program. 2005:118–122. 10.1182/asheducation-2005.1.118.

231. Kondo T, Tasaka T, Sano F, et al. Philadelphia chromosome-positive acute myeloid leukemia (Ph+AML) treated with imatinib mesylate (IM): a report with IM plasma concentration and bcr-abl transcripts. Leuk Res. 2009;33(9):e137–8. doi:10.1016/j.leukres.2009.03.017.

232. Thomas ED, Clift RA, Fefer A, et al. Marrow transplantation for the treatment of chronic myelogenous leukemia. Ann Intern Med. 1986;104(2):155–63.

233. Gratwohl A, Heim D. Current role of stem cell transplantation in chronic myeloid leukaemia. Best Pract Res Clin Haematol. 2009;22(3):431–43. doi:10.1016/j.beha.2009.05.002.

234. Radich JP, Gooley T, Bensinger W, et al. HLA-matched related hematopoietic cell transplantation for chronic-phase CML using a targeted busulfan and cyclophosphamide preparative regimen. Blood. 2003;102(1):31–5. doi:10.1182/blood-2002-08-2619.

235. Clift RA, Buckner CD, Thomas ED, et al. Marrow transplantation for patients in accelerated phase of chronic myeloid leukemia. Blood. 1994;84(12):4368–73.

236. Hansen JA, Gooley TA, Martin PJ, et al. Bone marrow transplants from unrelated donors for patients with chronic myeloid leukemia. N Engl J Med. 1998;338(14):962–8. doi:10.1056/NEJM199804023381405.

237. Pasquini MC, Wang Z. Current use and outcome of hematopoietic stem cell transplantation: CIBMTR Summary Slides. 2010. CIBMTR Web site. www.cibmtr.org. Updated 2010. Accessed 1 June 2011.

238. Radich J. Stem cell transplant for chronic myeloid leukemia in the imatinib era. Semin Hematol. 2010;47(4):354–61. doi:10.1053/j.seminhematol.2010.06.008.

239. Venepalli N, Rezvani K, Mielke S, Savani BN. Role of allo-SCT for CML in 2010. Bone Marrow Transplant. 2010;45(11):1579–86. doi:10.1038/bmt.2010.138.

240. Cortes J, Talpaz M, Bixby D, et al. A phase 1 trial of oral ponatinib (AP24534) in patients with refractory chronic myelogenous leukemia (CML) and other hematologic malignancies: emerging safety and clinical response findings. Blood (ASH Annu Meeting Abstr). 2010;116(21):210. http://abstracts.hematologylibrary.org/cgi/content/abstract/ashmtg;116/21/210.

241. Oehler VG, Gooley T, Snyder DS, et al. The effects of imatinib mesylate treatment before allogeneic transplantation for chronic myeloid leukemia. Blood. 2007;109(4):1782–9. doi:10.1182/blood-2006-06-031682.

242. Lee SJ, Kukreja M, Wang T, et al. Impact of prior imatinib mesylate on the outcome of hematopoietic cell transplantation for chronic myeloid leukemia. Blood. 2008;112(8):3500–7. doi:10.1182/blood-2008-02-141689.

243. Shimoni A, Leiba M, Schleuning M, et al. Prior treatment with the tyrosine kinase inhibitors dasatinib and nilotinib allows stem cell transplantation (SCT) in a less advanced disease phase and does not increase SCT toxicity in patients with chronic myelogenous leukemia and Philadelphia positive acute lymphoblastic leukemia. Leukemia. 2009;23(1):190–4. doi:10.1038/leu.2008.160.

244. Weisser M, Schleuning M, Haferlach C, Schwerdtfeger R, Kolb HJ. Allogeneic stem-cell transplantation provides excellent results in advanced stage chronic myeloid leukemia with

major cytogenetic response to pre-transplant imatinib therapy. Leuk Lymphoma. 2007;48(2):295–301. doi:10.1080/10428190601078464.

245. Deininger M, Schleuning M, Greinix H, et al. The effect of prior exposure to imatinib on transplant-related mortality. Haematologica. 2006;91(4):452–9.

246. Gratwohl A, Hermans J, Goldman JM, et al. Risk assessment for patients with chronic myeloid leukaemia before allogeneic blood or marrow transplantation. Chronic Leukemia Working Party of the European Group for Blood and Marrow Transplantation. Lancet. 1998;352(9134): 1087–92.

247. Passweg JR, Walker I, Sobocinski KA, et al. Validation and extension of the EBMT risk score for patients with chronic myeloid leukaemia (CML) receiving allogeneic haematopoietic stem cell transplants. Br J Haematol. 2004;125(5):613–20. doi:10.1111/j.1365-2141. 2004.04955.x.

248. Clift RA, Buckner CD, Appelbaum FR, et al. Allogeneic marrow transplantation in patients with chronic myeloid leukemia in the chronic phase: a randomized trial of two irradiation regimens. Blood. 1991;77(8):1660–5.

249. Kerbauy FR, Storb R, Hegenbart U, et al. Hematopoietic cell transplantation from HLA-identical sibling donors after low-dose radiation-based conditioning for treatment of CML. Leukemia. 2005;19(6):990–7. doi:10.1038/sj.leu.2403730.

250. Or R, Shapira MY, Resnick I, et al. Nonmyeloablative allogeneic stem cell transplantation for the treatment of chronic myeloid leukemia in first chronic phase. Blood. 2003;101(2):441–5. doi:10.1182/blood-2002-02-0535.

251. Crawley C, Szydlo R, Lalancette M, et al. Outcomes of reduced-intensity transplantation for chronic myeloid leukemia: an analysis of prognostic factors from the Chronic Leukemia Working Party of the EBMT. Blood. 2005;106(9):2969–76. doi:10.1182/blood-2004-09-3544.

252. Bensinger WI, Martin PJ, Storer B, et al. Transplantation of bone marrow as compared with peripheral-blood cells from HLA-identical relatives in patients with hematologic cancers. N Engl J Med. 2001;344(3):175–81. doi:10.1056/NEJM200101183440303.

253. Couban S, Simpson DR, Barnett MJ, et al. A randomized multicenter comparison of bone marrow and peripheral blood in recipients of matched sibling allogeneic transplants for myeloid malignancies. Blood. 2002;100(5):1525–31. doi:10.1182/blood-2002-01-0048.

254. Oehler VG, Radich JP, Storer B, et al. Randomized trial of allogeneic related bone marrow transplantation versus peripheral blood stem cell transplantation for chronic myeloid leukemia. Biol Blood Marrow Transplant. 2005;11(2):85–92. doi:10.1016/j.bbmt.2004.09.010.

255. Sanz J, Sanz GF. Umbilical cord blood transplantation from unrelated donors in adult patients with chronic myeloid leukemia. Best Pract Res Clin Haematol. 2010;23(2):217–22. doi:10.1016/j.beha.2010.05.001.

256. Olavarria E, Siddique S, Griffiths MJ, et al. Posttransplantation imatinib as a strategy to postpone the requirement for immunotherapy in patients undergoing reduced-intensity allografts for chronic myeloid leukemia. Blood. 2007;110(13):4614–7. doi:10.1182/blood-2007-04-082990.

257. DeAngelo DJ, Hochberg EP, Alyea EP, et al. Extended follow-up of patients treated with imatinib mesylate (Gleevec) for chronic myelogenous leukemia relapse after allogeneic transplantation: durable cytogenetic remission and conversion to complete donor chimerism without graft-versus-host disease. Clin Cancer Res. 2004;10(15):5065–71. doi:10.1158/1078-0432.CCR-03-0580.

258. Hess G, Bunjes D, Siegert W, et al. Sustained complete molecular remissions after treatment with imatinib-mesylate in patients with failure after allogeneic stem cell transplantation for chronic myelogenous leukemia: results of a prospective phase II open-label multicenter study. J Clin Oncol. 2005;23(30):7583–93. doi:10.1200/JCO.2005.01.3110.

259. Kolb HJ, Schattenberg A, Goldman JM, et al. Graft-versus-leukemia effect of donor lymphocyte transfusions in marrow grafted patients. Blood. 1995;86(5):2041–50.

260. Savani BN, Montero A, Kurlander R, Childs R, Hensel N, Barrett AJ. Imatinib synergizes with donor lymphocyte infusions to achieve rapid molecular remission of CML relapsing after allogeneic stem cell transplantation. Bone Marrow Transplant. 2005;36(11):1009–15. doi:10.1038/sj.bmt.1705167.

261. Silver RT, Cortes J, Waltzman R, Mone M, Kantarjian H. Sustained durability of responses and improved progression-free and overall survival with imatinib treatment for accelerated phase and blast crisis chronic myeloid leukemia: long-term follow-up of the STI571 0102 and 0109 trials. Haematologica. 2009;94(5):743–4. doi:10.3324/haematol.2009.006999.

262. Novartis Pharmaceuticals Corporation. Gleevec (imatinib mesylate): prescribing information (online). http://www.pharma.us.novartis.com/product/pi/pdf/gleevec_tabs.pdf. Accessed 26 May 2011.

263. Novartis Pharmaceuticals Corporation. Tasigna (nilotinib): prescribing information (online). http://www.pharma.us.novartis.com/product/pi/pdf/tasigna.pdf. Accessed 27 May 2011.

264. Bristol Myers Squibb Corporation. Sprycel (dasatinib): prescribing information (online). http://packageinserts.bms.com/pi/pi_sprycel.pdf. Accessed 25 May 2011.

265. Ramar K, Potti A, Mehdi SA. Uncommon syndromes and treatment manifestations of malignancy: Case 4. Periorbital edema and imatinib mesylate therapy for chronic myelogenous leukemia. J Clin Oncol. 2003;21(1):172–3.

266. Porkka K, Khoury HJ, Paquette RL, Matloub Y, Sinha R, Cortes JE. Dasatinib 100 mg once daily minimizes the occurrence of pleural effusion in patients with chronic myeloid leukemia in chronic phase and efficacy is unaffected in patients who develop pleural effusion. Cancer. 2010;116(2):377–86. doi:10.1002/cncr.24734.

267. Quintas-Cardama A, Kantarjian H, O'Brien S, et al. Pleural effusion in patients with chronic myelogenous leukemia treated with dasatinib after imatinib failure. J Clin Oncol. 2007;25(25):3908–14. doi:10.1200/JCO.2007.12.0329.

268. Deininger MW, O'Brien SG, Ford JM, Druker BJ. Practical management of patients with chronic myeloid leukemia receiving imatinib. J Clin Oncol. 2003;21(8):1637–47. doi:10.1200/JCO.2003.11.143.

269. Deremer DL, Ustun C, Natarajan K. Nilotinib: a second-generation tyrosine kinase inhibitor for the treatment of chronic myelogenous leukemia. Clin Ther. 2008;30(11):1956–75. doi:10.1016/j.clinthera.2008.11.014.

270. Cortes JE, Hochhaus A, le Coutre PD, et al. Minimal cross-intolerance with nilotinib in patients with chronic myeloid leukemia in chronic or accelerated phase who are intolerant to imatinib. Blood. 2011;117(21):5600–6. http://bloodjournal.hematologylibrary.org/content/early/2011/04/04/blood-2010-11-318949.abstract. 10.1182/blood-2010-11-318949.

271. Keller G, Schafhausen P, Brummendorf TH. Bosutinib. Recent Results Cancer Res. 2010;184:119–27. doi:10.1007/978-3-642-01222-8_9.

272. Quintas-Cardama A, Kantarjian H, Cortes J. Imatinib and beyond – exploring the full potential of targeted therapy for CML. Nat Rev Clin Oncol. 2009;6(9):535–43. doi:10.1038/nrclinonc.2009.112.

273. Quintas-Cardama A, Kantarjian H, Cortes J. Homoharringtonine, omacetaxine mepesuccinate, and chronic myeloid leukemia circa 2009. Cancer. 2009;115(23):5382–93. doi:10.1002/cncr.24601.

274. Konig H, Hartel N, Schultheis B, et al. Enhanced Bcr-Abl-specific antileukemic activity of arsenic trioxide (Trisenox) through glutathione-depletion in imatinib-resistant cells. Haematologica. 2007;92(6):838–41.

275. Cortes-Franco J, Dombret H, Schafhausen P, et al. Danusertib hydrochloride (PHA-739358), a multi-kinase aurora inhibitor, elicits clinical benefit in advanced chronic myeloid leukemia and Philadelphia chromosome positive acute lymphoblastic leukemia. Blood (ASH Annu Meeting Abstr). 2009;114(22):864. http://abstracts.hematologylibrary.org/cgi/content/abstract/ashmtg;114/22/864.

276. Irvine DA, Zhang B, Allan EK, et al. Combination of the hedgehog pathway inhibitor LDE225 and nilotinib eliminates chronic myeloid leukemia stem and progenitor cells. Blood. 2009;114(22):1428. http://abstracts.hematologylibrary.org/cgi/content/abstract/ashmtg;114/22/1428.

277. Van Etten RA, Chan WW, Zaleskas VM, et al. Switch pocket inhibitors of the ABL tyrosine kinase: distinct kinome inhibition profiles and in vivo efficacy in mouse models of CML and

B-lymphoblastic leukemia induced by BCR-ABL T315I. Blood. 2008;112(11):576. http://abstracts.hematologylibrary.org/cgi/content/abstract/ashmtg;112/11/576.

278. Lapenna S, Giordano A. Cell cycle kinases as therapeutic targets for cancer. Nat Rev Drug Discov. 2009;8(7):547–66. doi:10.1038/nrd2907.

279. Zhang J, Adrian FJ, Jahnke W, et al. Targeting Bcr-Abl by combining allosteric with ATP-binding-site inhibitors. Nature. 2010;463(7280):501–6. doi:10.1038/nature08675.

280. O'Brien S, Kantarjian H, Keating M, et al. Homoharringtonine therapy induces responses in patients with chronic myelogenous leukemia in late chronic phase. Blood. 1995;86(9):3322–6.

281. O'Brien S, Kantarjian H, Koller C, et al. Sequential homoharringtonine and interferon-alpha in the treatment of early chronic phase chronic myelogenous leukemia. Blood. 1999;93(12):4149–53. http://bloodjournal.hematologylibrary.org/cgi/content/abstract/bloodjournal;93/12/4149.

282. O'Hare T, Shakespeare WC, Zhu X, et al. AP24534, a pan-BCR-ABL inhibitor for chronic myeloid leukemia, potently inhibits the T315I mutant and overcomes mutation-based resistance. Cancer Cell. 2009;16(5):401–12. doi:10.1016/j.ccr.2009.09.028.

283. Talpaz M, Cortes JE, Deininger MW, et al. Phase I trial of AP24534 in patients with refractory chronic myeloid leukemia (CML) and hematologic malignancies. ASCO Meeting Abstr. 2010;28(15):6511. http://meeting.ascopubs.org/cgi/content/abstract/28/15_suppl/6511.

284. Milojkovic D, Nicholson E, Apperly JF, et al. Early prediction of success or failure of treatment with second-generation tyrosine kinase inhibitors in patients with chronic myeloid leukemia. Haematologica. 2010;95(2):224–231. 10.3324/haematol. 2009.012781.

Chapter 5
Myelodysplastic Syndromes (MDS)

Bart Lee Scott

Abstract The hematopoietic disorders referred to as myelodysplastic syndromes (MDS) are a heterogeneous collection of marrow diseases unified by a similar presentation of peripheral blood cytopenias. The incidence rate of MDS in the USA for 2001–2003 was 3.3/100,000, and the overall 3-year survival for MDS was 45%. The incidence increases with age, and the median age at diagnosis is 70–75 years. Men have a significantly higher incidence rate than women (4.5 vs. 2.7 per 100,000/year). The majority of patients with MDS have macrocytic anemia with or without additional cytopenias present at time of diagnosis.

Keywords Myelodysplastic syndrome • Leukemia • Marrow • Peripheral blood cytopenia • Macrocytic anemia • Cytogenic testing • Hematopoietic disorder • Iron chelation

Introduction

The hematopoietic disorders referred to as myelodysplastic syndromes (MDS) are a heterogeneous collection of marrow diseases unified by a similar presentation of peripheral blood cytopenias. The incidence rate of MDS in the USA for 2001–2003 was 3.3/100,000, and the overall 3-year survival for MDS was 45% [1]. The incidence increases with age, and the median age at diagnosis is 70–75 years. Men have a significantly higher incidence rate than women (4.5 vs. 2.7 per 100,000/year) [2].

B.L. Scott, M.D. (✉)
Clinical Research Division, Fred Hutchinson Cancer Research Center,
1100 Fairview Ave N, D1-100, 98109, Seattle, WA, USA

Department of Medicine, University of Washington Medical Center, Seattle, WA, USA
e-mail: bscott@fhcrc.org

E.H. Estey and F.R. Appelbaum (eds.), *Leukemia and Related Disorders:*
Integrated Treatment Approaches, Contemporary Hematology,
DOI 10.1007/978-1-60761-565-1_5, © Springer Science+Business Media, LLC 2012

The majority of patients with MDS have macrocytic anemia with or without additional cytopenias present at time of diagnosis. The differential diagnosis includes other causes of macrocytic anemia such as vitamin B12 and folate deficiencies, alcohol consumption, and thyroid disorders. Initial laboratory workup includes blood cell counts, serum ferritin levels, total iron binding capacity, serum iron, reticulocyte counts, vitamin B12, RBC folate, and thyroid stimulating hormone levels. Persistent unexplained cytopenias warrant additional investigation with bone marrow aspiration and biopsy including cytogenetic testing and iron stains.

Diagnosis

The diagnosis of MDS is based upon the recently updated World Health Organization (WHO) criteria (Table 5.1) [3]. The WHO diagnostic schema now includes the presence of recurrent cytogenetic abnormalities as presumptive evidence of MDS even in the absence of significant dysplasia (Table 5.2). Other important differences include the incorporation of multilineage dysplasia, which has been shown to impart an inferior prognosis, and the incorporation of isolated deletion of chromosome 5q, which is associated with prolonged life expectancy. The WHO classification is help-

Table 5.1 World Health Organization (WHO) diagnostic classification of myelodysplastic syndromes [3]

Disease	Blood findings	BM findings
Refractory cytopenia with unilineage dysplasia (RCUD): refractory anemia [RA], refractory neutropenia [RN], refractory thrombocytopenia [RT]	Unicytopenia or bicytopenia[a] No or rare blasts (<1%)[b]	Unilineage dyplasia: ≥10% of the cells in one myeloid lineage <5% blasts <15% of erythroid precursors are ring sideroblasts
Refractory anemia with ring sideroblasts (RARS)	Anemia No blasts	≥15% of erythroid precursors are ring sideroblasts Erythroid dysplasia only <5% blasts
Refractory cytopenia with multilineage dysplasia (RCMD)	Cytopenia(s) No or rare blasts (<1%)[b] No Auer rod <1 × 10⁹/L monocytes	Dysplasia in ≥10% of the cells in ≥2 myeloid lineages (neutrophil and/or erythroid precursors and/or megakaryocytes) <5% blasts in marrow No Auer rods ± 15% ring sideroblasts

(continued)

Table 5.1 (continued)

Disease	Blood findings	BM findings
Refractory anemia with excess blasts-1 (RAEB-1)	Cytopenia(s) <5% blasts[b] No Auer rods <1 × 10⁹/L monocytes	Unilineage or multilineage dysplasia 5–9% blasts[b] No Auer rods
Refractory anemia with excess blasts-2 (RAEB-2)	Cytopenia(s) 5–19% blasts[c] Auer rods ±[c] <1 × 10⁹/L monocytes	Unilineage or multilineage dysplasia 10–19% blasts[c] Auer rods ±[c]
Myelodysplastic syndrome – unclassified (MDS-U)	Cytopenias <1% blasts[b]	Unequivocal dysplasia in <10% of cells in 1 or more myeloid lineages when accompanied by a cytogenic abnormality considered as presumptive evidence for diagnosis of MDS <5% blasts
MDS associated with isolated del (5q)	Anemia. Usually normal or increased platelet No or rare blasts (<1%)	Normal to increased megakaryocytes with hypolobulated nuclei <5% blasts Isolated del (5q) cytogenic abnormality No Auer rods

[a]Bicytopenia may occasionally be observed. Cases with pancytopenia should be classified as MDS-U

[b]If the marrow myeloblast percentage is <5%, but there are 2–4% myeloblasts in the blood, the diagnostic classification is RAEB-1. Cases of RCUD and RCMD with 1% myeloblasts in the blood should be classified as MDS-U

[c]Cases with Auer rods and <5% myeloblasts in the blood and less than 10% in the marrow should be classified as RAEB-2. Although the finding of 5–19% blasts in the blood is, in itself, diagnostic of RAEB-2, cases of RAEB-2 may have <5% blasts in the blood if they have Auer rods or 10–19% blasts in the marrow or both. Similarly, cases of RAEB-2 may have <10% blasts in the marrow but may be diagnosed by the other 2 findings, Auer rod + and/or 5–19% blasts in the blood

Table 5.2 Recurrent chromosomal abnormalities considered sufficient for a presumptive diagnosis of MDS even in the absence of significant dysplasia

Unbalanced abnormalities	Balanced abnormalities
−7 or del(7q)	T(11;16)(q23;p13.3)
−5 or del(5q)	T(3;21)(q26.2;q22.1)
i(17q) or t(17p)	T(1;3)(p36.3;q21.1)
−13 or del(13q)	T(2;11)(p21;q23)
del(11q)	inv(3)(q31 q26.2)
del(12q) or t(12p)	t(6;9)(p23;q34)
del(9q)	
Idic(X) (q13)	

Complex karyotype (3 or more chromosomal abnormalities) involving one or more of the above abnormalities

ful for both prognostication [4] and in selection of therapy [5]. Despite advancements in classification schemata, there is often discordance among pathologists in diagnosing lesser degrees of dysplasia, and the diagnosis may be delayed for months following initial presentation.

Prognosis

The international prognostic scoring system (IPSS) was developed on the basis of findings in 816 patients with primary MDS [6]. Marrow myeloblast percentage, cytogenetic status, and number of low blood cell counts offered prognostic information (Table 5.3). The IPSS divided patients into four risk groups (low, intermediate-1, intermediate-2, and high) and reliably discriminated between these groups in regards to expected survival and AML progression (Fig. 5.1). Limitations of the IPSS are the exclusion of patients with secondary MDS and the inability to estimate the real-time risk as only variables present at the time of diagnosis were included in the analysis. Transfusion burden and high ferritin levels have also been associated with inferior survival in MDS patients [7]. On the basis of this finding, a new prognostic system, termed WHO classification-based prognostic scoring system (WPSS), incorporated the WHO classification, transfusion dependence, and IPSS cytogenetic status (Table 5.4) [9]. Again, patients with secondary MDS were excluded from the WPSS, and the impact of cytogenetics may be underestimated in this classification [8]. The advantage of the WPSS is that it provides a real-time assessment of prognosis (Fig. 5.2). The WPSS has been validated in an external data base and subsequently been shown to offer an advantage over IPSS particularly in patients considered to have low-risk MDS [10, 11]. Low platelet counts, high ferritin levels, elevated β2-microglobulin levels, elevated LDH, and presence of marrow fibrosis are also associated with inferior survival [12–14]. A validated flow cytometric scoring system (FCSS) adds information regarding prognosis particularly in patients who are otherwise thought to be low risk [15, 16]. Flow cytometry may be helpful with both diagnosis and prognosis, particularly in patients with minimal evidence of dysplasia by morphology.

Table 5.3 IPSS classification criteria [7]

	Score value				
Prognostic variable	0	0.5	1.0	1.5	2.0
BM blasts (%)	<5	5–10	–	11–20	21–30
Karyotype[a]	Good	Intermediate	Poor		
Cytopenias	0/1	2/3			

Score for risk groups are as follows: low, 0; int-1, 0.5–1.0; int-2, 1.5–2.0; and high, ≥2.5
[a]Good, normal, -Y, del(5q), del(20q); poor, complex (≥3 abnormalities or chromosome 7 anomalies); intermediate, other abnormalities

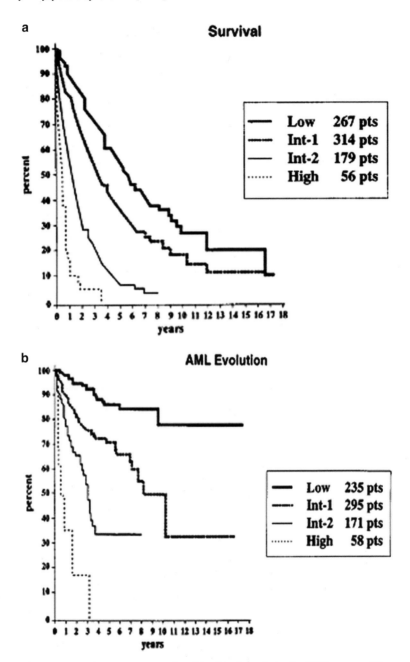

Fig. 5.1 (**a**) Survival by IPSS category. (**b**) Risk of AML evolution by IPSS category [7]

Table 5.4 WPSS prognostic system [8]

Variable	0	1	2	3
WHO category	RA, RARS, 5q-	RCMD, RCMD-RS	RAEB-1	RAEB-2
Karyotype[a]	Good	Intermediate	Poor	–
Transfusion requirement[b]	No	Regular	–	–

Note: Risk groups were as follows: very low score (score = 0), low (score = 1), intermediate (score = 2), high (score = 3–4), and very high score (score = 5–6). *MDS* myelodysplastic syndrome, *RA* refractory anemia, *RARS* refractory anemia with ringed sideroblasts, *5q-* myelodysplastic syndrome with isolated del (5q) and marrow blasts less than 5%, *RCMD* refractory cytopenia with multilineage dysplasia, *RCMD-RS* refractory cytopenia with multilineage dysplasia and ringed sideroblasts, *RAEB-1* refractory anemia with excess of blasts-1, *RAEB-2* refractory anemia with excess of blasts-2

[a]Karyotype was as follows: good: normal, -Y, del (5q), del (20q); poor: complex (≥3 abnormalities, chromosome 7 anomalies); and intermediate: other abnormalities

[b]RBC transfusion dependency was defined as having at least one RBC transfusion every 8 weeks over a period of 4 months

Treatment of MDS

MDS comprises a disparate group of disorders with impaired hematopoiesis, variable prognosis, and likely multiple pathogenic causes. Therefore, there is no routine method of care for all patients with MDS. The appropriate therapeutic choices are influenced by patient-related factors (preference, performance status, age, and cost) as well as disease-related factors (cytogenetic status, decline of peripheral cytopenias, bone marrow myeloblast count).

Supportive Care

Patients with low-risk disease and stable blood counts who are asymptomatic may not require any treatment. A review of a national MDS registry found that the majority of patients with MDS receive supportive therapy and relatively few receive more aggressive therapy [17]. We recommend that asymptomatic patients with low-risk disease have yearly marrow evaluations and, at least initially, monthly blood cell counts. Patients who have symptomatic cytopenias with coexisting medical illnesses that would prevent compliance with therapy may benefit from limited transfusion support and antibiotics (as indicated). There is no single hemoglobin cutoff at which red blood cell (RBC) transfusion support should be offered to patients. Rather, decisions regarding RBC transfusions should be made on an individual basis in accordance with the patients' self assessment. At our center, we offer platelet transfusions when the platelet count is <10,000/μL, but do adjust this practice on the basis of individual risk factors and bleeding tendencies. MDS are associated with decreased production and abnormal function of cells, and patients may have symptoms which appear to be out of proportion to the level of cytopenia [18, 19].

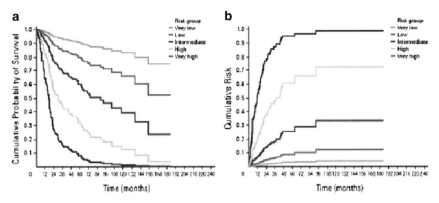

Fig. 5.2 (**a**) Survival and (**b**) risk of AML by WPSS in the German cohort by time-dependent analysis [8]

Iron Chelation

Iron chelation remains a controversial topic in MDS. While increased ferritin levels are associated with inferior survival [7], it is not clear that reduction in ferritin leads to improved survival. Cohort studies have demonstrated improved survival in patients who received iron chelation [20, 21]. However, there likely was a selection bias operating in these cohort studies since many patients were selected to receive iron chelation because they were expected to have a longer life expectancy. The current NCCN (National Cancer Center Network) guidelines recommend considering iron chelation in patients who have received >20–30 U of RBC transfusions with low- or int-1-risk disease (or who have reached ferritin levels of >2,500 ng/mL) and in potential stem cell transplant candidates. Since complications from iron overload may take years to develop, some experts argue that patients with short life expectancies (<1 year) are unlikely to benefit from iron chelation. Deferasirox (Exjade®) is FDA-approved for chronic iron overload due to RBC transfusions in patients who are older than 2 years. In patients who receive deferasirox, it is important to assess kidney and liver function monthly as nephrotoxicity and hepatotoxicity have been described in postmarketing surveillance reports. Auditory and ophthalmic disturbances have been reported <1% with deferasirox, and testing is recommended prior to and yearly in patients receiving deferasirox.

Hematopoietic Stimulating Agents

Granulocyte colony-stimulating factor (GCSF) may be useful in neutropenic patients with recurrent or resistant infections, but there are no data to support chronic use or use for routine infection prophylaxis [22]. Therefore, we typically only offer patients GCSF during period of active infection or in combination with erythroid stimulating agents (ESA), as discussed below [23].

Table 5.5 Predictive model for response to ESAs in MDS [24]

Patient criteria	Probability of response (%)
Transfusion need <2 U/month and serum EPO <500 U/L	74
Only one of the above criteria	23
Neither criteria	7

Although ESA are not FDA-approved for MDS, they are the most commonly used agents to treat patients with MDS [17]. A validated decision model uses baseline erythropoietin levels and previous RBC transfusion requirements to predict the probability of response to ESA (Table 5.5) [25]. ESA are most effective for low- or int-1-risk MDS patients with <5% myeloblasts [24, 26]. A phase III randomized, placebo-controlled study did not show a statistically significant improvement in hemoglobin values or reduction in RBC transfusion requirements with ESA + granulocyte-macrophage colony-stimulating factor (GMCSF) [23]; however, there were only 37 patients with an erythropoietin level of less than 500 mU/mL included. Therefore, the lack of significant improvement with ESA + GCSF is likely a reflection of the low power to detect a benefit rather than an absence of benefit. Another phase III randomized study in 110 patients with MDS did show significant improvements in hemoglobin levels and reduction in RBC transfusion requirements in patients treated with erythropoietin (EPO) at 150 U/kg/day (34% vs. 5.8%, $p = 0.001$) [27]. If patients did not respond to EPO, then GCSF at 1 μg/kg/day was added, and if there was no response to the addition of GCSF, then the dose of EPO was increased to 300 U/kg/day. After 4 months of treatment, this study allowed crossover from the placebo arm to the active treatment arm. There were no differences in overall survival or rate of leukemic transformation between the placebo and EPO treatment arms; however, any long-term interpretation of results is obviously impaired by the crossover design. Interestingly, 22% of subjects responded to the addition of GCSF to the EPO. Recently, two separate groups performed retrospective analyses comparing results in patients with MDS treated with ESA to MDS patients who received no treatment. These studies suggested a survival benefit in patients treated with ESA [26, 28]. The primary weaknesses of these analyses are the retrospective nature and the potential lack of comparability between the cohorts. This is highlighted by a previous retrospective study, which found no survival benefit when comparing ESA-treated patients to untreated patients [24]. Despite these conflicting results, we typically use ESA as first line therapy in patients who have symptomatic anemia with a low transfusion requirement, low serum erythropoietin level (≤500 mU/mL), and who do not have deletion 5q and are not candidates for clinical trials. The recommended dose of EPO is 40,000–60,000 U 1–3 times/week, and the recommended dose of darbopoietin is 150–300 mcg/week. Patients should receive ESA for at least 8 weeks before a decision is made regarding effectiveness. Whether or not GCSF adds anything to treatment with ESA alone remains controversial [26, 29]. At our center, we do not routinely combine GCSF with ESA.

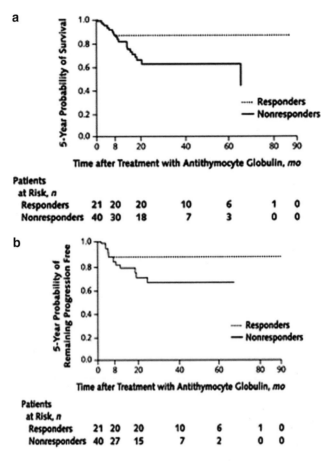

Fig. 5.3 (**a**) Overall survival and (**b**) progression-free duration in responders vs. nonresponders to ATG [31]

Antithymocyte Globulin (ATG)

In a phase II study, 61 patients with RBC transfusion dependent MDS received horse ATG, ATGAM® 40 mg/kg/day for 4 days [30]. Twenty-one (34%) became transfusion independent with a median time to response of 10 weeks. ATG responders had a longer survival and a lower risk of disease progression than nonresponders (Fig. 5.3). Younger age, presence of HLA-DR 15, and a shorter duration of RBC transfusion dependence was associated with response to ATG [31]. Other centers report that bone marrow hypocellularity and low IPSS scores are associated with response to ATG therapy [32]. In a randomized phase II study, horse ATG 15 mg/kg/day for 5 days was compared to rabbit ATG (Thymoglobulin®) 3.75 mg/kg/day for 5 days in MDS patients with clinically significant cytopenias [33]. There was no difference in response rates (42%). Recently, NHLBI investigators retrospectively compared patients treated with ATG to patients who received no therapy and showed that patients who received ATG were at a lower risk of dying (hazard rate (HR) 0.5, $p=0.002$) and a lower risk of progression to AML (HR 0.45, $p=0.092$) [34]. This analysis compared patients from different time periods and from different centers which may have influenced the findings. Trials at our center suggest that combining ATG with a short course of the soluble TNF receptor etanercept enhances the response rate [35].

Lenalidomide (Revlimid®)

Lenalidomide, a derivative of thalidomide, has a broad spectrum of effects, including immunomodulation [36]. It is FDA-approved for MDS patients with low- or int-1-risk disease by IPSS with associated deletion of 5q and who are transfusion dependent. In a multicenter phase II study, MDS patients with del (5q) were treated with 10 mg/day of lenalidomide given orally [37]. Patients with an absolute neutrophil count of less than 500/μL and a platelet count less than 50,000/μL were excluded. One hundred forty-eight patients were treated for 24 weeks, at which point disease assessment occurred with bone marrow aspiration, biopsy, and cytogenetic evaluation. The primary endpoint of the study was transfusion independence. The chief toxicities were neutropenia and thrombocytopenia; in fact, 79% of patients enrolled in this study required dose reductions secondary to hematopoietic toxicity. Thus, patients should have weekly blood counts for the first 8 weeks following initiation of lenalidomide. Among the 148 patients enrolled, 112 had reduced transfusion requirements, and 99 (67%) became transfusion independent with a median response time of 4.6 weeks. However, patients should be treated for at least 12 weeks before making a decision regarding effectiveness or lack thereof. The median duration of transfusion independence was not reached at the time of publication (Fig. 5.4), but a recent update shows a median duration of 2.2 years. In a simultaneous multicenter phase II study, 214 transfusion-dependent MDS patients with low- or int-1-risk MDS without del (5q) were treated with lenalidomide at 10 mg/day [38]. The most commonly observed grade 3 or 4 adverse events were thrombocytopenia (25%) and neutropenia (30%). Fifty-six patients (26%) achieved transfusion independence after a median of 4.8 weeks of treatment for a median duration of transfusion independence of 41 weeks. The use of lenalidomide in more advanced stages of MDS, such as patients with ≥10% myeloblasts, is an area of ongoing investigation. In a phase II study, 47 patients with int-2- or high-risk MDS and deletion 5q were treated with 10 mg/day of lenalidomide. Twenty-seven percent of patients achieved hematologic responses including seven complete remissions [39]. While lenalidomide has been shown to improve RBC transfusion requirements in MDS, there is no data to suggest it has any impact on survival.

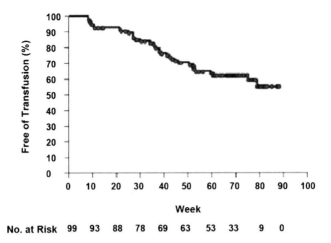

Fig. 5.4 Duration of transfusion independence in patients who responded to lenalidomide [38]

Azacitidine (Vidaza®)

The DNA methyltransferase inhibitor azacitidine was FDA-approved for all IPSS categories and all FAB subtypes of MDS, essentially based on a phase III multicenter trial which randomized 191 patients to receive azacitidine (75 mg/m²/day × 7 days every 28 days) or supportive care (transfusions and antibiotics) [40, 41]. The overall response rate was 60%, with 7% achieving complete remissions and 16% partial remissions. The major limitation of the study was the option for crossover, and approximately half of the patients (n = 49) initially randomized to supportive care crossed over to azacitidine within 6 months of enrollment. The study did not show a difference in overall survival; however, a landmark analysis showed a survival benefit with azacitidine when patients who crossed over to azacitidine prior to 6 months were excluded from the analysis (median survival 11 months vs. 18 months, p = 0.03). The major toxicity was myelosuppression with grades 3 or 4 granulocytopenia in 43% and thrombocytopenia in 52%. The median time to response was 64 days, and the median duration of response was 15 months. These results were confirmed in a phase III randomized study comparing azacitidine (75 mg/m²/day × 7 days every 28 days) to conventional care regimens (CCR) in 358 patients with int-2- or high-risk MDS as defined by IPSS and FAB [42]. The choices among CCR were best supportive care (transfusion, antibiotics, GCSF), low-dose cytarabine (20 mg/m²/day sc × 14 days every 28 days), or intensive chemotherapy (cytarabine 100–200 mg/m²/day × 7 days + anthracycline × 3 days). The study was unique in that selection of the three choices of CCR occurred before randomization. Two hundred twenty-two patients were selected for best supportive care, 94 patients for low-dose cytarabine, and 42 patients for intensive chemotherapy. All patients were subsequently randomized to receive either azacitidine or CCR. The median overall survival was 24.5 months in the azacitidine-treated patients compared to

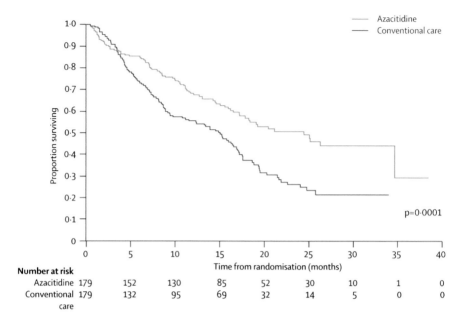

Fig. 5.5 Probability of overall survival azacitidine vs. supportive care [42]

15 months in the CCR-treated patients (Fig. 5.5). The hazard ratio for mortality was 0.58 (95% CI 0.43–0.77; $p=0.0001$) among the azacitidine-treated patients compared to CCR-treated patients. Time to leukemia progression was longer in the azacitidine arm, but there was no difference in time to leukemia progression in patients selected to receive low-dose cytarabine or intensive chemotherapy. The most common adverse event in all treatment groups was myelosuppression. Infection rates were significantly lower in patients who received azacitidine compared to patients who received CCR (relative risk 0.66, 95% CI 0.49–0.87, $p=0.0032$). Patients were to receive at least six cycles of azacitidine prior to deciding effectiveness/ineffectiveness. Blood cell counts may initially decline with azacitidine, particularly during the first two cycles, before an improvement in counts is observed.

Decitabine (Dacogen®)

Decitabine (differing from azacitidine only by a hydroxy group in the sugar moiety) is FDA-approved for int-1-, int-2-, and high-risk MDS patients of all FAB subtypes. In a phase III multicenter trial, 170 patients with MDS were randomized to decitabine (15 mg/m^2 every 8 h for 3 days every 6 weeks) or supportive care (transfusions, antibiotics, and growth factors) [43]. The overall response rate with decitabine was 17%, with 9% complete remissions and 13% hematologic improvements.

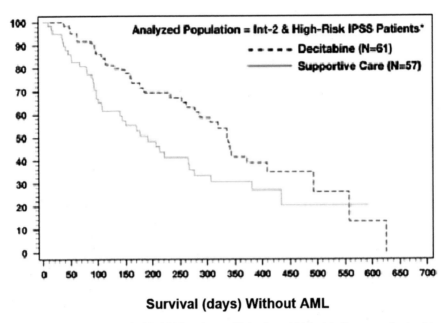

Fig. 5.6 Disease-free survival in MDS patients with int-2- and high-risk disease randomized to decitabine vs. supportive care [43]

Patients who received decitabine showed a trend toward delay in progression to AML or death (median 12.1 vs. 7.8 months, $p = 0.16$).This trend was significant in patients with int-2- or high-risk disease (median 12.6 vs. 9.4 months, $p = 0.03$) (Fig. 5.6). However, there was no difference between decitabine and supportive care in overall survival. A subsequent study randomized 95 MDS patients with int-1-, int-2-, or high-risk disease to decitabine 20 mg/m^2/day IV for 5 days, decitabine 20 mg/m^2/day subcutaneously for 5 days, or decitabine 10 mg/m^2/day IV for 10 days [44]. Notably, the FDA-approved dose was not included in this analysis. A Bayesian design was used for this protocol, allowing for adaptive randomization with a prior pretest probability distributed equally among the three regimens. Sixty-four patients received 20 mg/m^2/day IV for 5 day, 14 received 20 mg/m^2/day sc for 5 days, and 17 received 10 mg/m^2/day IV for 10 days. Decitabine 20 mg/m^2/day IV for 5 days was the optimal regimen with a complete remission rate of 39% vs. 21% vs. 24% ($p < 0.05$), respectively. Preliminary results of a randomized phase III trial comparing decitabine (15 mg/m^2 3 times a day for 3 days every 6 weeks) to best supportive care in 223 patients with advanced MDS or CMML(chronic myelomonocytic leukemia) were recently presented [45]. There was no significant difference in survival between the decitabine and supportive care arms. A major problem with this study was the discontinuation of decitabine already after two cycles following best response. Some critiques have also argued that the dose selected for the decitabine arm was not the optimal dose.

Intensive Chemotherapy

Very few published studies evaluating intensive chemotherapy are focused solely on MDS. Rather, most publications have evaluated AML and "high-risk" MDS together with variable definitions of "high-risk" MDS not based upon IPSS. Therefore, it is difficult to evaluate intensive chemotherapy in patients with MDS based upon published data. Investigators at M.D. Anderson Cancer Center have published data suggesting that topotecan-based chemotherapy may be preferable to other alternatives in patients with MDS [46]. In a retrospective analysis, 77 patients received topotecan-cytarabine, 270 idarubicin-cytarabine, 67 topotecan-cytarabine and cyclophosphamide, and 96 fludarabine-cytarabine. Topotecan-cytarabine regimens were equivalent to idarubicin-cytarabine regimens in regards to complete remission and survival rates but were associated with lower induction mortality rates.

An important current issue is how the introduction of hypomethylating agents affects the use of more conventional options of intensive chemotherapy. Proponents of hypomethylating agents argue that those have a lower toxicity profile and allow patients to receive therapy on an outpatient basis and that the lower complete remission rates do not necessarily translate into lower survival rates. This may be particularly relevant for older MDS patients who are at higher risk of morbidity (and mortality) from intensive chemotherapy. To date, there has been no prospective randomized study evaluating hypomethylating agents against intensive chemotherapy. However, a retrospective matched-cohort analysis indicated a survival advantage with decitabine ($n = 115$) in comparison to intensive chemotherapy ($n = 115$) (median survival 22 months vs. 12 months, $p < 0.001$) [47]. Matching parameters included age, chromosomal abnormalities, and IPSS risk group. The major limitation of this analysis was the retrospective nature and the lack of comparable time periods of treatment (2001–2003 for the decitabine cohort and 1995 and later for the intensive chemotherapy cohort). Another limitation was the use of a variety of regimens (topotecan, clofarabine, fludarabine, anthracyclines, etc.) in the intensive chemotherapy cohort. Despite these limitations, this study was the first attempt to address an emerging issue in the treatment of MDS patients. As discussed earlier, azacitidine has been compared to intensive chemotherapy in patients with int-2- or high-risk MDS including patients with RAEB-T, as defined by FAB [42]. In this subset analysis, there was no difference in overall survival between patients who received azacitidine ($n = 17$) or intensive chemotherapy ($n = 25$). There were very few subjects selected to receive intensive chemotherapy in this trial. At our center, we tend to use intensive chemotherapy regimens in MDS patients with >10% marrow myeloblasts who are candidates for stem cell transplantation.

Hematopoietic Cell Transplantation (HCT)

HCT has curative potential for patients with MDS (Fig. 5.7) [48]. Unfortunately, many patients with MDS are not eligible for HCT because of a lack of donor availability or because of advanced comorbidity scores [49]. The major limitation of

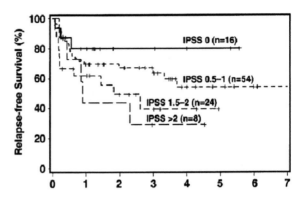

Fig. 5.7 Relapse-free survival by IPSS category following HCT [48]

HCT is the upfront treatment-related mortality which may be as high as 30% depending upon patient and donor specific factors. Since patients with low- or int-1-risk MDS may have life expectancies of many years without disease progression, some experts question the utility of HCT in MDS patients who historically have been considered "good risk." A multicenter retrospective analysis used a Markov decision model to evaluate the optimal timing of HCT for MDS patients [50]. This analysis suggested that low- or int-1-risk MDS patients did benefit, i.e., had longer life expectancy if HCT was delayed, whereas int-2- or high-risk MDS patients had the best outlook (i.e., longest life expectancy) if transplanted soon after diagnosis (Fig. 5.8). Reduced-intensity conditioning (RIC) regimens represent an emerging issue in the field of HCT. RIC regimens are less toxic but also have a higher relapse risk than more intensive regimens [51]. Retrospective analyses comparing conventional regimens to RIC regimens show no difference in survival [52]; however, no controlled prospective data are available.

Patients with secondary MDS are typically thought to have an inferior outcome as compared to patients with primary MDS and as such may particularly benefit from HCT. We observed in a recent analysis that patients with secondary MDS, unexpectedly, had a posttransplant prognosis comparable to patients with de novo MDS once the data were adjusted for cytogenetic risk [53]. Thus, the increased risk of posttransplant relapse historically seen in patients with secondary MDS was mainly due to the presence of poor risk cytogenetics. In addition to poor risk cytogenetic features, IPSS, WPSS, and WHO classification are associated with posttransplant outcomes [54]. Additional factors such as the presence of marrow fibrosis [55], elevated serum ferritin levels [56, 57], and pretransplant neutropenia [58] were found to negatively impact posttransplant outcomes.

Another topical issue in the field of HCT for MDS is the role of pretransplant induction chemotherapy. It is unclear whether patients with MDS benefit from cytoreductive given prior to conditioning for HCT with conventional high-dose regimens [59], although available data indicate that reduction of the tumor burden before transplantation is associated with improved outcome in patients conditioned with RIC regimens. In fact, we have speculated that in patients who are to be transplanted following RIC, pretransplant chemotherapy may improve outcome

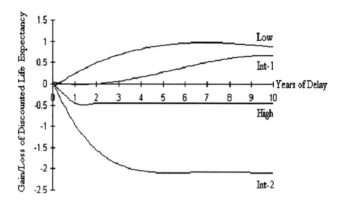

Fig. 5.8 Gain vs. loss in life expectancy with delay in HCT by IPSS category [50]

even in patients with "low-risk" MDS [52]. In any event, an overall management plan that incorporates the possibility of HCT should be developed for patients with MDS at the time of diagnosis.

Summary

Although advancements have been made in the therapy of MDS, there is still more work to be done. Among the currently FDA-approved agents for MDS, only one has been shown to improve survival and only on the order of approximately 9 months. Patients will be pleased but are not likely to be thrilled by this information. It is clear that treatment advances can only occur through carefully conducted, rigorously designed clinical trials. We are at a quandary at how we can improve accrual into clinical trials in MDS. There certainly does appear to be a "no treatment" bias in MDS, likely related to the advanced age of patients at the time of diagnosis. Treatments do not necessarily have to be toxic and, indeed, they may improve the quality of life of patients and extend their survival. At our center, we make a valid attempt to enroll all patients with MDS into clinical studies as we do not believe any current therapy should be considered the standard of care.

Acknowledgment Supported in part by grants HL084054, HL036444, and HL082941 from the National Institutes of Health, Bethesda, MD.

Disclosure Statement Bart Scott has served as a consultant for Novartis, Alexion, and Celgene.

References

1. Rollison DE, Howlader N, Smith MT, et al. Epidemiology of myelodysplastic syndromes and chronic myeloproliferative disorders in the United States, 2001–2004, using data from the NAACCR and SEER programs. Blood. 2008;112(1):45–52.

2. Ma X, Does M, Raza A, Mayne ST. Myelodysplastic syndromes: incidence and survival in the United States. Cancer. 2007;109(8):1538–42.
3. Vardiman JW, Thiele J, Arber DA, et al. The 2008 revision of the World Health Organization (WHO) classification of myeloid neoplasms and acute leukemia: rationale and important changes. Blood. 2009;114(5):937–51.
4. Malcovati L, Porta MG, Pascutto C, et al. Prognostic factors and life expectancy in myelodysplastic syndromes classified according to WHO criteria: a basis for clinical decision making. J Clin Oncol. 2005;23(30):7594–603.
5. Howe RB, Porwit-MacDonald A, Wanat R, Tehranchi R, Hellstrom-Lindberg E. The WHO classification of MDS does make a difference. Blood. 2004;103(9):3265–70.
6. Greenberg P, Cox C, LeBeau MM, et al. International scoring system for evaluating prognosis in myelodysplastic syndromes [erratum appears in Blood 1998 Feb 1;91(3):1100]. Blood. 1997;89(6):2079–88.
7. Malcovati L, Della Porta MG, Cazzola M. Predicting survival and leukemia evolution in patients with myelodysplastic syndrome. Haematologica. 2006;91(12):1588–90.
8. Haase D, Germing U, Schanz J, et al. New insights into the prognostic impact of the karyotype in MDS and correlation with subtypes: evidence from a core dataset of 2124 patients. Blood. 2007;110(13):4385–95.
9. Malcovati L, Germing U, Kuendgen A, et al. Time-dependent prognostic scoring system for predicting survival and leukemic evolution in myelodysplastic syndromes. J Clin Oncol. 2007;25(23):3503–10.
10. Kuendgen A, Gattermann N, Germing U. Improving the prognostic evaluation of patients with lower risk myelodysplastic syndromes. Leukemia. 2009;23(1):182–4.
11. Park MJ, Kim HJ, Kim SH, et al. Is International Prognostic Scoring System (IPSS) still standard in predicting prognosis in patients with myelodysplastic syndrome? External validation of the WHO Classification-Based Prognostic Scoring System (WPSS) and comparison with IPSS. Eur J Haematol. 2008;81(5):364–73.
12. Garcia-Manero G, Shan J, Faderl S, et al. A prognostic score for patients with lower risk myelodysplastic syndrome. Leukemia. 2008;22(3):538–43.
13. Buesche G, Teoman H, Wilczak W, et al. Marrow fibrosis predicts early fatal marrow failure in patients with myelodysplastic syndromes. Leukemia. 2008;22(2):313–22.
14. Germing U, Hildebrandt B, Pfeilstocker M, et al. Refinement of the international prognostic scoring system (IPSS) by including LDH as an additional prognostic variable to improve risk assessment in patients with primary myelodysplastic syndromes (MDS). Leukemia. 2005;19(12):2223–31.
15. Scott BL, Wells DA, Loken MR, Myerson D, Leisenring WM, Deeg HJ. Validation of a flow cytometric scoring system as a prognostic indicator for posttransplantation outcome in patients with myelodysplastic syndrome. Blood. 2008;112(7):2681–6.
16. van de Loosdrecht AA, Westers TM, Westra AH, Dräger AM, van der Velden VHJ, Ossenkoppele GJ. Identification of distinct prognostic subgroups in low- and intermediate-1-risk myelodysplastic syndromes by flow cytometry. Blood. 2008;111(3):1067–77.
17. Van Bennekom CM, Abel G, Anderson T, Stone RM, Kaufman DW. Patterns of treatment among patients with recently-diagnosed myelodysplastic syndromes in a national registry, 2006-2008. Blood. 2008;112(11):324, 324, #876. 11-16-2008. Ref Type: Abstract.
18. Yamaguchi N, Ito Y, Ohyashiki K. Increased intracellular activity of matrix metalloproteinases in neutrophils may be associated with delayed healing of infection without neutropenia in myelodysplastic syndromes. Ann Hematol. 2005;84(6):383–8.
19. Zeidman A, Sokolover N, Fradin Z, Cohen A, Redlich O, Mittelman M. Platelet function and its clinical significance in the myelodysplastic syndromes. Hematol J. 2004;5(3):234–8.
20. Rose C, Brechignac S, Vassilieff D, Beyne-Rauzy O, Stamatoulla A, Larbaa D, et al. Positive impact of iron chelation therapy (CT) in survival in regularly transfused MDS patients. A prospective analysis by the GFM. Blood. 2007;110((Part 1) [11]):80a–1, #249. 11-16-2007. Ref Type: Abstract.
21. Leitch HA, Leger CS, Goodman TA, et al. Improved survival in patients with myelodysplastic syndrome receiving iron chelation therapy. Clin Leuk. 2008;2(3):205–11.

22. Negrin RS, Haeuber DH, Nagler A, et al. Treatment of myelodysplastic syndromes with recombinant human granulocyte colony-stimulating factor. A phase I-II trial. Ann Intern Med. 1989;110(12):976–84.

23. Thompson JA, Gilliland DG, Prchal JT, et al. Effect of recombinant human erythropoietin combined with granulocyte/ macrophage colony-stimulating factor in the treatment of patients with myelodysplastic syndrome. Blood. 2000;95(4):1175–9.

24. Jädersten M, Montgomery SM, Dybedal I, Porwit-MacDonald A, Hellström-Lindberg E. Long-term outcome of treatment of anemia in MDS with erythropoietin and G-CSF. Blood. 2005;106(3):803–11.

25. Hellstrom-Lindberg E, Gulbrandsen N, Lindberg G, et al. A validated decision model for treating the anaemia of myelodysplastic syndromes with erythropoietin + granulocyte colony-stimulating factor: significant effects on quality of life. Br J Haematol. 2003;120(6):1037–46.

26. Park S, Grabar S, Kelaidi C, et al. Predictive factors of response and survival in myelodysplastic syndrome treated with erythropoietin and G-CSF: the GFM experience. Blood. 2008;111(2):574–82.

27. Greenberg PL, Sun Z, Miller KB, et al. Treatment of myelodysplastic syndrome patients with erythropoietin with or without granulocyte colony-stimulating factor: results of a prospective randomized phase 3 trial by the Eastern Cooperative Oncology Group (E1996). Blood. 2009;114(12):2393–400.

28. Jädersten M, Malcovati L, Dybedal I, et al. Erythropoietin and granulocyte-colony stimulating factor treatment associated with improved survival in myelodysplastic syndrome. J Clin Oncol. 2008;26(21):3607–13.

29. Hellstrom-Lindberg E, Ahlgren T, Beguin Y, et al. Treatment of anemia in myelodysplastic syndromes with granulocyte colony-stimulating factor plus erythropoietin: results from a randomized phase II study and long-term follow-up of 71 patients. Blood. 1998;92(1):68–75.

30. Molldrem JJ, Leifer E, Bahceci E, et al. Antithymocyte globulin for treatment of the bone marrow failure associated with myelodysplastic syndrome [summary for patients in Ann Intern Med. 2002 Aug 6;137(3):I-27]. Ann Intern Med. 2002;137(3):156–63.

31. Saunthararajah Y, Nakamura R, Wesley R, Wang QJ, Barrett AJ. A simple method to predict response to immunosuppressive therapy in patients with myelodysplastic syndrome. Blood. 2003;102(8):3025–7.

32. Lim ZY, Killick S, Germing U, et al. Low IPSS score and bone marrow hypocellularity in MDS patients predict hematological responses to antithymocyte globulin. Leukemia. 2007;21(7):1436–41.

33. Stadler M, Germing U, Kliche KO, et al. A prospective, randomised, phase II study of horse antithymocyte globulin vs. rabbit antithymocyte globulin as immune-modulating therapy in patients with low-risk myelodysplastic syndromes. Leukemia. 2004;18(3):460–5.

34. Sloand EM, Wu CO, Greenberg P, Young N, Barrett J. Factors affecting response and survival in patients with myelodysplasia treated with immunosuppressive therapy. J Clin Oncol. 2008;26(15):2505–11.

35. Deeg HJ, Jiang PYZ, Holmberg LA, Scott B, Petersdorf EW, Appelbaum FR. Hematologic responses of patients with MDS to antithymocyte globulin plus etanercept correlate with improved flow scores of marrow cells. Leuk Res. 2004;28:1177–80.

36. Richardson PG, Schlossman RL, Weller E, et al. Immunomodulatory drug CC-5013 overcomes drug resistance and is well tolerated in patients with relapsed multiple myeloma. Blood. 2002;100(9):3063–7.

37. List A, Dewald G, Bennett J, et al. Lenalidomide in the myelodysplastic syndrome with chromosome 5q deletion. N Engl J Med. 2006;355(14):1456–65.

38. Raza A, Reeves JA, Feldman EJ, et al. Phase 2 study of lenalidomide in transfusion-dependent, low-risk, and intermediate-1-risk myelodysplastic syndromes with karyotypes other than deletion 5q. Blood. 2008;111(1):86–93.

39. Adès L, Boehrer S, Prebet T, et al. Efficacy and safety of lenalidomide in intermediate-2 or high-risk myelodysplastic syndromes with 5q deletion: results of a phase 2 study [see comment]. Blood. 2009;113(17):3947–52.

40. Silverman LR, Demakos EP, Peterson BL, et al. Randomized controlled trial of azacitidine in patients with the myelodysplastic syndrome: a study of the cancer and leukemia group B. J Clin Oncol. 2002;20(10):2429–40.

41. Silverman LR, McKenzie DR, Peterson BL, et al. Further analysis of trials with azacitidine in patients with myelodysplastic syndrome: studies 8421, 8921, and 9221 by the Cancer and Leukemia Group B. J Clin Oncol. 2006;24(24):3895–903.

42. Fenaux P, Mufti GJ, Hellstrom-Lindberg E, et al. Efficacy of azacitidine compared with that of conventional care regimens in the treatment of higher-risk myelodysplastic syndromes: a randomised, open-label, phase III study. Lancet Oncol. 2009;10(3):223–32.

43. Kantarjian H, Issa JP, Rosenfeld CS, et al. Decitabine improves patient outcomes in myelodysplastic syndromes: results of a phase III randomized study. Cancer. 2006;106(8):1794–803.

44. Kantarjian H, Oki Y, Garcia-Manero G, et al. Results of a randomized study of 3 schedules of low-dose decitabine in higher-risk myelodysplastic syndrome and chronic myelomonocytic leukemia. Blood. 2007;109(1):52–7.

45. Wijermans P, Suciu S, Baila L, Platzbecker U, Giagounidis A, Selleslag D, et al. Low dose decitabine versus best supportive care in elderly patients with intermediate or high risk MDS not eligible for intensive chemotherapy: final results of the randomized phase III study (06011) of the EORTC Leukemia and German MDS Study Groups. Blood. 2008;112(11):90, #226. 11-16-2008. Ref Type: Abstract.

46. Kantarjian H, Beran M, Cortes J, et al. Long-term follow-up results of the combination of topotecan and cytarabine and other intensive chemotherapy regimens in myelodysplastic syndrome. Cancer. 2006;106(5):1099–109.

47. Kantarjian HM, O'Brien S, Huang X, et al. Survival advantage with decitabine versus intensive chemotherapy in patients with higher risk myelodysplastic syndrome: comparison with historical experience. Cancer. 2007;109(6):1133–7.

48. Deeg HJ, Storer B, Slattery JT, et al. Conditioning with targeted busulfan and cyclophosphamide for hematopoietic stem cell transplantation from related and unrelated donors in patients with myelodysplastic syndrome. Blood. 2002;100(4):1201–7.

49. Sorror ML, Sandmaier BM, Storer BE, et al. Comorbidity and disease status-based risk stratification of outcomes among patients with acute myeloid leukemia or myelodysplasia receiving allogeneic hematopoietic cell transplantation. J Clin Oncol. 2007;25(27):4246–54.

50. Cutler CS, Lee SJ, Greenberg P, et al. A decision analysis of allogeneic bone marrow transplantation for the myelodysplastic syndromes: delayed transplantation for low-risk myelodysplasia is associated with improved outcome. Blood. 2004;104(2):579–85.

51. Martino R, Iacobelli S, Brand R, et al. Retrospective comparison of reduced-intensity conditioning and conventional high-dose conditioning for allogeneic hematopoietic stem cell transplantation using HLA-identical sibling donors in myelodysplastic syndromes. Blood. 2006; 108(3):836–46.

52. Scott BL, Sandmaier BM, Storer B, et al. Myeloablative vs. nonmyeloablative allogeneic transplantation for patients with myelodysplastic syndrome or acute myelogenous leukemia with multilineage dysplasia: a retrospective analysis. Leukemia. 2006;20:128–35.

53. Chang CK, Storer BE, Scott BL, et al. Hematopoietic cell transplantation in patients with myelodysplastic syndrome or acute myeloid leukemia arising from myelodysplastic syndrome: similar outcomes in patients with de novo disease and disease following prior therapy or antecedent hematologic disorders. Blood. 2007;110(4):1379–87.

54. Alessandrino EP, Della Porta MG, Bacigalupo A, et al. WHO classification and WPSS predict posttransplantation outcome in patients with myelodysplastic syndrome: a study from the Gruppo Italiano Trapianto di Midollo Osseo (GITMO). Blood. 2008;112(3):895–902.

55. Scott BL, Storer BE, Greene JE, Hackman RC, Appelbaum FR, Deeg HJ. Marrow fibrosis as a risk factor for post-transplant outcome in patients with advanced MDS or AML with multilineage dysplasia. Biol Blood Marrow Transplant. 2007;13(3):345–54.

56. Armand P, Kim HT, Cutler CS, et al. Prognostic impact of elevated pretransplantation serum ferritin in patients undergoing myeloablative stem cell transplantation. Blood. 2007;109(10): 4586–8.

57. Platzbecker U, Bornhäuser M, Germing U, et al. Red blood cell transfusion dependence and outcome after allogeneic peripheral blood stem cell transplantation in patients with de novo myelodysplastic syndrome (MDS). Biol Blood Marrow Transplant. 2008;14:1217–25.
58. Scott BL, Park JY, Deeg HJ, et al. Pre-transplant neutropenia is associated with poor-risk cytogenetic features and increased infection-related mortality in patients with myelodysplastic syndromes. Biol Blood Marrow Transplant. 2008;14:799–806.
59. Scott BL, Storer B, Loken M, Storb R, Appelbaum FR, Deeg HJ. Pretransplantation induction chemotherapy and posttransplantation relapse in patients with advanced myelodysplastic syndrome. Biol Blood Marrow Transplant. 2005;11:65–73.

Chapter 6
Myeloablative Transplant (HCT)

Gunnar Bjarni Ragnarsson and Paul J. Martin

Abstract Initial attempts to use allogeneic bone marrow to reconstitute hematopoiesis after myeloablative treatment for hematologic malignancies began in the late 1930s but were unsuccessful. Advance in the knowledge of histocompatibility, conditioning, prevention, and treatment of graft-versus-host disease and supportive care in the late 1960s and early 1970s enabled successful outcomes after allogeneic hematopoietic cell transplantation (HCT) for treatment of hematologic malignancies and certain nonmalignant diseases, such as immune deficiencies. Treatment with myeloablative or nonmyeloablative conditioning regimens followed by allogeneic HCT is now used routinely in the management of several hematologic malignancies, including acute and chronic leukemia and high-risk myelodysplastic syndrome (MDS).

Keywords Myeloablative transplant • Allogeneic bone marrow • Leukemia • Hematopoiesis • Cell transplantation • Immune deficiency • High risk myelodysplastic syndrome

G.B. Ragnarsson, M.Sc., M.D. (✉)
Clinical Research Division, Fred Hutchinson Cancer Research Center,
1100 Fairview Ave N, D3-100, 98109 Seattle, WA, USA

Department of Clinical Research, University of Washington Medical Center, Seattle, WA, USA
e-mail: gunnib@fhcrc.org

P.J. Martin, M.D.
Clinical Research Division, Fred Hutchinson Cancer Research Center,
1100 Fairview Ave N, D3-100, 98109 Seattle, WA, USA
e-mail: pmartin@fhcrc.org

E.H. Estey and F.R. Appelbaum (eds.), *Leukemia and Related Disorders:*
Integrated Treatment Approaches, Contemporary Hematology,
DOI 10.1007/978-1-60761-565-1_6, © Springer Science+Business Media, LLC 2012

Introduction

Initial attempts to use allogeneic bone marrow to reconstitute hematopoiesis after myeloablative treatment for hematologic malignancies began in the late 1930s but were unsuccessful. Advance in the knowledge of histocompatibility, conditioning, prevention, and treatment of graft-versus-host-disease and supportive care in the late 1960s and early 1970s enabled successful outcomes after allogeneic hematopoietic cell transplantation (HCT) for treatment of hematologic malignancies and certain nonmalignant diseases, such as immune deficiencies. Treatment with myeloablative or nonmyeloablative conditioning regimens followed by allogeneic HCT is now used routinely in the management of several hematologic malignancies, including acute and chronic leukemia and high-risk myelodysplastic syndrome (MDS) [1].

High-dose treatment with radiation and/or chemotherapy is given with the goal of eradicating malignant cells, but this treatment also ablates normal hematopoietic stem cells. To restore normal bone marrow function, patients are given hematopoietic cells from related or unrelated donors by infusing bone marrow, growth factor-mobilized blood cells, or umbilical cord blood cells. Reconstitution of hematopoiesis and innate immunity occurs within weeks, while reconstitution of adaptive T and B cell immunity occurs gradually over a longer period of time. Recipient T cells can reject the allogeneic donor cells (host-versus-graft), thereby causing graft failure, while donor T cells can react against recipient cells, resulting in graft-versus-host disease (GVHD). At the same time, donor T cells can also produce beneficial graft-versus-leukemia (GVL) effects by recognizing and eradicating malignant cells in the recipient. Polymorphic HLA antigens that differ from one individual to the next have a critical role in triggering the immune responses that lead to graft rejection or GVHD. Therefore, donors are selected so that their HLA antigens are closely matched with those of the recipient. Other polymorphic antigens can also cause immune responses leading to graft rejection or GVHD. Since it is not feasible to match donors and recipients for these non-HLA antigens, immunosuppressive therapy must be used to decrease the risks of graft rejection and GVHD, even when the donor and recipient are HLA identical.

In the following sections, we review the historical advances that have led to the current state of the art in using myeloablative conditioning regimens and allogeneic HCT for treatment of acute myeloid leukemia (AML) [2, 3]. We review advances in pretransplant conditioning regimens, the advantages and disadvantages of different sources of hematopoietic stem cells, methods for prevention and treatment of GVHD, and current approaches for management of recurrent malignancy after allogeneic HCT. We conclude with an overview of improvements during the past decade.

Myeloablative Conditioning Before Allogeneic Hematopoietic Cell Transplantation

The goal of myeloablative conditioning before allogeneic HCT is to eradicate malignant cells in the recipient and to prevent rejection of the graft. The intensity of conditioning therapy is limited by toxicities in nonhematopoietic organs. The choice of conditioning therapy can therefore be influenced by both the underlying disease and by any pretransplant comorbidity in the recipient.

Radiation therapy has been an important part of the conditioning regimen from the beginning of allogeneic HCT and is usually provided as a systemic therapy in the form of total body irradiation (TBI). Radiation therapy can be effective for treatment of AML that is refractory to chemotherapy and has the advantage of penetrating sites that are inaccessible to chemotherapy, for example, in the central nervous system. Higher radiation exposures have increased antileukemic efficacy but increase the risk of toxicity, especially in the liver, lungs, and gastrointestinal tract. Fractionation is used to decrease the risk of toxicity while maintaining efficacy. Exposures from 10 to 16 Gy have been evaluated in several trials, often in combination with high-dose cyclophosphamide (CY) [4]. Clift et al. [5] compared results for patients who received 15.75 Gy ($n=37$) or 12.0 Gy ($n=34$) fractionated TBI in combination with CY (60 mg/kg on each of 2 successive days) before allogeneic HCT with HLA-identical sibling donors for treatment of AML in first remission. The 3-year probability of relapse was 12% in the 15.75 Gy group and 35% in the 12.0 Gy group ($p=0.06$). The 3-year probability of transplant-related mortality was 32% in the 15.75 Gy group and 12% in the 12.0 Gy group ($p=0.04$), and the probability of moderate to severe acute GVHD was 48% in the 15.75 Gy group vs. 12% in the 12.0 Gy group. The projected 3-year relapse-free survival rate was 59% in the 15.75 Gy group and 58% in the 12 Gy group. Similar results were seen in patients who had HCT for treatment of chronic myeloid leukemia in chronic phase [6].

At our center, TBI is now delivered by linear accelerator at 150–200 cGy/fraction twice daily for a total exposure of 12 Gy in adults before administration of chemotherapy. To decrease pulmonary toxicity, the lungs are usually shielded for at least part of the TBI so that the lung exposure does not to exceed 750 cGy. Recent studies have indicated that radiolabeled antibodies can be used to increase the efficacy and decrease toxicities of radiation therapy. CD45 is expressed by most hematologic malignancies but is not expressed in organs outside the hematopoietic system. Pagel et al. [7] reported results for 58 patients older than 50 years of age who were given ^{131}I-radiolabeled CD45-specific antibody in combination with fludarabine and 2 Gy TBI before allogeneic HCT for treatment of advanced AML or high-risk MDS. In this phase I–II study, all patients had a complete response, and survival at 1 year was projected at 41%.

Chemotherapy agents are generally given with TBI before allogeneic HCT. A widely used regimen is CY at 60 mg/kg on each of 2 successive days with 12 Gy fractionated TBI. McDonald et al. [8] measured plasma levels of CY and its metabolites in 147 patients who were treated with CY and 12 Gy TBI before allogeneic HCT. The results showed that high exposure to carboxyethylphosphoramide mustard (CEPM), a toxic metabolite of CY, was associated with liver injury and poor patient outcome. In a subsequent phase II study, 50 patients were treated with 12 Gy fractionated TBI followed by CY 45 mg/kg on the fourth day and a personalized dose of CY on the fifth day, calibrated to avoid excessive CEPM exposure based on results from the fourth day. Patients who received personalized CY dosing had significantly lower risks of hepatic and renal toxicity with similar nonrelapse mortality and overall survival as compared to results for 100 patients who received the standard regimen of 120 mg/kg CY and 12 Gy TBI [9].

Long-term effects of irradiation can be avoided by replacing TBI with chemotherapy, potentially providing more effective conditioning and making myeloablative therapy feasible in places where TBI is not available. Busulfan (BU) is an alkylating agent that has been used as a substitute for TBI in combination with CY. BU is available in oral form, but absorption varies from one patient to the next, resulting in significant interpatient variability in efficacy and toxicity, especially in the liver [10]. Dose adjustments to maintain a targeted steady-state BU plasma concentration during conditioning have been used successfully to reduce toxicities and increase efficacy [11]. The use of intravenous (iv) BU produces less variable blood concentrations, and first pass through the pulmonary circulation after parenteral administration may decrease the risk of hepatic toxicity in comparison to first pass through the liver after oral administration [12].

McCune et al. [13] suggested that giving BU before CY may deplete hepatic glutathione and potentiate liver toxicity caused by CY. Rezvani et al. [14] and unpublished data tested the hypothesis that administration of CY before BU would decrease the risk of toxicity. Fifty of the 51 patients with myelofibrosis, AML, or MDS who enrolled in the trial were alive at 100 days after HCT. Cantoni et al. [15] also compared outcomes in patients who were treated with BU-CY ($n = 16$) and CY-BU ($n = 59$) and showed that patients in the BU-CY group had higher incidence of transplant-related mortality (45% vs. 17% at 2 years after HCT) and liver toxicity manifested as sinusoidal obstruction syndrome (12.5% vs. 0%). In some regimens, CY has been replaced with other chemotherapeutic agents. For example, De Lima et al. [16] used iv BU (130 mg/m^2) and fludarabine (40 mg/m^2) in patients who had HCT after myeloablative conditioning for treatment of AML ($n = 74$) and MDS ($n = 22$). This regimen had a very favorable toxicity profile, and only two patients had liver toxicity manifested as sinusoidal obstruction syndrome.

During the past two decades, investigators at our center have decreased the intensity of myeloablative conditioning regimens, and conditioning regimens have been adapted to accommodate the needs and limitations of individual groups of patients. These strategies have produced improved outcomes, as discussed below [3].

Replacement of Hematopoietic Stem Cells

Normal hematopoietic stem cells are destroyed and must be replaced after myeloablative treatment. The probability of HLA-matching with any given sibling is 25%. The probability of finding at least one HLA-matched sibling depends on the number of siblings in the family. HLA-matched siblings have been identified for approximately one third of patients in the United States. The availability of large registries of volunteers who are willing to donate marrow or growth factor–mobilized blood cells has made it possible to find suitably matched unrelated donors for approximately 60–70% of patients of patients with Northern European ancestry in the United States. The success rate in finding a suitably matched unrelated donor is lower for patients with ancestry outside of Northern Europe [17]. Advances in the use of HLA-haploidentical donors and umbilical cord blood cells as alternative sources of hematopoietic cells have increased the availability of allogeneic HCT for patients with hematologic malignancies, as discussed in Chap. 8.

Initially, bone marrow (BM) collected by multiple aspirations from the posterior iliac crests was used as the source of hematopoietic cells for transplantation. Hematopoietic cells can be mobilized from the marrow into the blood by administration of granulocyte colony-stimulating factor (G-CSF) and other agents, making it feasible to use apheresis as an alternative method for collecting the numbers of cells needed for allogeneic HCT. This approach has gained increased popularity and is now used for most HCT recipients. Umbilical cord blood (UCB) cells can also be used for allogeneic HCT. The feasibility of this approach has been advanced through the development of repositories containing large numbers of cryopreserved cord blood units. The various sources of hematopoietic cells differ in several ways. Hematopoietic reconstitution is fastest with mobilized blood and slowest with UCB, reflecting the lower numbers of hematopoietic cells in cord blood units. Cord blood cells have less propensity to cause GVHD, but this advantage is offset by the higher frequency of HLA mismatching as compared to other graft sources [18–20].

After stem cells are infused, they enter the pulmonary vasculature and accumulate in the lungs before reaching the systemic circulation. A portion of the cells adhere to the vascular endothelium in the marrow and extravasate into stromal niches that support hematopoietic stem cell repopulation and functional engraftment. Neutrophil recovery (absolute neutrophil count >500/μL) occurs at a median of 14 days after transplantation of mobilized blood cells, and platelet recovery (platelet count >20,000/μL) occurs approximately 1 week later [18]. Recovery of innate immunity (e.g., NK-cells, monocytes-macrophages) occurs in conjunction with neutrophil recovery, while recovery of adaptive immunity (T cells and B cells) takes longer and is delayed in patients with chronic GVHD. For example, immunoglobulin levels approach the normal range at approximately 6–12 months after HCT in patients without chronic GVHD [2].

Adhesion molecules and chemoattraction play an important role in homing and engraftment. For example, SDF-1 is a chemoattractant that is secreted by bone marrow stromal cells. This ligand binds to CXCR4 expressed on the surface of several cell types including hematopoietic stem cells [21]. Dipeptidyl-peptidase IV (DPP-IV) is a membrane-bound exopeptidase that inactivates SDF-1 by cleaving the N-terminal region [22]. These observations have raised the interesting prospect that homing of hematopoietic stem cells and engraftment of cord blood cells could be enhanced by inhibiting DPP-IV activity with gliptins, a class of medications used in treatment of diabetes (Clinical trial NCT00862719) [23].

Graft-Versus-Host Disease

Acute GVHD and the immunosuppression needed to prevent or treat GVHD remain as major causes of transplant-related toxicity and mortality. Donor T cells that recognize recipient alloantigens can attack normal recipient cells and cause GVHD. Tissue damage induced by the conditioning regimen can aggravate the inflammatory response by increasing the expression of recipient alloantigens or the availability of inflammatory cytokines [24]. Grade II–IV acute GVHD develops in more than 50% of HCT recipients [25]. Factors that have been implicated as risk factors for acute GVHD include disparity of HLA and minor histocompatibility antigens between the recipient and donor, use of female donors for male recipients, donor parity, recipient age, use of mobilized blood cell grafts, high numbers of CD8+ and low numbers of regulatory T cells in the graft, and intensity of the conditioning regimen [26].

GVHD can be prevented by reducing the number or activity of donor T cells that recognize recipient alloantigens either by depleting donor T cells from the graft or through pharmacologic management with immunosuppressive medications. Methotrexate (MTX) is a folate acid antagonist that selectively kills donor T cells that proliferate after stimulation by recipient alloantigens. Calcineurin inhibitors (CNI) include cyclosporine (CSP) and tacrolimus (TAC). CNI block the calcium-dependent T cell receptor-induced activation of T cells and subsequent production of interleukin-2 (IL-2) [27]. MTX and CNI have comparable efficacy as single drugs in preventing GVHD. In three prospective trials, Storb et al. [28] compared the use of CSP vs. MTX for patients receiving a bone marrow transplant after myeloablative conditioning for treatment of acute nonlymphoblastic leukemia (ANL) in first remission ($n=75$), CML ($n=48$), or advanced leukemia ($n=56$). In the combined results from the three studies, the rates of acute GVHD and chronic GVHD were 40% and 42%, respectively, in the CSP group, compared to 55% and 48% in the MTX group ($p=0.13$ for acute GVHD; $p=0.67$ for chronic GVHD). The risk of leukemic relapse and the probability of long-term survival were comparable in the two groups.

In a subsequent study, Storb et al. [29] randomized patients undergoing patients with ANL in first remission ($n=38$) and CML ($n=55$) to receive either single-agent CSP or the combination of MTX and CSP. Patients who received only CSP had 2.1-fold higher risk of developing acute GVHD than those who received MTX and

CSP ($p=0.014$). The incidence of chronic GVHD was not different between the two groups. Survival at 3 years was 65% in the MTX/CSP group and 54% in the CSP group ($p=0.08$). As a result, the combination of MTX and CNI is still the most frequently used regimen for preventing GVHD in patients who have allogeneic HCT after myeloablative conditioning. No prospective randomized trials have shown that replacing MTX with sirolimus or mycophenolate mofetil (MMF) is superior to the standard regimen of MTX and CNI. Another approach now being explored in clinical trials at our center and elsewhere is to administer high-dose CY on days 3 and 4 after HCT transplant to eradicate T cells that are proliferating after activation by recipient alloantigens. Studies are in progress to determine whether treatment with CY alone is sufficient to prevent GVHD or whether other immuno-suppressive medications must be added [30–32].

In vitro depletion of donor T cells from the donor graft can prevent acute GVHD but has been associated with higher risks of graft rejection, infections, and relapse. Wagner et al. [33] compared MTX/CSP vs. T cell depletion (TCD) plus CSP to prevent GVHD in 405 patients who received HLA-matched unrelated marrow grafts after myeloablative conditioning for treatment of hematologic malignancies. The conditioning regimen in the TCD group was modified to minimize the risk of rejection, and the methods used for T cell depletion were designed to yield a 90% reduction in the number of T cells in the graft. The incidence of grades III–IV acute GVHD was significantly lower in the TCD group (18% vs. 37%), but the risks of chronic GVHD and primary and secondary graft failure showed no statistically significant differences between the two groups. The TCD group experienced a higher incidence of life-threatening or fatal infections during the first year (44% vs. 32%, $p=0.012$).

The study showed no statistically significant differences in the 3-year cumulative incidence of deaths attributed to acute GVHD, chronic GVHD, infection without GVHD, or organ toxicity and no difference in the 3-year incidence of treatment-related mortality (49% in both groups). The overall 3-year disease-free survival rate was 27% in the TCD group and 34% in the MTX/CSP group ($p=0.016$). For patients with AML, CML, and ALL, respectively, the 3-year disease-free survival rates were 29%, 25%, and 28% in the TCD group and 34%, 40%, and 35% in the MTX/CSP group. CML patients in the TCD arm experienced a significantly higher risk of relapse than in the MTX/CSP arm (20% vs. 7%, $p=0.009$), reflecting the importance of GVL effects in CML.

Selective depletion of T cell subsets is an alternative strategy that can be used to prevent GVHD. Laboratory studies have indicated that the donor T cells responsible for initiating acute GVHD arise primarily from the naïve T cell population (T_N) and not from the memory T cell pool. Thus, removal of T_N from the graft has been effective in preventing GVHD in rodent models [34, 35]. This hypothesis is now being tested in a clinical trial at our center.

GVHD can also be prevented by in vivo depletion of T cells with the use of T cell-specific antibodies. In a recent prospective and randomized trial, Finke et al. [36] compared CSP/MTX with ($n=103$) or without ($n=98$) rabbit anti-Jurkat anti-thymocyte globulin-Fresenius (ATG-F) in patients who received HLA-matched unrelated grafts after myeloablative conditioning for treatment of acute leukemia, CML, MDS, or myelofibrosis. The primary endpoint was severe acute GVHD or death during the first 100 days after HCT. In the ATG-F group, 21.4% of patients died or had severe acute GVHD during the first 100 days, compared to 33.7% in the control group (adjusted odds ratio 0.59, 95% CI 0.30–1.17; $p=0.13$). The cumulative incidence rates of grade III–IV acute GVHD and chronic extensive GVHD were 11.7% and 12.2%, respectively, in the ATG-F group, compared to 24.5% and 42.6% in the control group (adjusted hazard ratio [HR] 0.50 and 0.22; $p=0.054$ and <0.0001, respectively). No significant differences were observed in the risks of relapse, nonrelapse mortality or death from infections, or in overall survival.

Corticosteroids serve as the mainstay of treatment for acute GVHD. Since long-term steroid treatment causes considerable toxicity, efforts have been made to limit the exposure of patients to systemic glucocorticoid treatment. In a prospective randomized trial, Van Lint et al. [37] compared the use of methylprednisolone of 2 versus 10 mg/kg/day for treatment of 94 patients with grade II–IV acute GVHD and showed no benefit of the higher dose. McDonald et al. [38] randomized 60 patients with anorexia and poor oral intake because of intestinal GVHD to receive prednisone (1 mg/kg) plus either oral beclomethasone, a topically active oral steroid, or placebo. The initial treatment response at day 10 was 71% in the beclomethasone group and 55% in the placebo group. The incidence of durable response at day 30 was 71% and 41%, respectively ($p=0.02$), indicating that the use of topical steroids might allow more rapid withdrawal of systemic glucocorticoid treatment. In a subsequent trial, 129 patients with gastrointestinal GVHD were randomized to receive prednisone and either oral beclomethasone or placebo for 50 days [39]. Prednisone doses were tapered rapidly if GVHD improved by day 10. The risk of treatment failure by day 80 was significantly reduced in the beclomethasone group (HR 0.55; $p=0.02$). Day 200 and 1 year mortality were significantly reduced in the beclomethasone group (HR 0.33, $p=0.03$ and HR 0.54; $p=0.04$, respectively).

Mielcarek et al. [40] retrospectively compared outcomes of patients treated with glucocorticoids at a prednisone-equivalent dose of 2 mg/kg/day ($n=386$) or 1 mg/kg/day ($n=347$). The study showed no statistically significant differences in overall mortality, relapse, and nonrelapse mortality between the two groups. A multivariate analysis showed a decreased risk of invasive fungal infections in the low-dose group. These results suggest that prednisone doses lower than 2 mg/kg can be used successfully to treat patients with acute GVHD.

At our center, mild skin acute GVHD is either observed or treated topically. Mild GVHD of the stomach and intestines is typically treated with prednisone at 1 mg/kg/day and topical steroids (beclomethasone for the upper gut and budesonide for lower gut). Prednisone doses are tapered starting at day 10 in patients with a good response. More severe acute GVHD is treated with methylprednisolone at 2 mg/kg/day with reevaluation at day 3–5 for consideration of secondary therapy in patients with steroid-refractory acute GVHD or taper of prednisone doses at day 5 in patients with clinical improvement. ATG is frequently used as a secondary therapy of acute GVHD and can produce durable improvement of 20–30% of patients, but this treatment is very immunosuppressive and is associated with increased risks of opportunistic infection. A wide variety of other therapies have been tested for treatment of steroid-refractory acute GVHD, including pharmacologic agents (e.g., MMF, CNI, sirolimus), antibodies targeting T cells, and photosensitization with 8-methoxypsoralen and UVA irradiation. Results have been disappointing, and the prognosis for patients with steroid-refractory acute GVHD remains very poor [41].

Extensive chronic GVHD (chronic GVHD) can develop in about 30–60% of patients [25] and is a major cause of morbidity and mortality after HCT [42] but has also been associated with GVL effects [43]. Mild chronic GVHD can be treated with topical glucocorticoids, but extensive chronic GVHD is typically treated initially with prednisone at 1.0 mg/kg/day, with or without a CNI. The median duration of treatment for chronic GVHD exceeds 2 years, and good management requires a multidisciplinary approach.

Graft-Versus-Leukemia Effects and Treatment of Relapse After HCT

Despite many advances in the field of HCT [3], relapse after HCT continues to pose a major challenge. The relapse rate in patients with MDS or AML with poor prognostic features is ~25% at 3 months and ~40% at 1 year after myeloablative conditioning and HCT from HLA-identical siblings [44–48]. Relapse of AML and MDS after allogeneic HCT is typically rapidly progressive and nonresponsive to chemotherapy, and >75% of patients die within a year [49, 50].

Relapse after HCT can be managed with supportive care, cytotoxic therapy, or interventions to induce GVL effects. Remission can be induced with chemotherapy in approximately one third of cases, but long-term survival is very rare [50]. Cytoreductive therapy in conjunction with induction of GVL can provide more durable responses. Withdrawal of immunosuppressive therapy (WIS) to induce GVL effects by donor cells is frequently the first action taken when recurrent AML is detected after HCT. Although remission can be induced by WIS, the remission duration is typically very short [51]. If GVHD does not occur after WIS, donor lymphocyte infusion (DLI) can be used to provide more potent GVL effects. DLI as a sole therapy for relapsed AML yields an overall complete response rate of 15–29% [52, 53].

In two prospective clinical trials, cytoreductive chemotherapy was followed by growth factor–stimulated DLI as a treatment for relapsed AML after HCT. In the study by Choi et al. [54], 10 of 16 patients had a complete remission. Relapse at 6 months or later after HCT was associated with a higher probability of remission (8 of 11) and disease-free survival at 2 years (4 of 11), as compared to relapse <6 months after HCT (2 of 5 and 0 of 5, respectively). Grade III–IV acute GVHD developed in 8 of 13 evaluated patients, and chronic GVHD developed in 8 of 9 evaluated patients. Nonrelapse mortality was 25% at 2 months after DLI. Levine et al. [55] reported outcomes after DLI in 65 patients with relapsed myeloid malignancy after HCT. Complete response was induced in 27 of 57 evaluated patients

(47%) and was more frequent in patients with relapse beyond 6 months after HCT than in those with relapse during the first 6 months. One-year overall survival in patients with complete response was 51% but <5% in those without complete response. Overall survival at 2 years for the entire cohort was 19%. The risk of non-relapse mortality was 23% at 5 months after DLI, and 28% of the patients had grade III–IV acute GVHD. A retrospective analysis of 399 patients with recurrent AML after HCT showed 21% overall survival at 2 years for the 228 patients who were treated with DLI and 9% for those who were not treated with DLI [56]. Better outcome was associated with lower age and onset of relapse more than 5 months after HCT, and better response in DLI recipients was associated with lower tumor burden and favorable cytogenetics.

Second allogeneic HCT has been explored as a way of treating AML that has relapsed after HCT. In a retrospective analysis, 85 patients with relapsed AML after HCT patients received myeloablative HCT. Treatment-related mortality was 46%, and the actuarial risk of relapse was 59%, but 25% were disease free at 5 years [57]. CR at the time of second HCT and a longer interval time from HCT to relapse were associated with better outcome. In an attempt to decrease the toxicity associated with second HCT, Baron et al. [58] treated 35 AML or MDS patients who had relapsed after HCT with reduced intensity HCT and reported a 32% risk of TRM and 29% survival at 3 years.

Mielcarek et al. [59] analyzed outcomes in 307 patients with recurrent AML ($n=244$), CML in blast phase ($n=28$), or advanced MDS ($n=35$) after allogeneic HCT at our center. Patients were treated with WIS, DLI, or chemotherapy. The overall remission rate was 30%, and remission was associated with a median survival prolongation of 9.5 months. The remission rate was 18% in patients with the onset of relapse during the first 100 days, compared to 33% in those with relapse at 100–200 days and 40% in those with relapse at later time points. Overall survival at 2 years in the three groups was 3%, 9%, and 19%, respectively.

One way to harness the GVL activity of T cells and reduce toxicity might be to target the leukemia cells with CD8+ cytotoxic T cells (CTL) specific for antigens expressed by the malignant cells. Warren et al. [60] treated seven patients who had recurrent leukemia after HCT by infusing donor-derived ex vivo expanded minor histocompatibility antigen-specific CTL clones. Four of six patients with relapse had transient CR after WIS, chemotherapy, and T cell infusion, including three patients who had blasts persisting after chemotherapy. Three patients had pulmonary toxicity which correlated with the level of expression of the target genes in the lungs. Three patients experienced GVHD, although it was more likely related to rapid WIS before the study therapy and not to the CTL infusion. In this approach, the different antigens targeted in each patient can result in variable clinical response or toxicities.

Another approach for management of recurrent AML after HCT is to target a well-defined tumor-associated antigen with specific T cells. WT1, a transcription factor that can promote the malignant phenotype, is overexpressed in myeloid leukemia [61–64]. Preclinical studies have shown that WT1-specific CTL can recognize and kill WT1-expressing leukemia cells without affecting normal cells both in vitro and in vivo [65–69]. Detection of WT1-specific CD8+ T cells in patients with myeloid or lymphoblastic leukemia has been associated with beneficial GVL effects [70–73]. Clinical vaccine trials with WT1 peptide have shown that WT1-specific CD8[+] T cells can be induced, and development of a WT1-specific CTL response has been associated with antileukemic activity in some patients [74–79]. In an ongoing clinical trial at our center, Ragnarsson et al. [80] are evaluating adoptively transferred donor-derived WT1-specific CD8[+] T cells for treatment of relapsed acute leukemia after HCT.

T cell-based adoptive immunotherapy is a promising treatment for leukemia, but several factors currently limit the efficacy and broad application of this approach. In vitro stimulation and expansion of T cells can promote the terminal differentiation of responding CD8[+] cells, thereby limiting the persistence and proliferation of the transferred T cells in vivo [81]. Also, isolation of high affinity T cells that recognize relevant tumor-associated antigens poses a major challenge. It is now possible to transfer T cell receptor (TCR) genes into primary T cells as an alternative strategy to impart specificity for a desired target antigen. This approach provides the opportunity to introduce TCR that have been selected based on high affinity into T cell subtypes with high proliferative potential and ability to home preferentially to tumor sites in vivo [82]. Strategies to increase the efficacy of adoptive T cell therapy include the coadministration of cytokines, including IL-2 and IL-15, to increase the persistence and antitumor activity of transferred T cells [83–85]. CTLA4 and PD-1 are receptors on T cells that have an inhibitory effect on T cell activation, and monoclonal antibodies that neutralize these receptors have demonstrated activity as single agents in clinical trials for patients with various metastatic malignancies [86, 87]. Coadministration of these antibodies with tumor-specific T cells is being investigated as a potential means to increase the therapeutic efficacy of adoptive T cell therapy.

Relapsed AML after allogeneic HCT carries a poor prognosis. Relapse early after HCT carries an especially poor prognosis, probably reflecting the aggressive biology of disease, together with the decreased ability of patients to tolerate additional intensive therapy. Palliation or participation in clinical trials should therefore be strongly considered in this patient group. The probability of durable response after therapy to induce GVL effects is higher when the onset of relapse occurs beyond the first 3–6 months after HCT, if chemotherapy can reduce the burden of disease, but currently available approaches carry a high toxicity rate and a low chance of cure. Therapies that amplify GVL effects and minimize toxicities such as GVHD might improve outcomes in this patient group.

Progress Made in Myeloablative Allogeneic HCT

Gooley et al. [3] compared outcomes for patients undergoing allogeneic HCT at the FHCRC from 1993 to 1997 ($n = 1,418$) and from 2003 to 2007 ($n = 1,169$) and analyzed the frequency and severity of GVHD and hepatic, renal, pulmonary, and infectious complications. The Pretransplant Assessment of Mortality (PAM) score was used to adjust for differences in the severity of illness at transplant. Patients in the more recent group were older (median age 47.5 years vs. 37.4 years) and less frequently had CML (9% vs. 33%) or low-risk disease (15% vs. 31%). In 2003–2007, the proportion of unrelated donors was higher (59% vs. 42%), and mobilized blood cells were used for 76% of patients, whereas marrow grafts were used for 87% of patients in 1993–1997.

Very-high-dose myeloablative regimens (defined as CY and TBI > 12 Gy; BU, CY, and TBI; carmustine, CY, and etoposide; and nontargeted BU and CY) were used less frequently in the more recent group (10% vs. 70%). Less intensive myeloablative regimens (CY and TBI ≤ 12 Gy; targeted BU and CY; and fludarabine and BU or treosulfan) were used more frequently used in 2003–2007 (66% vs. 30%), and reduced-intensity regimens were also more frequently used in 2003–2997 (24% vs. <1%).

After adjusting for differences in PAM scores, the 2003–2007 group had a 61% decreased risk of day 200 nonrelapse mortality (NRM), a 52% decreased risk of overall NRM, a 21% decreased risk of relapse or disease progression, and a 41% decreased risk of overall mortality. If the patients who received reduced intensity regimens were excluded, the risks of day 200 NRM, overall NRM, relapse, and overall mortality was reduced by 56%, 52%, 18%, and 39%, respectively.

The authors also assessed the incidence and severity of certain complications of HCT associated with poor outcomes. The frequency of mild, moderate, and severe acute GVHD was decreased in the 2003–2007 group. Thirty percent of patients developed grade III–IV acute GVHD in the 1993–1997 group, compared to 14% in the 2003–2007 group, with 67% decrease in odds after adjusting for the PAM score. This improvement occurred despite the increased use of mobilized blood cells and unrelated donors, with no significant change in GVHD prophylaxis. The reasons may be related to improved HLA matching and decreased intensity of conditioning regimens with less tissue damage. The use of ursodiol could have decreased the risk of liver GVHD, and the use of topically active steroids for treatment of gut GVHD could have improved the response rate. The use of systemic glucocorticoids decreased by 48% and could have reduced the risk of other serious complications, such as severe infections.

Liver toxicity was reduced in the 2003–2007 period as marked by a >70% decrease in the odds of clinical and deep jaundice and a decrease in the average peak serum bilirubin concentration from 7.6 to 3.3 mg/dL. The improvement was similar if patients who received reduced intensity regimens were excluded. The improvement was attributed to the use of less intensive conditioning regimens, the use of ursodiol to prevent cholestasis, and to lower incidence of bacteremia and GVHD. The use of alternative conditioning therapies in patients at higher risk of liver injury could further decrease the risk of regimen-related toxicities in the future [16].

The risk of early CMV disease was reduced by 49% (47% in the myeloablative group). The hazard of developing gram-negative bacteremia was reduced by 39%, invasive mold infection by 51%, and invasive Candida infection by 88%. Results were similar for patients who received myeloablative conditioning. This benefit could result from earlier neutrophil and immune recovery, decreased tissue damage from less intensive conditioning, decreased use of systemic glucocorticoids, less frequent GVHD, and decreased numbers of patients developing multiorgan failure. Also, antimicrobial prophylaxis and preemptive therapy for CMV has been improved in the more recent period.

The risk of developing of acute kidney injury (serum creatinine concentration > twofold higher than baseline) was decreased in the more recent group (adjusted HR 0.44, $p = 0.0001$ both for all patients and patients receiving myeloablative HCT), and the adjusted maximum creatinine difference was 0.54 mg/dL lower in the 2003–2007 group. The hazard of respiratory failure was reduced by 37%, with a similar difference seen in the myeloablative group. The lower risk of pulmonary and renal complications could be related to decreased use of high-intensity conditioning regimens, decreased incidence or severity of liver disease, GVHD, gram-negative bacteremia and fungal infections, and a wider choice of less toxic antimicrobials.

Reduced intensity of the conditioning regimen has decreased toxicities without sacrificing efficacy of treatment for the underlying malignancy. Improvements in the treatment or prevention of transplant-related complications have contributed to better patient outcomes after myeloablative HCT. More accurate assessment of comorbidity, for example, by using the HCT comorbidity index (HCT-CI) score published by Sorror et al. [88] and tailored conditioning therapy and supportive care for each patient will likely decrease treatment-related toxicities further in the future. The use of more narrowly targeted antileukemic therapy based on individual leukemic phenotypes should also lead to further improvement in outcome.

Conclusions

Myeloablative allogeneic stem cell transplantation remains an important therapeutic option for many otherwise incurable hematologic malignancies, including AML. Improvement in therapy has lead to better outcomes after HCT, and further improvement is expected with increased understanding of transplantation biology. Awareness of potent effects mediated by the immune system has prompted the use of nonmyeloablative conditioning regimens for patients who could not tolerate high-dose conditioning regimens. Targeted therapies with leukemia-specific T cells to harness the GVL response may lead to advances in care of patient with hematologic malignancies.

References

1. Thomas E. A history of allogeneic hematopoietic cell transplantation. In: Appelbaum FR, Forman SJ, Negrin RS, Blume KG, editors. Thomas' hematopoietic cell transplantation. Oxford, England: Wiley-Blackwell Publishing; 2009. p. 3–7.
2. Barrett J. Essential biology of stem cell transplantation. In: Treleaven J, Barrett J, editors. Hematopoietic stem cell transplantation in clinical practice. 1st ed. Edinburgh: Churchill Livingstone; 2009. p. 9–21.

3. Gooley TA, Chien JW, Pergam SA, et al. Reduced mortality after allogeneic hematopoietic-cell transplantation. N Engl J Med. 2010;363(22):2091–101.
4. Bensinger WI. High-dose preparatory regimens. In: Appelbaum FR, Forman SJ, Negrin RS, Blume KG, editors. Thomas' hematopoietic cell transplantation. Oxford, England: Wiley-Blackwell Publishing; 2009. p. 316–31.
5. Clift RA, Buckner CD, Appelbaum FR, et al. Allogeneic marrow transplantation in patients with acute myeloid leukemia in first remission: a randomized trial of two irradiation regimens. Blood. 1990;76(9):1867–71.
6. Clift RA, Buckner CD, Appelbaum FR, et al. Allogeneic marrow transplantation in patients with chronic myeloid leukemia in the chronic phase: a randomized trial of two irradiation regimens. Blood. 1991;77(8):1660–5.
7. Pagel JM, Gooley TA, Rajendran J, et al. Allogeneic hematopoietic cell transplantation after conditioning with 131I-anti-CD45 antibody plus fludarabine and low-dose total body irradiation for elderly patients with advanced acute myeloid leukemia or high-risk myelodysplastic syndrome. Blood. 2009;114(27):5444–53.
8. McDonald GB, Slattery JT, Bouvier ME, et al. Cyclophosphamide metabolism, liver toxicity, and mortality following hematopoietic stem cell transplantation. Blood. 2003;101(5):2043–8.
9. McCune JS, Batchelder A, Guthrie KA, et al. Personalized dosing of cyclophosphamide in the total body irradiation-cyclophosphamide conditioning regimen: a phase II trial in patients with hematologic malignancy. Clin Pharmacol Ther. 2009;85(6):615–22.
10. Grochow LB. Busulfan disposition: the role of therapeutic monitoring in bone marrow transplantation induction regimens. Semin Oncol. 1993;20(4 Suppl 4):18–25; quiz 26.
11. Radich JP, Gooley T, Bensinger W, et al. HLA-matched related hematopoietic cell transplantation for chronic-phase CML using a targeted busulfan and cyclophosphamide preparative regimen. Blood. 2003;102(1):31–5.
12. Kashyap A, Wingard J, Cagnoni P, et al. Intravenous versus oral busulfan as part of a busulfan/cyclophosphamide preparative regimen for allogeneic hematopoietic stem cell transplantation: decreased incidence of hepatic venoocclusive disease (HVOD), HVOD-related mortality, and overall 100-day mortality. Biol Blood Marrow Transplant. 2002;8(9):493–500.
13. McCune JS, Batchelder A, Deeg HJ, et al. Cyclophosphamide following targeted oral busulfan as conditioning for hematopoietic cell transplantation: pharmacokinetics, liver toxicity, and mortality. Biol Blood Marrow Transplant. 2007;13(7):853–62.
14. Rezvani AR, McCune JS, Batchelder A, Storer BE, McDonald GB, Deeg J. Low toxicity and mortality with reversed-order conditioning (cyclophosphamide followed by targeted intravenous busulfan) in allogeneic hematopoietic cell transplantation: preliminary results of a prospective clinical trial (Abstract #1175). Paper presented at: 51st American Society of Hematology (ASH) annual meeting 2009, New Orleans, 2009.
15. Cantoni N, Gerull S, Heim D, et al. Order of application and liver toxicity in patients given BU and CY containing conditioning regimens for allogeneic hematopoietic SCT. Bone Marrow Transplant. 2010;46(3):344–9.
16. de Lima M, Couriel D, Thall PF, et al. Once-daily intravenous busulfan and fludarabine: clinical and pharmacokinetic results of a myeloablative, reduced-toxicity conditioning regimen for allogeneic stem cell transplantation in AML and MDS. Blood. 2004;104(3):857–64.
17. Aversa F, Reisner Y, Martelli MF. Hematopoietic stem cell transplantation from alternative sources in adults with high-risk acute leukemia. Blood Cells Mol Dis. 2004;33(3):294–302.
18. Group SCTC. Allogeneic peripheral blood stem-cell compared with bone marrow transplantation in the management of hematologic malignancies: an individual patient data meta-analysis of nine randomized trials. J Clin Oncol. 2005;23(22):5074–87.
19. Ringden O, Labopin M, Bacigalupo A, et al. Transplantation of peripheral blood stem cells as compared with bone marrow from HLA-identical siblings in adult patients with acute myeloid leukemia and acute lymphoblastic leukemia. J Clin Oncol. 2002;20(24):4655–64.
20. Rocha V, Labopin M, Sanz G, et al. Transplants of umbilical-cord blood or bone marrow from unrelated donors in adults with acute leukemia. N Engl J Med. 2004;351(22):2276–85.

21. Mohle R, Bautz F, Rafii S, Moore MA, Brugger W, Kanz L. The chemokine receptor CXCR-4 is expressed on CD34+ hematopoietic progenitors and leukemic cells and mediates transendothelial migration induced by stromal cell-derived factor-1. Blood. 1998;91(12):4523–30.

22. Christopherson 2nd KW, Hangoc G, Mantel CR, Broxmeyer HE. Modulation of hematopoietic stem cell homing and engraftment by CD26. Science. 2004;305(5686):1000–3.

23. Mielcarek M, Storb R, Georges GE, Golubev L, Nikitine A, Hwang B, Nash RA, Torok-Storb B. Mesenchymal stromal cells fail to prevent acute graft-versus-host disease and graft rejection after dog leukocyte antigen-haploidentical bone marrow transplantation. Biol Blood Marrow Transplant. 2011;17(2):214–25. Epub 2010 Oct 30.

24. Deeg HJ. How I treat refractory acute GVHD. Blood. 2007;109(10):4119–26.

25. Mielcarek M, Martin PJ, Leisenring W, et al. Graft-versus-host disease after nonmyeloablative versus conventional hematopoietic stem cell transplantation. Blood. 2003;102(2):756–62.

26. Cutler C, Antin J. Manifestation and treatment of acute graft-versus-host disease. In: Appelbaum FR, Forman SJ, Negrin RS, Blume KG, editors. Thomas' hematopoietic cell transplantation. Oxford, England: Wiley-Blackwell Publishing; 2009. p. 1287–303.

27. Chao NJ, Sullivan KM. Pharmacologic prevention of acute graft-versus-host disease. In: Appelbaum FR, Forman SJ, Negrin RS, Blume KG, editors. Thomas' hematopoietic cell transplantation. Oxford, England: Wiley-Blackwell Publishing; 2009. p. 1257–74.

28. Storb R, Deeg HJ, Fisher L, et al. Cyclosporine v methotrexate for graft-v-host disease prevention in patients given marrow grafts for leukemia: long-term follow-up of three controlled trials. Blood. 1988;71(2):293–8.

29. Storb R, Deeg HJ, Pepe M, et al. Methotrexate and cyclosporine versus cyclosporine alone for prophylaxis of graft-versus-host disease in patients given HLA-identical marrow grafts for leukemia: long-term follow-up of a controlled trial. Blood. 1989;73(6):1729–34.

30. Luznik L, Bolanos-Meade J, Zahurak M, et al. High-dose cyclophosphamide as single-agent, short-course prophylaxis of graft-versus-host disease. Blood. 2010;115(16):3224–30.

31. Luznik L, O'Donnell PV, Symons HJ, et al. HLA-haploidentical bone marrow transplantation for hematologic malignancies using nonmyeloablative conditioning and high-dose, posttransplantation cyclophosphamide. Biol Blood Marrow Transplant. 2008;14(6):641–50.

32. O'Donnell PV, Luznik L, Jones RJ, et al. Nonmyeloablative bone marrow transplantation from partially HLA-mismatched related donors using posttransplantation cyclophosphamide. Biol Blood Marrow Transplant. 2002;8(7):377–86.

33. Wagner JE, Thompson JS, Carter SL, Kernan NA. Effect of graft-versus-host disease prophylaxis on 3-year disease-free survival in recipients of unrelated donor bone marrow (T-cell Depletion Trial): a multi-centre, randomised phase II-III trial. Lancet. 2005;366(9487): 733–41.

34. Anderson BE, McNiff J, Yan J, et al. Memory CD4+ T cells do not induce graft-versus-host disease. J Clin Invest. 2003;112(1):101–8.

35. Chen BJ, Cui X, Sempowski GD, Liu C, Chao NJ. Transfer of allogeneic CD62L-memory T cells without graft-versus-host disease. Blood. 2004;103(4):1534–41.

36. Finke J, Bethge WA, Schmoor C, et al. Standard graft-versus-host disease prophylaxis with or without anti-T-cell globulin in haematopoietic cell transplantation from matched unrelated donors: a randomised, open-label, multicentre phase 3 trial. Lancet Oncol. 2009;10(9): 855–64.

37. Van Lint MT, Uderzo C, Locasciulli A, et al. Early treatment of acute graft-versus-host disease with high- or low-dose 6-methylprednisolone: a multicenter randomized trial from the Italian Group for Bone Marrow Transplantation. Blood. 1998;92(7):2288–93.

38. McDonald GB, Bouvier M, Hockenbery DM, et al. Oral beclomethasone dipropionate for treatment of intestinal graft-versus-host disease: a randomized, controlled trial. Gastroenterology. 1998;115(1):28–35.

39. Hockenbery DM, Cruickshank S, Rodell TC, et al. A randomized, placebo-controlled trial of oral beclomethasone dipropionate as a prednisone-sparing therapy for gastrointestinal graft-versus-host disease. Blood. 2007;109(10):4557–63.

40. Mielcarek M, Storer BE, Boeckh M, et al. Initial therapy of acute graft-versus-host disease with low-dose prednisone does not compromise patient outcomes. Blood. 2009;113(13): 2888–94.
41. Deeg HJ, Flowers M. Acute graft-versus-host disease. In: Treleaven J, Barrett J, editors. Hematopoietic stem cell transplantation in clinical practice. Edinburgh: Churchill Livingstone; 2009. p. 387–400.
42. Goerner M, Gooley T, Flowers ME, et al. Morbidity and mortality of chronic GVHD after hematopoietic stem cell transplantation from HLA-identical siblings for patients with aplastic or refractory anemias. Biol Blood Marrow Transplant. 2002;8(1):47–56.
43. Sullivan KM, Weiden PL, Storb R, et al. Influence of acute and chronic graft-versus-host disease on relapse and survival after bone marrow transplantation from HLA-identical siblings as treatment of acute and chronic leukemia. Blood. 1989;73(6):1720–8.
44. Appelbaum FR. Allogeneic hematopoietic stem cell transplantation for acute leukemia. Semin Oncol. 1997;24(1):114–23.
45. Clift RA, Buckner CD, Appelbaum FR, et al. Allogeneic marrow transplantation during untreated first relapse of acute myeloid leukemia. J Clin Oncol. 1992;10(11):1723–9.
46. Deeg HJ, Storer B, Slattery JT, et al. Conditioning with targeted busulfan and cyclophosphamide for hemopoietic stem cell transplantation from related and unrelated donors in patients with myelodysplastic syndrome. Blood. 2002;100(4):1201–7.
47. de Witte T, Hermans J, Vossen J, et al. Haematopoietic stem cell transplantation for patients with myelo-dysplastic syndromes and secondary acute myeloid leukaemias: a report on behalf of the Chronic Leukaemia Working Party of the European Group for Blood and Marrow Transplantation (EBMT). Br J Haematol. 2000;110(3):620–30.
48. Walter RB, Pagel JM, Gooley TA, et al. Comparison of matched unrelated and matched related donor myeloablative hematopoietic cell transplantation for adults with acute myeloid leukemia in first remission. Leukemia. 2010;24(7):1276–82.
49. Frassoni F, Barrett AJ, Granena A, et al. Relapse after allogeneic bone marrow transplantation for acute leukaemia: a survey by the E.B.M.T. of 117 cases. Br J Haematol. 1988;70(3):317–20.
50. Mortimer J, Blinder MA, Schulman S, et al. Relapse of acute leukemia after marrow transplantation: natural history and results of subsequent therapy. J Clin Oncol. 1989;7(1):50–7.
51. Elmaagacli AH, Beelen DW, Trenn G, Schmidt O, Nahler M, Schaefer UW. Induction of a graft-versus-leukemia reaction by cyclosporin A withdrawal as immunotherapy for leukemia relapsing after allogeneic bone marrow transplantation. Bone Marrow Transplant. 1999; 23(8):771–7.
52. Collins Jr RH, Shpilberg O, Drobyski WR, et al. Donor leukocyte infusions in 140 patients with relapsed malignancy after allogeneic bone marrow transplantation. J Clin Oncol. 1997;15(2):433–44.
53. Kolb HJ, Schattenberg A, Goldman JM, et al. Graft-versus-leukemia effect of donor lymphocyte transfusions in marrow grafted patients. European Group for Blood and Marrow Transplantation Working Party Chronic Leukemia. Blood. 1995;86(5):2041–50.
54. Choi SJ, Lee JH, Lee JH, et al. Treatment of relapsed acute myeloid leukemia after allogeneic bone marrow transplantation with chemotherapy followed by G-CSF-primed donor leukocyte infusion: a high incidence of isolated extramedullary relapse. Leukemia. 2004;18(11):1789–97.
55. Levine JE, Braun T, Penza SL, et al. Prospective trial of chemotherapy and donor leukocyte infusions for relapse of advanced myeloid malignancies after allogeneic stem-cell transplantation. J Clin Oncol. 2002;20(2):405–12.
56. Schmid C, Labopin M, Nagler A, et al. Donor lymphocyte infusion in the treatment of first hematological relapse after allogeneic stem-cell transplantation in adults with acute myeloid leukemia: a retrospective risk factors analysis and comparison with other strategies by the EBMT acute leukemia working party. J Clin Oncol. 2007;25(31):4938–45.
57. Bosi A, Laszlo D, Labopin M, et al. Second allogeneic bone marrow transplantation in acute leukemia: results of a survey by the European cooperative group for blood and marrow transplantation. J Clin Oncol. 2001;19(16):3675–84.

58. Baron F, Storb R, Storer BE, et al. Factors associated with outcomes in allogeneic hematopoietic cell transplantation with nonmyeloablative conditioning after failed myeloablative hematopoietic cell transplantation. J Clin Oncol. 2006;24(25):4150–7.
59. Mielcarek M, Storer BE, Flowers ME, Storb R, Sandmaier BM, Martin PJ. Outcomes among patients with recurrent high-risk hematologic malignancies after allogeneic hematopoietic cell transplantation. Biol Blood Marrow Transplant. 2007;13(10):1160–8.
60. Warren EH, Fujii N, Akatsuka Y, et al. Therapy of relapsed leukemia after allogeneic hematopoietic cell transplantation with T cells specific for minor histocompatibility antigens. Blood. 2010;115(19):3869–78.
61. Yamagami T, Sugiyama H, Inoue K, et al. Growth inhibition of human leukemic cells by WT1 (Wilms tumor gene) antisense oligodeoxynucleotides: implications for the involvement of WT1 in leukemogenesis. Blood. 1996;87(7):2878–84.
62. Tsuboi A, Oka Y, Ogawa H, et al. Constitutive expression of the Wilms' tumor gene WT1 inhibits the differentiation of myeloid progenitor cells but promotes their proliferation in response to granulocyte-colony stimulating factor (G- CSF). Leuk Res. 1999;23(5):499–505.
63. Cilloni D, Gottardi E, Messa F, et al. Significant correlation between the degree of WT1 expression and the International Prognostic Scoring System Score in patients with myelodysplastic syndromes. J Clin Oncol. 2003;21(10):1988–95.
64. Menssen HD, Renkl HJ, Rodeck U, et al. Presence of Wilms' tumor gene (wt1) transcripts and the WT1 nuclear protein in the majority of human acute leukemias. Leukemia. 1995;9(6):1060–7.
65. Ohminami H, Yasukawa M, Fujita S. HLA class I-restricted lysis of leukemia cells by a CD8(+) cytotoxic T- lymphocyte clone specific for WT1 peptide. Blood. 2000;95(1):286–93.
66. Oka Y, Elisseeva OA, Tsuboi A, et al. Human cytotoxic T-lymphocyte responses specific for peptides of the wild-type Wilms' tumor gene (WT1) product. Immunogenetics. 2000;51(2):99–107.
67. Gao L, Bellantuono I, Elsasser A, et al. Selective elimination of leukemic CD34(+) progenitor cells by cytotoxic T lymphocytes specific for WT1. Blood. 2000;95(7):2198–203.
68. Oka Y, Udaka K, Tsuboi A, et al. Cancer immunotherapy targeting Wilms' tumor gene WT1 product. J Immunol. 2000;164(4):1873–80.
69. Tsuboi A, Oka Y, Ogawa H, et al. Cytotoxic T-lymphocyte responses elicited to Wilms' tumor gene WT1 product by DNA vaccination. J Clin Immunol. 2000;20(3):195–202.
70. Rezvani K, Brenchley JM, Price DA, et al. T-cell responses directed against multiple HLA-A*0201-restricted epitopes derived from Wilms' tumor 1 protein in patients with leukemia and healthy donors: identification, quantification, and characterization. Clin Cancer Res. 2005;11(24):8799–807.
71. Rezvani K, Grube M, Brenchley JM, et al. Functional leukemia-associated antigen-specific memory CD8+ T cells exist in healthy individuals and in patients with chronic myelogenous leukemia before and after stem cell transplantation. Blood. 2003;102(8):2892–900.
72. Rezvani K, Yong ASM, Savani BN, et al. Graft-versus-leukemia effects associated with detectable Wilms tumor-1 specific T lymphocytes following allogeneic stem cell transplantation for acute lymphoblastic leukemia (ALL). Blood. 2007;110(6):1924–32:blood-2007-2003-076844.
73. Scheibenbogen C, Letsch A, Thiel E, et al. CD8 T-cell responses to Wilms tumor gene product WT1 and proteinase 3 in patients with acute myeloid leukemia. Blood. 2002;100(6):2132–7.
74. Mailander V, Scheibenbogen C, Thiel E, Letsch A, Blau IW, Keilholz U. Complete remission in a patient with recurrent acute myeloid leukemia induced by vaccination with WT1 peptide in the absence of hematological or renal toxicity. Leukemia. 2004;18(1):165–6.
75. Oka Y, Tsuboi A, Murakami M, et al. Wilms tumor gene peptide-based immunotherapy for patients with overt leukemia from myelodysplastic syndrome (MDS) or MDS with myelofibrosis. Int J Hematol. 2003;78(1):56–61.
76. Oka Y, Tsuboi A, Taguchi T, et al. Induction of WT1 (Wilms' tumor gene)-specific cytotoxic T lymphocytes by WT1 peptide vaccine and the resultant cancer regression. Proc Natl Acad Sci USA. 2004;101(38):13885–90.

77. Maslak PG, Dao T, Krug LM, et al. Vaccination with synthetic analog peptides derived from WT1 oncoprotein induces T-cell responses in patients with complete remission from acute myeloid leukemia. Blood. 2010;116(2):171–9.
78. Keilholz U, Letsch A, Busse A, et al. A clinical and immunologic phase 2 trial of Wilms tumor gene product 1 (WT1) peptide vaccination in patients with AML and MDS. Blood. 2009; 113(26):6541–8.
79. Zhou J, Shen X, Huang J, Hodes RJ, Rosenberg SA, Robbins PF. Telomere length of transferred lymphocytes correlates with in vivo persistence and tumor regression in melanoma patients receiving cell transfer therapy. J Immunol. 2005;175(10):7046–52.
80. Ragnarsson G, Nguyen H, Chaney C, Ho B, Greenberg P. Adoptive T cell therapy targeting WT1 in leukemia and MDS patients. J Immunol. 2009;182(1_MeetingAbstracts):41.34.
81. Sallusto F, Geginat J, Lanzavecchia A. Central memory and effector memory T cell subsets: function, generation, and maintenance. Annu Rev Immunol. 2004;22(1):745–63.
82. Berger C, Jensen MC, Lansdorp PM, Gough M, Elliott C, Riddell SR. Adoptive transfer of effector CD8+ T cells derived from central memory cells establishes persistent T cell memory in primates. J Clin Invest. 2008;118(1):294–305.
83. Berger C, Berger M, Hackman RC, et al. Safety and immunological effects of IL-15 administration in nonhuman primates. Blood. 2009;114:2417–26:blood-2008-2012-189266.
84. Klebanoff CA, Finkelstein SE, Surman DR, et al. IL-15 enhances the in vivo antitumor activity of tumor-reactive CD8+ T cells. Proc Natl Acad Sci USA. 2004;101(7):1969–74.
85. Yee C, Thompson JA, Byrd D, et al. Adoptive T cell therapy using antigen-specific CD8+ T cell clones for the treatment of patients with metastatic melanoma: in vivo persistence, migration, and antitumor effect of transferred T cells. Proc Natl Acad Sci USA. 2002; 99(25):16168–73.
86. Hodi FS, Mihm MC, Soiffer RJ, et al. Biologic activity of cytotoxic T lymphocyte-associated antigen 4 antibody blockade in previously vaccinated metastatic melanoma and ovarian carcinoma patients. Proc Natl Acad Sci USA. 2003;100(8):4712–7.
87. Brahmer JR, Topalian SL, Powderly J, et al. Phase II experience with MDX-1106 (Ono-4538), an anti-PD-1 monoclonal antibody, in patients with selected refractory or relapsed malignancies. J Clin Oncol. 2009;27(15S):3018 (Meeting Abstracts).
88. Sorror ML, Storer B, Storb RF. Validation of the hematopoietic cell transplantation-specific comorbidity index (HCT-CI) in single and multiple institutions: limitations and inferences. Biol Blood Marrow Transplant. 2009;15(6):757–8.

Chapter 7
Reduced-Intensity and Non-Myeloablative Conditioning Followed by Hematopoietic Cell Transplantation

Aravind Ramakrishnan and Brenda M. Sandmaier

Abstract Hematopoietic cell transplantation (HCT) is the only curative modality for the majority of hematologic malignancies. Initial approaches to treat leukemia began in the 1960s and were based on the premise that high-dose chemotherapy and/or radiation would eradicate the underlying malignancy, and patients could subsequently be rescued by infusion of allogeneic marrow which would reestablish normal hematopoiesis. Subsequently, clinical observations made in the late 1970s and early 1980s confirmed prior observations in animal models that the allograft itself had antileukemic properties.

Keywords Hematopoietic cell transplantation • Leukemia • Allogeneic marrow • Hematopoiesis • Nonmyeloablative conditioning • Allograft • Relapse

Introduction

Hematopoietic cell transplantation (HCT) is the only curative modality for the majority of hematologic malignancies. Initial approaches to treat leukemia began in the 1960s and were based on the premise that high-dose chemotherapy and/or radiation would eradicate the underlying malignancy, and patients could subsequently be rescued by infusion of allogeneic marrow which would reestablish normal hematopoiesis [1]. Subsequently, clinical observations made in the late 1970s and early 1980s confirmed prior observations in animal models that the allograft itself

A. Ramakrishnan, M.D. (✉) • B.M. Sandmaier, M.D.
Department of Medicine, University of Washington School of Medicine, Seattle, WA, USA

Clinical Research Division, Fred Hutchinson Cancer Research Center,
1100 Fairview Ave N, Research Div, 98109 Seattle, WA, USA
e-mail: aramakri@fhcrc.org; bsandmai@fhcrc.org

E.H. Estey and F.R. Appelbaum (eds.), *Leukemia and Related Disorders:*
Integrated Treatment Approaches, Contemporary Hematology,
DOI 10.1007/978-1-60761-565-1_7, © Springer Science+Business Media, LLC 2012

had antileukemic properties. Weiden et al. first observed that patients who developed chronic graft-versus-host disease (GVHD) had the lowest rates of relapse [2–4]. Over the last two decades, there has been considerable data that show that this "graft-versus-tumor" effect (GVT) after allogeneic HCT is mediated by donor T-cells that are contained in the allograft. The strongest evidence for the GVT effect came from the observations that recipients of T-cell depleted grafts had a higher risk of relapse, and patients who relapsed after HCT could achieve remission after donor lymphocyte infusion (DLI) [5–8]. Further clinical data over the last few decades have also revealed that escalation of conditioning intensity only leads to increased toxicity without impacting overall survival [9, 10].

These clinical observations have led to a significant paradigm shift in the field of HCT with recent efforts focused on harnessing the power of GVT to eradicate malignancy while minimizing toxicity [11]. A successful allograft must overcome two immunological barriers both mediated by T-cells: (1) host-versus-graft (HVG) and (2) graft-versus-host (GVH) reactions. The high-intensity chemotherapy and/or irradiation included in high-dose conditioning regimens have the dual effect of providing disease control as well as overcoming HVG reactions. After HCT, the GVH reactions are controlled by providing immunosuppressive agents that target the donor T-cells with the goal of establishing graft-host tolerance. However, the organ toxicities associated with intensive conditioning regimens have limited this curative modality to younger patients. Given that the majority of patients with hematologic malignancies tend to be elderly and have other medical comorbidities, they are generally not good candidates for high-dose transplants.

The development of reduced-intensity approaches has also allowed the extension of HCT to an older population of patients who were previously deemed ineligible for this lifesaving therapy due to the morbidity and mortality associated with high-dose chemotherapy/radiation. Current approaches have focused on designing conditioning regimens that are minimally toxic but provide sufficient immunosuppression to prevent HVG reactions and achieve engraftment of donor hematopoietic cells; GVH reactions are controlled by postgrafting immunosuppression [12]. Unlike high-dose transplants, most patients initially develop a state of mixed hematopoietic chimerism where there is mutual graft-host tolerance, and hematopoiesis is derived from both host and donor cells. While mixed chimerism is likely to correct any deficiencies from genetic diseases, full donor chimerism is generally required to eradicate hematologic malignancies through GVT provided by donor T-cells. In this chapter, we will discuss the clinical results with reduced-intensity approaches to transplantation.

What Constitutes a Reduced-Intensity Regimen

Over the last 15 years, a number of conditioning regimens of varying intensity have been introduced ranging from very low, to moderate, to very high. This has led to some controversy, and what exactly constitutes a reduced-intensity regimen has remained somewhat arbitrary. There has been general agreement that reduced-intensity regimens cause reversible myelosuppression that does not require hematopoietic cell support and will result in a state of mixed chimerism after hematopoietic cell transplantation [12]. Most reduced-intensity conditioning regimens have combined a purine analog that provides potent immunosuppression along with varying doses of alkylating agents to provide cytotoxic antitumor effects to control the malignancy until the occurrence of GVT. In an effort to further decrease toxicity, the Seattle group has developed a nonmyeloablative conditioning regimen based on results in a preclinical canine model [13]. This regimen consists of 2 Gy TBI with or without fludarabine and postgrafting cyclosporine (CSP) or tacrolimus (Tac) and mycophenolate mofetil (MMF) all of that provide enough immunosuppression to overcome HVG reactions. In contrast to reduced-intensity regimens which can offer some antitumor effect, this nonmyeloablative approach relies entirely on GVT to eradicate the underlying malignancy [14].

Given this spectrum of conditioning regimens with varying intensity, there has been great interest in generating a classification system for defining conditioning intensity so that communication can be uniform within the transplant community, and retrospective studies can be analyzed appropriately. Initial efforts by the Center for International Blood and Marrow Transplantation (CIBMTR) defined reduced-intensity regimens as any regimen that met the following criteria: (1) a total body irradiation dose (TBI) of ≤ 5 Gy if given as a single fraction or 8 Gy if given in a fractionated manner, (2) a busulfan dose of ≤ 9 mg/kg, (3) a melphalan dose ≤ 140 mg/m^2, (4) a thiotepa dose ≤ 10 mg/kg, and (5) the BEAM regimen (carmustine, etoposide, cytarabine, and melphalan) [15]. Although these definitions were useful, there were still problems with this system in that there was no distinction between truly nonmyeloablative regimens.

In an effort to further refine these definitions, the CIBMTR convened an expert panel which recently proposed a new classification system for conditioning regimens [16]. This system now proposes three categories of conditioning regimens based on the duration of pancytopenia and requirement for hematopoietic cell support: (1) *myeloablative*, defined as a regimen that produces profound pancytopenia within 1–3 weeks of administration and which is generally thought to be irreversible without hematopoietic cell rescue; (2) *nonmyeloablative*, defined as a regimen that causes minimal pancytopenia which is quickly reversible without hematopoietic cell support; and (3) *reduced-intensity*, defined as any regimen that cannot be classified as myeloablative or nonmyeloablative. Reduced-intensity regimens differ from the other two categories in that they do cause significant cytopenias, and although autologous recovery can occur, it can be quite prolonged such that in practice hematopoietic cell rescue is necessary to decrease morbidity and mortality. The expert panel also introduced the concept of *immunoablation*, the main principle behind nonmyeloablative approaches [16]. Examples of these various regimens are shown in Table 7.1 and Fig. 7.1 [17]. The use of this classification system for future clinical trials will allow for better standardization and analysis of data.

Table 7.1 Reduced-intensity regimens

Myeloablative	Nonmyeloablative	Reduced-intensity
Cy120/TBI 12 Gy ± VP16	TBI 2 Gy ± Fludarabine	Flu/Bu ± ATG
Bu 16/CY120	TLI + ATG	Flu/Mel
	Flu/Cy ± ATG	Thiotepa/Cy
		Cy200/ATG

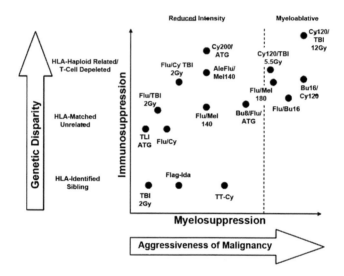

Fig. 7.1 Commonly used conditioning regimens in relation to their immunosuppressive and myelosuppressive properties. Abbreviations: *Ale* alemtuzumab, *ATG* antithymocyte globulin, *Bu8* busulfan 8 mg/kg, *Bu16* busulfan 16 mg/kg, *Cy* cyclophosphamide, *Cy120* cyclophosphamide 120 mg/kg, *Cy200* cyclophosphamide 200 mg/kg, *Flu* fludarabione, *Flag-Ida* fludarabine; cytarabine; idarubicin, *Mel140* melphalan 140 mg/m^2, *Mel180* melphalan 180 mg/m^2, *TBI* total body irradiation, *TLI* total lymphoid irradiation, *TT* thiotepa (Adapted with permission from Storb et al. [17]. Copyright 2001 by American Society of Hematology (ASH). Reproduced with permission of American Society of Hematology (ASH)© 2001)

Engraftment and Kinetics

In contrast to myeloablative regimens where upon recovery hematopoiesis is derived entirely from donor cells, nonmyeloablative and reduced-intensity regimens generally result in a state of mixed chimerism. This is especially true for nonmyeloablative transplants. Reduced-intensity regimens also result in a state of mixed chimerism, but these are generally proportional to the intensity of the conditioning regimen [18–20]. The overall goal is to achieve high levels of donor T-cell chimerism early after stem cell transplantation as this has been associated with a lower risk of graft rejection and relapse [14, 20, 21].

Investigators at our center have evaluated the engraftment kinetics of various donor cell populations in 120 patients with hematologic malignancies who received hematopoietic cell transplants after 2 Gy TBI ± fludarabine conditioning followed by postgrafting immunosuppression with CSP and MMF [21]. Although the majority of patients rapidly developed high degrees of donor cell chimerism, there were many patients that remained mixed chimeras for up to 6 months posttransplant. Generally, patients achieved complete donor myeloid chimerism early, while conversion to complete donor T-cell chimerism took several months [21]. Several studies have also shown that patients who fail to achieve high levels of donor NK and T-cell chimerism early after transplantation are at high risk for graft rejection [14, 21, 22]. Other factors that are associated with more rapid engraftment of donor T-cells include the intensity of conditioning regimen and postgraft immunosuppression [23–25] and use of peripheral blood hematopoietic cells with high numbers of CD34+ cells and T-cells compared to a marrow source [26–28]. Patients who received myelosuppressive chemotherapy before transplantation also had a more rapid engraftment of donor T-cells. This is likely due to the immunosuppression provided by chemotherapy which weakened HVG reactions [21, 26].

An association between high levels of donor T-cell chimerism and the appearance of GVHD has been observed by several investigators. Childs et al. noted that full donor chimerism preceded the development of acute GVHD in patients conditioned with fludarabine and cyclophosphamide [20]. Other studies, in contrast, have found that the majority of patients were mixed chimeras at the time of development of acute GVHD [21, 29]. However, when chimerism was analyzed as a continuous linear variable, higher levels of donor T-cell chimerism 1 month posttransplant were associated with an increased risk for the development of grades II–IV acute GVHD [14, 21, 27]. Patients who subsequently achieved full donor chimerism had the lowest risk of relapse [21]. A recent study also evaluated the impact of early (days 14, 28, and 42) donor T-cell and NK cell engraftment on HCT outcomes in 282 patients with hematologic malignancies given nonmyeloablative conditioning. When modeling chimerism levels as a continuous linear variable, only high early donor T-cell chimerism was significantly associated with acute GVHD. In contrast, only high early donor NK cell chimerism was significantly associated with lower relapse rates [30].

Toxicities Associated with Nonmyeloablative/ Reduced-Intensity Conditioning

Myeloablative conditioning is associated with significant nonrelapse mortality due to nonhematologic organ toxicities and infectious complications. These include a number of transplant specific organ toxicities such as hepatic veno-occlusive disease/ sinusoidal obstruction syndrome (VOD/SOS) and idiopathic pneumonia syndrome (IPS). In a retrospective analysis of 193 patients who received nonmyeloablative conditioning, no cases of VOD/SOS were noted [31]. Similarly, a retrospective analysis also revealed that the incidence of IPS was only 2.2% in patients undergoing nonmyeloablative conditioning compared to 8.4% in patients undergoing myeloablative conditioning [32]. Furthermore, patients who underwent myeloablative conditioning had a significantly higher risk of experiencing a >20% per year reduction in their forced expiratory volume (FEV1) when compared to patients undergoing nonmyeloablative conditioning [33]. A retrospective analysis also revealed that the incidence of renal failure is significantly reduced in patients undergoing reduced-intensity conditioning compared to high-intensity conditioning [34].

A number of retrospective analyses have evaluated infectious complications and have also shown that many of these are decreased with reduced-intensity and particularly nonmyeloablative transplants. Patients conditioned with decreasing intensity typically have shorter periods of cytopenias, and this has translated to fewer complications. Patients undergoing nonmyeloablative transplants experience fewer episodes of bacteremia during the first month, 9% compared to 27% in patients undergoing myeloablative transplants [35]. There is no difference in the incidence of fungal infections, but there is a decreased incidence of severe CMV infections, although overall CMV disease rate are not different [35–37]. A recent analysis also revealed that lower tract respiratory viral infections during the 100 days after transplantation were much less common after nonmyeloablative conditioning when compared to myeloablative conditioning [38]. Retrospective analyses also show a decreased requirement for transfusion support and inpatient hospitalizations for patients undergoing nonmyeloablative conditioning [39–41]. Overall, the data suggest that, as expected, causes of nonhematologic organ toxicity are reduced and are related to the degree of conditioning intensity. Although bacterial infections are decreased, other infectious complications such as fungal infections remain a problem due to the profound immunosuppression associated with all allogeneic transplant modalities.

Comorbidities and Their Impact in Selecting Conditioning Regimens

As most patients that develop hematologic malignancies tend to be elderly, they often have other coexisting medical problems that can lead to increased nonrelapse mortality after transplantation. Although commonly used comorbidity indices, such as the Charleston Comorbidity Index (CCI), are useful in predicting nonrelapse mortality after transplantation, they do have limitations [42–44]. For example, some comorbidities in the CCI were rarely found in the transplant patient population, whereas other common comorbidities found in transplant patients were not captured by the CCI. To overcome these limitations, Sorror et al. have modified the CCI and developed a hematopoietic cell transplantation-specific comorbidity index (HCT-CI) which better predicts for survival when compared to the CCI (see Fig. 7.2) [45]. The HCT-CI has now been used to compare outcomes among patients undergoing allogeneic transplant for many diseases including acute leukemia, myelodysplastic

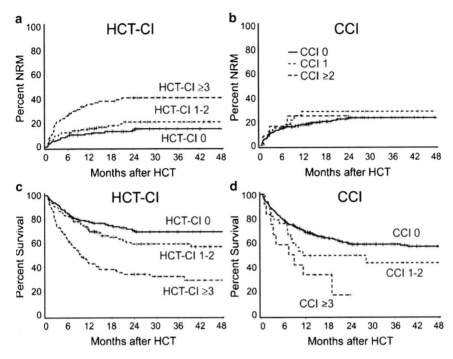

Fig. 7.2 Panels (**a**) and (**b**): Nonrelapse mortality as stratified by the HCT-CI or CCI. Panel (**c**) and (**d**): Kaplan-Meier estimates of survival as stratified by the HCT-CI or CCI. The HCT-CI better predicts for nonrelapse mortality and overall survival when compared to the CCI (This research was originally published in Sorror et al. [45] © the American Society of Hematology)

syndrome, and lymphomas [46–49]. Consistently, patients with very low HCT-CI scores have similar overall survivals after either myeloablative or nonmyeloablative conditioning. These patients would be ideal candidates for prospective trials that compare the intensity of conditioning on outcomes. However, patients with high HCT-CI scores have better overall survival when undergoing nonmyeloablative conditioning [49]. Thus, the HCT-CI has become a useful tool and maybe helpful in selecting the optimal intensity of a conditioning regimen.

GVHD and GVT After Nonmyeloablative and Reduced-Intensity Conditioning

As discussed above, the major focus of reduced-intensity and nonmyeloablative regimens is to rely on the donor immune system to eradicate the underlying malignancy via GVT. Historically, in patients transplanted with conventional conditioning, the appearance of GVHD was associated with GVT [3, 4]. This raised several questions regarding GVHD and GVT after reduced-intensity and nonmyeloablative conditioning as the biology of immune reconstitution is different when compared to high-dose conditioning. First, most patients develop a state of mixed chimerism after reduced-intensity transplantation, establishing the potential for immunologic tolerance which may lead to lower rates of GVHD. The tissue injury that results from high-dose conditioning has been implicated in the pathophysiology of acute GVHD by leading to direct interactions between cellular components of both the donor and host as well as the release of a number of inflammatory cytokines [50, 51]. As patients that undergo reduced-intensity conditioning have minimal tissue damage, one would anticipate that the donor T-cells are not exposed to this inflammatory environment, and GVHD would be reduced. However, reduced-intensity regimens have less toxicity on host antigen presenting cells which have been implicated in the initiation of GVHD, and one might expect higher rates of GVHD [52].

Several retrospective studies have sought to answer these questions regarding GVHD and GVT after reduced-intensity conditioning. The majority of these studies have shown lower rates of acute GVHD and similar or lower rates of chronic GVHD after reduced-intensity conditioning [42, 44, 53, 54]. In 2005, the NIH sponsored a consensus conference that proposed new guidelines for the diagnosis and classification of GVHD based on the clinical manifestations rather than time from transplantation [55]. A syndrome of "late" acute GVHD does occur in some patients after day 100 after reduced-intensity conditioning, and this should be taken into account in future prospective studies [53, 56].

Given that historically the appearance of GVHD was associated with GVT, several groups have also performed retrospective studies to evaluate the impact of GVT after reduced-intensity conditioning. Martino et al. evaluated outcomes in 37 patients with AML and MDS who underwent reduced-intensity conditioned allografts and noted that patients who experienced acute or chronic GVHD have significantly lower rates of relapse [57]. Another analysis of 120 myeloma patients who underwent reduced-intensity conditioned allografts revealed that only patients who developed chronic GVHD had lower rates of relapse, while the occurrence of acute GVHD had no impact on relapse [58]. An EBMT analysis of myeloma patients also revealed that chronic GVHD was associated with lower rates of relapse [59]. Similar observations were made by Blaise et al. who evaluated 33 patients with AML who underwent reduced-intensity conditioning, and a landmark analysis starting on day 100 revealed that the development of chronic GVHD was associated with reduced relapse risk and higher leukemia-free survival [60]. Investigators at the FHCRC evaluated 322 patients with various malignancies who underwent nonmyeloablative conditioned transplants and found similar results. However, in this analysis, the development of grades II–IV acute GVHD was associated with increased rates of nonrelapse mortality and lower progression-free survival [61]. Only the occurrence of chronic GVHD was associated with lower rates of relapse and higher progression-free survival without an increase in nonrelapse mortality (see Fig. 7.3) [62]. Collectively, these data suggest that transplant protocols that aim to minimize rates of acute GVHD without affecting GVT effects associated with chronic GVHD may improve outcomes.

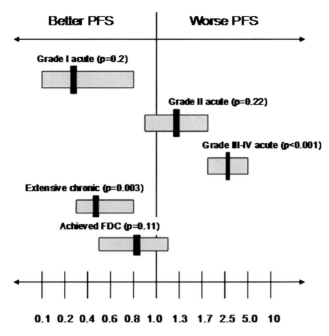

Fig. 7.3 *Impact of acute and chronic GVHD on outcomes in patients given nonmyeloablative conditioning.* Only chronic GVHD and grade I acute GVHD were associated with improved progression free survival (PFS). Grades III–IV acute GVHD were associated with nonrelapse mortality and worse progression-free survival [62] (Adapted from Baron and Sandmaier [62]. With kind permission Springer Science+Business Media). FDC = Full Donor Chimerism

Clinical Results

Tables 7.2 [63–82] and 7.3 [59, 83–91] show results of some of the large studies of reduced-intensity and nonmyeloablative conditioned transplants in patients with lymphoid malignancies, myeloma, and myeloid malignancies. These data suggest that reduced-intensity and nonmyeloablative transplantation can be very effective in controlling disease. However, this seems to be limited to early stage disease. The best results were seen in patients with AML in complete remission, low-grade MDS with less than 5% blasts, indolent or low-grade NHL, CML in first chronic phase, and CLL. In patients with more aggressive disease, such as leukemia not in remission, advanced MDS, high-grade NHL, and advanced CML, results are poor with the major problem being high relapse rates. There are several reasons for these poor results in advanced disease. First, in contrast to high-dose regimens where some disease control is provided by the conditioning regimen, reduced-intensity and nonmyeloablative approaches rely more heavily on GVT for disease eradication. After reduced-intensity and nonmyeloablative conditioning, the maximum GVT does not occur immediately, and thus rapidly proliferating diseases may relapse early.

Table 7.2 Recent results in lymphoid malignancies and myeloma

Study	Disease	Regimen	Pts	Median age	Donor	Grades III–IV acute GVHD (%)	Chronic GVHD (%)	Relapse (%)	NRM (%)	Median follow-up	Survival
Seattle Consortium [66]	CLL	2 Gy TBI±Flu	82	56	MRD	16	51	38	23	5 years	5-year OS 50% 5-year PFS 39%
Seattle Consortium [67]	Aggressive NHL	2 Gy TBI±Flu	32	52	(n=52)	19	47	45	25	45 months	3-year OS 45% 3-year PFS 35%
Seattle Consortium [68]	Hodgkin	2 Gy TBI±Flu	38	33	MUD	16	50	56	21	25 months	2-year OS 53% 2-year PFS 23%
Seattle Consortium [68]	Hodgkin	2 Gy TBI±Flu	24	28	(n=30)	8	63	63	8	25 months	2-year OS 58% 2-year PFS 29%
Seattle Consortium [68]	Hodgkin	2 Gy TBI±Flu	28	32	MRD	11	35	40	9	25 months	2-year OS 58% 2-year PFS 51%
Seattle Consortium [69]	Relapsed or transformed indolent NHL	2 Gy TBI±Flu	62	54	(n=21)	18	47	20	42	36.6 months	3-year OS 43% 3-year PFS 38%
Seattle Consortium [70]	Mantle cell	2 Gy TBI+Flu	33	53	MUD	30	64	9	24	24.6 months	2-year OS 65% 5-year DFS 27%
Seattle Consortium [71]	ALL	2 Gy TBI+Flu	50	56	(n=8)	8	53	38	31	31 months	5-year OS 37%

Study	Disease	Conditioning			Donor					Follow-up	Outcomes
Seattle Consortium [72]	Myeloma	2 Gy TBI±Flu	102	52	MMUD	5	74	50	18	6.3 years	5-year OS 64% / 5-year PFS 36%
GITMO [73]	Myeloma	2 Gy TBI	100	54	(n=3)	NR	50	41	11	5 years	5-year OS 68% / 5-year EFS 39%
EBMT [63]	Follicular NHL	Various	87	51	MRD	NR	48	20	33	36 months	3-year OS 53% / 3-year PFS 49%
EBMT [64]	Hodgkin	Various	285	31	(n=38)	12	38	53	21	26 months	3-year OS 43% / 3-year PFS 25%
EBMT [74]	CLL	Various	77	54	MUD	16	57	31	18	18 months	2-year OS 72% / 2-year EFS 56%
EBMT [75]	HL/NHL	Various	188	40	(n=24)	NR	16	24	34	283 days	2-year OS 50% / 2-year PFS 21%
EBMT [76]	ALL	Various	97	38	Haplo	12	37	61	8	2.8 years	2-year OS 31% / 2-year LFS 30%
EBMT [77]	Myeloma	Various	320	51	(n=28)	NR	50	54	24	36 months	3-year OS 38% / 3-year PFS 19%
CIBMTR [78]	HL	Various	143	30	MRD	40	69	47	33	25 months	2-year OS 37% / 2-year PFS 20%
CIBMTR [65]	F-NHL	Various	88	51	(n=34)	21	62	17	28	50 months	3-year OS 69% / 3-year PFS 55%
MDACC [79]	HL	Flu/Mel	58	32	MUD	NR	73	55	15	24 months	2-year OS 64% / 2-year PFS 32%
MDACC [80]	Mantle	Cis/Flu/AraC Flu/Cy/Rituxan	35	58	(n=28)	0	60	31	20	56 months	6 year OS 53% / 6 year PFS 46%
MDACC [81]	Follicular	Flu/Cy/Rituxan±ATG	47	53	MRD	2	60	4	15	60 months	5-year OS 85% / 5-year PFS 83%
MDACC [82]	CLL	Flu/Cy/Rituxan	39	57	(n=16)	NR	48	10	18	27 months	4-year OS 48% / 4-year PFS 44%

Table 7.3 Recent results in myeloid malignancies

Study	Disease	Regimen	Pts	Median age	Donor	Grades III–IV acute GVHD (5)	Chronic GVHD (%)	Relapse (%)	NRM (%)	Median follow-up	Survival
Seattle Consortium [83]	MDS MPD	2 Gy TBI±Flu	148	59	MRD (n=75) MRD (n=73)	11	37	41	32	47 months	3-year OS 27% 3-year RFS 27%
Seattle Consortium [84]	AML	2 Gy TBI±Flu	122	58	MRD (n=58) MUD (n=42) MMRD (n=22)	12	36	39	16	44 months	2-year OS 48% 2-year DFS 44%
Seattle Consortium [85]	CML	2 Gy TBI±Flu	24	58	MRD (n=24)	12	32	25	21	36 months	3-year OS 54%
EBMT [87]	MDS	Various	833	59	NR	NR	NR	41	32	NR	4-year OS 32%
EBMT [88]	AML	Various	315	57	NR	8	48	41	18	14 months	2-year OS 47% 2-year LFS 40%
EBMT [91]	MPD	Various	103	55	MRD (n=33) MUD (n=70)	11	43	22	16	33 months	5-year OS 67% 5-year EFS 51%
EBMT [86]	CML	Various	186	50	MRD (n=125) MMRD (n=8) MUD (n=47) MMUD (n=5)	9	43	47	23	35 months	3-year OS 58% 3-year PFS 37%
MDACC [89]	AML/MDS	Flu/Mel	112	55	RD (n=59) UD (n=53)	NR	49	25	20	29.4 months	2-year OS 44%
MDACC [90]	CML	Various	64	52	MRD (n=30) MMRD (n=4) MUD (n=30)	10	28	34	48	7 years	5-year OS 33% 5-year PFS 20%

This was confirmed by a study from the Seattle consortium that evaluated the relapse risk in 834 patients with various hematologic malignancies treated with HCT after nonmyeloablative conditioning [92]. Relapse rates per patient year-at-risk adjusted for follow-up and competing NRM were calculated for 29 different diseases. Patients with CLL, myeloma, and low-grade NHL in complete remission or partial remissions had the lowest relapse rates per patient year (0–0.24). In contrast, patients with advanced myeloid or aggressive lymphoid malignancies had a very high rate of relapse (0.52) [92]. Second, it does appear that some malignancies are more susceptible to the GVT than others. CML, low-grade NHL, and CLL all seem very sensitive to GVL effects. AML, MDS, and myeloma seem to have intermediate sensitivity, while high-grade lymphomas seem to have the least sensitivity to GVT, or the kinetics of the disease outpaces the GVT effect. Several approaches are now underway to improve outcomes in more advanced disease.

Salvage Reduced-Intensity Allografts After Failed Auto/Allografts and After Graft Rejection

Patients who relapse after a prior autologous transplant or develop a secondary myelodysplastic syndrome generally have poor outcomes. Although a second high-dose transplant can be curative in this setting, this is associated with very high rates of nonrelapse mortality of over 50% [93]. The use of a reduced-intensity conditioning regimen is quite attractive in this setting, and several groups have evaluated this approach.

Investigators at the Haddasah University Hospital treated 12 patients, median age 33, with a reduced-intensity regimen consisting of fludarabine, busulfan, and ATG. One patient died due to nonrelapse mortality, and 3-year OS and DFS were 56% and 50%, respectively [94]. Investigators in Boston treated 13 patients, median age 38, transplanted patients from HLA-matched related donors after conditioning with Cytoxan and ATG with or without thymic irradiation. Patients also received donor lymphocyte infusion 5–6 weeks posttransplant to facilitate full donor chimerism. The 2-year OS and DFS were 45% and 38%, respectively [95]. Investigators from the City of Hope Cancer Center reported results on 28 patients, median age 47, who received transplants from HLA-matched related ($n=14$) or HLA-matched unrelated ($n=14$) donors after conditioning with fludarabine and melphalan ($n=24$) or fludarabine and 2 Gy TBI. Nonrelapse mortality was 21%, and 2-year OS and DFS were 57% and 41%, respectively [96]. The Seattle consortium evaluated 147 patients, median age 46, who failed autologous ($n=135$), allogeneic ($n=10$), or syngeneic ($n=2$) transplants. These patients received HLA-matched related ($n=62$) and HLA-matched unrelated ($n=85$) transplants after conditioning with 2 Gy TBI with or without fludarabine. The 3-year incidences of NRM, relapse, and OS were 32%, 48%, and 27%, respectively, for related donors and 28%, 44%, and 44%, respectively, for unrelated donors. Factors associated with better outcomes included having minimal disease at the time of transplant, developing chronic GVHD, having a low comorbidity score, and lack of acute GVHD [97].

A retrospective analysis from the United Kingdom evaluated 71 patients who received a second allogeneic transplant using reduced-intensity conditioning after relapse after a first allogeneic transplant [98]. A variety of fludarabine-based conditioning regimens were used, and the majority of patients had either AML or MDS. There were nine patients that had a lymphoproliferative disorder, two patients with myeloma, and three patients with a MPD. After a median follow-up of 906 days, the 1-year incidence of NRM, relapses, and OS were 23%, 48%, and 42%, respectively. In subgroup analysis, OS was significantly better in patients who relapsed 11 months after the first transplant when compared to those that relapsed before 6 months. The presence of full donor chimerism and chronic GVHD were also significantly associated with improved survival [98].

Investigators at the FHCRC have also evaluated salvage reduced-intensity allografts after graft failure [99]. Results were reported in 38 patients, median age 56, with hematologic malignancies ($n=35$), aplastic anemia ($n=2$), and renal cell carcinoma ($n=1$) who developed graft rejection following allogeneic transplant. In 24 patients, a new donor was used, while in 14 patients, the same donor was reused. Conditioning consisted of fludarabine with 3 or 4 Gy TBI. Thirty-three patients had sustained engraftment, while five patients had graft rejection, four of whom had advanced myelofibrosis. NRM was 24%, and after 2 years of follow-up; OS and DFS were 49% and 36%, respectively [99].

Collectively, these studies demonstrate that patients who relapse after prior high-dose therapy or have graft failure can be successfully salvaged with a reduced-intensity or nonmyeloablative allograft. Again, patients with more advanced disease at the time of transplant appeared to have inferior outcomes.

Myeloablative Versus Reduced-Intensity Conditioning: Does Conditioning Intensity Affect Outcomes?

Over the past decade, the number of patients undergoing reduced-intensity transplantation has increased considerably. This has led a number of investigators to ask the question whether the intensity of the conditioning regimen affects outcomes. In the past several years, a number of large retrospective studies have compared the outcomes between high-dose and reduced-intensity conditioning in several diseases, and the results are summarized in Table 7.4 [63, 65, 77, 87, 100–105]. In general, the patients in these studies undergoing reduced-intensity conditioning were typically older and had more comorbidities. Despite this fact, all studies consistently found that NRM was significantly decreased with the use of reduced-intensity conditioning. However, relapse rates were also consistently higher with the use of reduced-intensity conditioning. Therefore, overall survival was not significantly different for most diseases. The exception was an EBMT analysis of follicular lymphoma and Hodgkin lymphoma where reduced-intensity conditioning was associated with improved survival [63, 105]. This may be explained by the biology of these diseases, where patients can live for many months after relapse, allowing time for

Table 7.4 Recent comparisons of conditioning intensity

Study	Disease		Conditioning	Pts	Median age	Grades III–IV acute GVHD (%)	Chronic GVHD (%)	Relapse (%)	NRM (%)	Survival	Conclusion
AML/MDS											
DFCI [100]	AML/MDS		M	97	43	13	18	38	33	2-year OS 34% 2-year PFS 31%	There was no difference in OS or PFS NM associated with decreased NRM but negated by increased rate of relapse
			NM	39	56	21	33	61	26	2-year OS 28% 2-year PFS 20%	
EBMT [101]	AML	Age <50	M	149	36	NR	38	30	27	2-year LFS 43%	In patients <50, NRM and LFS was the same between M and RIC, but relapse higher with RIC
			RIC	972	39		31	38	25	2-year LFS 37%	
		Age >50	M	182	54	NR	46	29	39	2-year LFS 33%	In patients >50, relapse and LFS same between M and RIC, but NRM decreased in RIC
			RIC	252	57		36	42	25	2-year LFS 34%	
EBMT [87]	MDS/AML		M	500	54	NR		33	44	4-year OS 32%	RIC was associated with decreased NRM but increased relapse. Disease stage at transplant and not age or intensity of conditioning was the most important factor affecting survival
			RIC	833	59			41	32	4-year OS 30%	
FHCRC [102]	AML/MDS		M	112	53	21	64	23	32	3-year OS 48% 3-year PFS 44%	There was no difference between the groups. OS and PFS were similar for patients who had chemotherapy induced remissions regardless of conditioning intensity
			NM	38	62	22	55	31	15	3-year OS 28% 3-year PFS 27%	
CLL/NHL											
FHCRC [103]	CLL/NHL		M	68	46	NR		35		3-year OS 45%	Patients without comorbidity had comparable NRM and OS. Patients with comorbidities had significantly lower NRM and OS with NM
			NM	152	60			25		3-year OS 53%	

(continued)

Table 7.4 (continued)

Study	Disease	Conditioning	Pts	Median age	Grades III–IV acute GVHD (%)	Chronic GVHD (%)	Relapse (%)	NRM (%)	Survival	Conclusion
EBMT [63]	Follicular NHL	M	44	42	NR	42	20	37	3-year OS 47% 3-year PFS 43%	RIC was associated with lower NRM and a significantly longer PFS and OS compared to M
		RIC	87	51		48	20	33	3-year OS 53% 3-year PFS 49%	
CIBMTR [65]	Follicular NHL	M	120	44	13	46	8	23	3-year OS 71% 3-year PFS 67%	There was no difference in survival, and RIC was associated with increased relapse risk
		RIC	88	51	21	62	17	23	3-year OS 62% 3-year PFS 55%	
EBMT [104]	CLL	M	82	45	NR	45	11	26	2-year OS 70% 2-year EFS62%	There was no difference in OS or EFS. RIC was associated with reduced NRM but also with higher relapse
		RIC	73	53		55	28	19	2-year OS 70% 2-year EFS58%	
Hodgkin										
EBMT [105]	Hodgkin	M	79	31	12	38	30	46	5-year OS 22% 5-year PFS20%	RIC was associated with less NRM and better OS. There was a trend for better PFS survival with RIC as well
		RIC	89	30	10	40	57	23	5-year OS 28% 5-year PFS18%	
Myeloma										
EBMT [77]	Myeloma	M	196	45	NR	50	27	37	2-year OS 51% 2-year PFS 34%	RIC was associated with decreased NRM but also with increased relapse. No difference in OS or PFS between groups
		RIC	320	51		50	54	24	2-year OS 38% 2-year PFS 19%	

GVT or other therapies. This is in contrast to more aggressive diseases like AML, where relapse can be fatal within a few weeks. One interesting note is that in a subgroup analysis by Scott et al. patients with AML who were in a complete remission at the time of transplant had no difference in progression-free survival or relapse [102]. This suggests that GVT maybe more critical in preventing disease recurrence than conditioning intensity in this group of patients. Only future randomized trials can definitively address this issue. For patients with aggressive malignancies who have residual disease at the time of transplant, relapse with reduced-intensity conditioning remains a problem. Several strategies are being studied to improve outcomes in this population and are discussed below.

Consolidated Reduced-Intensity Allografts Following Planned Autografts

In rapidly progressive diseases such as aggressive lymphomas and myelomas, the GVT effect can be outpaced by the rapid growth of the malignancy. One strategy that has been employed to overcome this problem is to initially perform an autologous transplant with the purpose of debulking and providing disease control. Subsequently, a reduced-intensity allogeneic transplant is performed with the purpose of disease eradication. This approach was first evaluated by Carella et al. [106] where 15 patients with refractory lymphoma were first given an autologous transplant, and after a median of 61 days after engraftment were subsequently given an allograft from an HLA-matched sibling donor after reduced-intensity conditioning. This group saw encouraging results with this approach as ten patients were alive and in remission after a median follow-up of 337 days. Further studies are underway using this approach for the treatment of aggressive lymphoma.

The same tandem transplant approach has also been studied in multiple myeloma, and initial results were encouraging with high rates of complete response. Long-term follow-up on two of the largest studies investigating this tandem approach were published recently [72, 73]. Investigators at the FHCRC have recently reported results on 102 patients with myeloma who initially underwent an autologous transplant with high-dose melphalan and, after recovery, received an allograft from an HLA-matched sibling after nonmyeloablative conditioning. The rates of acute and chronic GVHD were 42% and 74%, respectively. Median time to progression was 5 years. Although this approach was quite effective at achieving a high response with 59 patients achieving a complete response, long-term disease control remained a problem [72]. Similarly, the Gruppo Italiano Trapianti di Midollo recently reported results on 100 patients with newly diagnosed myeloma. Patients initially received induction with VAD (vincristine, doxorubicin, and dexamethasone) chemotherapy followed by high-dose therapy with melphalan and autologous stem cell rescue. After recovery, all patients received an allograft from an HLA-matched related donor after nonmyeloablative conditioning. Again, this approach was very effective in achieving a high rate of complete remission (53%), and after a median follow-up of 5 years, event-free survival was 37 months. The rates of acute and chronic graft-versus-host disease (GVHD) were 38% and 50%, respectively. However, in this cohort, chronic GVHD was not associated with complete remission or response duration [73]. Current studies are underway in which novel agents such as bortezomib and lenalidomide are being incorporated into posttransplant regimens in an effort to provide both antimyeloma therapy as well as eliciting a stronger graft-versus-myeloma effect [107, 108].

HLA-Mismatched Related Donor Transplantation

Data from animal models suggest that a stronger GVT effect can be seen when there is greater MHC mismatching between the donor and the host. Since each patient shares an HLA haplotype with their parents and children, and since there is a 75% chance that a full sibling will share a haplotype with the patient, an HLA-haploidentical donor can be identified for most individuals. One method that has been studied to eliminate the high relapse rates after HCT associated with aggressive malignancies is to harness the potentially more powerful GVT from a haploidentical donor. Two major issues to overcome after haploidentical HCT both due to MHC mismatching have been graft rejection and GVHD. The Johns Hopkins group has recently developed a reduced-intensity conditioning regimen based on data from a murine model where high-dose cyclophosphamide is used after HCT to inhibit graft rejection and GVHD [109]. This conditioning regimen consists of pre-transplant fludarabine 150 mg/m^2, cyclophosphamide 29 mg/m^2 and TBI 2 Gy followed by an infusion of marrow. Posttransplant immunosuppression consists of cyclophosphamide, 50–100 mg/kg, tacrolimus, and mycophenolate mofetil. A recent study reported the results of 68 patients with various hematologic malignancies transplanted at Johns Hopkins and the FHCRC. The only difference between patients treated at these two centers was that patients at Johns Hopkins received 100 mg/kg of posttransplant cyclophosphamide divided equally on days +3 and +4, whereas patients at the FHCRC received only 50 mg/kg given on day +3. The rates of graft failure, grades II–IV acute GVHD, and grades III–IV acute GVHD were 13%, 35%, and 6%, respectively. The only difference between the two centers was that patients who received 50 mg/kg of posttransplant cyclophosphamide at the FHCRC had higher rates of chronic GVHD at 25% compared to 5% in the group at Johns Hopkins that received 100 mg/kg. The overall and event-free survivals at 2 years after HCT were 36% and 27%, respectively [109].

A subsequent analysis was also performed comparing outcomes of reduced-intensity HCT for patients with relapsed or refractory Hodgkin disease based on donor stem cell source (see Table 7.2) [68]. This analysis included 90 patients who received an allograft from HLA-matched related ($n=38$), unrelated ($n=24$), or haploidentical ($n=28$) donors. The risks of relapse and NRM were significantly decreased for patients who underwent an HLA-haploidentical HCT compared to HLA-matched related and unrelated donors. The rates of grades II–IV acute GVHD and chronic GVHD were 16%/50% (HLA-matched), 8%/64% (unrelated), and 11%/35% (HLA-haploidentical) [68].

These data together suggest that reduced-intensity conditioning followed by an HLA-haploidentical HCT can be effective at eradicating malignancy with acceptable rates of GVHD and graft rejection. Interestingly, the results in Hodgkin disease appear quite favorable after HLA-haploidentical HCT when compared to HLA-matched related and unrelated donors. Further clinical trials will be needed to confirm these encouraging results.

Optimizing Conditioning Regimens

As discussed above, although reduced-intensity conditioning followed by allogeneic transplantation is effective at eradicating hematologic malignancies, results in more advanced disease remain poor. One current effort to improve outcomes has focused on optimizing the conditioning regimen to provide disease control while limiting nonrelapse mortality. This has included the incorporation of new methods of delivering old agents as well as the addition of novel agents and targeted therapies into conditioning regimens.

One myelotoxic drug that has been linked to organ toxicity is busulfan. Oral busulfan leads to varying levels of plasma concentrations due to differences in bioavailability and pharmacokinetics. Patients who have low concentrations have a higher risk for relapse/graft rejection, and those with higher levels have more toxicity. A study from the FHCRC identified that targeting of oral busulfan to a level of 900 ng/ml yielded better results [110]. Similarly, the use of intravenous busulfan has been reported to reduce hepatotoxicity, and many transplant centers have now switched to the IV formulation [111]. The novel alkylating drug treosulfan has significant cytotoxicity against malignant myeloid cells while having limited nonhematologic toxicities, and it has a more predictable pharmacologic profile [112]. Current studies are underway in the use of this drug in conditioning regimens in a variety of malignancies [112–115]. Most reduced-intensity and nonmyeloablative regimens are now incorporating the purine analog fludarabine due to its potent immunosuppressive properties and favorable toxicity profile [116–119].

Targeted therapies are also being added to conditioning in the hope that these agents will decrease relapse rates without increasing NRM. Investigators at the FHCRC have pioneered the use of radiolabeled antibodies as part of reduced-intensity conditioning regimens. The use of radiolabeled antibodies targeted against CD45 for myeloid disease and CD20 for lymphoid disease is an attractive strategy as it provides effective disease control without incurring the risks of traditional high-dose regimens [120]. Disease control that is provided by this approach allows time for a robust GVT effect to develop before there is progression of disease. The FHCRC recently reported results with a reduced-intensity conditioning regimen of 2 Gy TBI, fludarabine, and I-131 radiolabeled anti-CD45 antibody in elderly patients with high- risk leukemia or myelodysplasia [121]. The use of this radiola-beled antibody allowed for the delivery of very high-intensity therapy to the target organ, while sparing toxicity in nonhematopoietic tissues. This regimen was used to transplant 58 patients (median age 63) with advanced MDS and AML from HLA-matched related ($n=22$) and unrelated ($n=36$) donors. Twenty patients (35%) had refractory disease that either was primary refractory ($n=8$) or was in relapse after prior remission ($n=12$) at the time of transplant. According to SWOG criteria, 55% of the patients had high-risk cytogenetic abnormalities. The maximum toler-ated dose of the antibody was estimated to be 24 Gy delivered to the liver, which allowed the delivery of an average of 36 Gy to the marrow space and 102 Gy to the spleen. After a median follow-up of 2.6 years, the 1-year probability of OS, RFS, and NRM are 41%, 40%, and 22% in this very high-risk population of elderly patients, which is very encouraging [121]. A similar approach is being studied in patients with NHL where I-131 and Yitrrium-90-labeled CD20 antibodies are being used, and preliminary data are promising even in aggressive lymphomas [122, 123]. Similarly, investigators at MDACC have incorporated gemtuzumab ozogamicin (GO), a monoclonal antibody against the CD33 antigen, conjugated to calicheami-cin into a reduced-intensity conditioning regimen of fludarabine and melphalan, and early results show some promise [124]. Further preclinical studies are also testing a variety of radioisotope/toxin conjugates, pretargeting strategies, and com-bining antibodies against two different targets to identify more effective therapies [125–128].

The addition of small molecule compounds that target common mutations in hematologic malignancies are also being incorporated into reduced-intensity regi-mens. The best example of this is in CML, where the use of tyrosine kinase inhibi-tors is clearly effective in patients who have relapsed postallogeneic transplant in controlling disease [129–131]. As discussed previously, the maximal GVT effect does not occur immediately after reduced-intensity conditioned transplantation, and rapidly proliferative diseases may relapse early. The use of tyrosine kinase inhibi-tors can modify the kinetics of the disease posttransplant until the GVT effect can occur. One recent study from the United Kingdom reported results on 22 patients transplanted with a reduced-intensity conditioning regimen on fludarabine/busulfan/Campath followed by 11 months of posttransplant imatinib [132]. The rate of acute GVHD was 5%; there was no chronic GVHD seen with NRM of 4% at 1 year. Of the 21 patients who completed 11 months of imatinib, 15 patients relapsed and required DLI. With a median follow-up of 3 years, OS was 87% [132]. There have also been anecdotal reports on the effectiveness of the Flt3 inhibitor sorafenib in patients with Flt3 + AML who relapse posttransplant ([133] and Eli Estey personal communication). This has led to the research protocols design to study the effective-ness of various Flt3 inhibition after reduced-intensity transplant. Novel drugs such as JAK2 inhibitors and aurora kinase inhibitors have also shown activity in a variety of hematologic malignancies [134, 135]. The incorporation of such targeted thera-pies into reduced-intensity transplant regimens hold great promise, but further stud-ies are needed to determine the optimal drug and the length of treatment time needed for optimal outcomes.

Separating GVT from GVHD

As discussed earlier, the first evidence of a GVT effect in humans was shown in the late 1970s [3]. There is also considerable data that acute GVHD is associated with higher NRM but does not influence relapse rates [61]. Consequently, attempts to minimize severe acute GVHD without affecting GVT may decrease NRM even further without impacting survival when using reduced-intensity conditioning.

Several groups have attempted to decrease rates of acute GVHD by manipulating the cellular content of the allograft. The most common methods used to decrease acute GVHD are the use of antibodies targeted against donor T-cells such as ATG or alemtuzumab [136]. Many studies have shown that these targeted agents are quite effective at decreasing the rate of acute GVHD; unfortunately, these agents also seem to target T-cells that mediate GVT as rates or relapse/disease progression are also higher [59, 86, 137, 138]. Also, the use of these agents is associated with higher rates of certain infectious complications, particularly CMV infection with the use of alemtuzumab [139].

The Stanford group has pioneered the use of total lymphoid irradiation of 8 Gy combined with ATG based on results from the murine studies where the use of this regimen prevented acute GVHD by increasing the proportion of regulatory NK-T-cells [140]. A recent publication from this group reported results on 111 patients with various hematologic and lymphoid malignancies who were conditioned with 8 Gy total lymphoid irradiation combined with ATG followed by allografts from HLA-matched related and unrelated donors. The rates of acute GVHD were very low, 2% for related and 10% for unrelated donors. The incidence of chronic GVHD was 27%, and NRM at 1 year was 4%. The 36-month probability of OS and RFS were 60% and 40% [141]. Although these results suggest that this regimen is associated with very low of GVHD while apparently preserving GVT, the follow-up period is relatively short, and further studies and follow-up will be necessary.

Another area of active research is the use of pharmacologic agents to enhance GVT while minimizing GVHD. The calcineurin inhibitors, methotrexate and mycophenolate mofetil, are currently the most commonly used agents for GVHD prophylaxis [142]. Although these drugs are effective, GVHD continues to be a problem. In a recent retrospective analysis, the use of rapamycin as GVHD prophylaxis after reduced-intensity conditioning was associated with improved survival in patients with lymphoma [143]. In addition to direct antitumor effects, rapamycin may also affect regulatory T-cells, and further studies with this drug are currently underway [144]. The proteasome inhibitor bortezomib and the histone deacetylase inhibitor SAHA have both been studied in murine models of transplantation and have been shown to reduce GVHD without compromising GVT [145, 146]. The combination of bortezomib, tacrolimus, and methotrexate was used for GVHD prophylaxis after HLA-mismatched HCT in a recent Phase I study, and the rates of acute GVHD was very low at 13% [147]. A recent retrospective analysis from our center also identified that the use of statin drugs by the donor was associated with a decreased risk of grades III–IV acute GVHD. Statin use by the recipient was not associated with any decreased risk of GVHD [148]. These results suggest a novel strategy to prevent severe acute GVHD without compromising GVT by treating donors with drugs that are immunomodulatory. These data are quite promising, but further studies with these agents in human trials will be needed to show their efficacy.

Conclusion

The development of reduced-intensity and nonmyeloablative conditioning regimens has allowed older patients with hematologic malignancies to benefit from the curative potential of hematopoietic cell transplantation. Although there is significant data to confirm that these less toxic conditioning regimens are associated with decreased NRM, relapse remains a problem, especially in patients with aggressive malignancies. Future efforts to optimize conditioning regimen with the addition of targeted therapies and posttransplant maintenance strategies hold great promise. Other efforts directed at preventing acute GVHD and harnessing the power of GVT will hopefully improve the effectiveness of reduced-intensity and nonmyeloablative transplantation.

Acknowledgments The authors would like to thank Helen Crawford, Bonnie Larson, and Sue Carbonneau who provided invaluable help in preparation of this manuscript. The authors are grateful for research funding from the National Institutes of Health, Bethesda, MD grants K08DK082783, P01HL036444, P01CA078902, P01CA018029, and R01CA118940. The content is solely the responsibility of the authors and does not necessarily represent the official views of the National Institutes of Health nor its subsidiary Institutes and Centers.

References

1. Thomas ED. A history of allogeneic hematopoietic cell transplantation. In: Appelbaum FR, Forman SJ, Negrin RS, Blume KG, editors. Thomas' hematopoietic cell transplantation. Oxford: Wiley-Blackwell; 2009. p. 3–7.
2. Weiden PL, Flournoy N, Sanders JE, Sullivan KM, Thomas ED. Antileukemic effect of graft-versus-host disease contributes to improved survival after allogeneic marrow transplantation. Transplant Proc. 1981;13(1):248–51.
3. Weiden PL, Flournoy N, Thomas ED, et al. Antileukemic effect of graft-versus-host disease in human recipients of allogeneic-marrow grafts. N Engl J Med. 1979;300:1068–73.
4. Weiden PL, Sullivan KM, Flournoy N, Storb R, Thomas ED, the Seattle Marrow Transplant Team. Antileukemic effect of chronic graft-versus-host disease. Contribution to improved survival after allogeneic marrow transplantation. N Engl J Med. 1981;304:1529–33.
5. Martin PJ, Hansen JA, Buckner CD, et al. Effects of in vitro depletion of T cells in HLA-identical allogeneic marrow grafts. Blood. 1985;66:664–72.
6. Maraninchi D, Gluckman E, Blaise D, et al. Impact of T-cell depletion on outcome of allogeneic bone-marrow transplantation for standard-risk leukaemias. Lancet. 1987;2:175–8.
7. Kolb HJ, Mittermüller J, Clemm Ch, et al. Donor leukocyte transfusions for treatment of recurrent chronic myelogenous leukemia in marrow transplant patients. Blood. 1990;76:2462–5.

8. Kolb HJ, Schattenberg A, Goldman JM, et al. Graft-versus-leukemia effect of donor lymphocyte transfusions in marrow grafted patients. European Group for Blood and Marrow Transplantation Working Party Chronic Leukemia. Blood. 1995;86(5):2041–50.

9. Clift RA, Buckner CD, Appelbaum FR, et al. Allogeneic marrow transplantation in patients with acute myeloid leukemia in first remission: a randomized trial of two irradiation regimens. Blood. 1990;76(9):1867–71.

10. Clift RA, Buckner CD, Appelbaum FR, et al. Allogeneic marrow transplantation in patients with chronic myeloid leukemia in the chronic phase: a randomized trial of two irradiation regimens. Blood. 1991;77:1660–5.

11. Sandmaier BM, Storb R. Reduced-intensity conditioning followed by hematopoietic cell transplantation for hematologic malignancies. In: Appelbaum FR, Forman SJ, Negrin RS, Blume KG, editors. Thomas' hematopoietic cell transplantation. Oxford: Wiley-Blackwell; 2009. p. 1043–58.

12. Giralt S, Ballen K, Rizzo D, et al. Reduced-intensity conditioning regimen workshop: defining the dose spectrum. Report of a workshop convened by the Center for International Blood and Marrow Transplant Research. Biol Blood Marrow Transplant. 2009;15:367–9.

13. Storb R, Yu C, Wagner JL, et al. Stable mixed hematopoietic chimerism in DLA-identical littermate dogs given sublethal total body irradiation before and pharmacological immunosuppression after marrow transplantation. Blood. 1997;89(8):3048–54.

14. McSweeney PA, Niederwieser D, Shizuru JA, et al. Hematopoietic cell transplantation in older patients with hematologic malignancies: replacing high-dose cytotoxic therapy with graft-versus-tumor effects. Blood. 2001;97(11):3390–400.

15. Giralt S, Logan B, Rizzo D, et al. Reduced-intensity conditioning for unrelated donor progenitor cell transplantation: long-term follow-up of the first 285 reported to the National Marrow Donor Program. Biol Blood Marrow Transplant. 2007;13:844–52.

16. Bacigalupo A, Ballen K, Rizzo D, et al. Defining the intensity of conditioning regimens: working definitions. Biol Blood Marrow Transplant. 2009;15(12):1628–33.

17. Storb RF, Champlin R, Riddell SR, Murata M, Bryant S, Warren EH. Non-myeloablative transplants for malignant disease. In: Schechter GP, Broudy VC, Williams ME, editors. Hematology 2001: American society of hematology education program book. Washington, DC: The American Society of Hematology; 2001. p. 375–91.

18. Baron F, Little M-T, Storb R. Kinetics of engraftment following allogeneic hematopoietic cell transplantation with reduced-intensity or nonmyeloablative conditioning. Blood Rev. 2005;19:153–64.

19. Dey BR, McAfee S, Colby C, et al. Impact of prophylactic donor leukocyte infusions on mixed chimerism, graft-versus-host disease, and antitumor response in patients with advanced hematologic malignancies treated with nonmyeloablative conditioning and allogeneic bone marrow transplantation. Biol Blood Marrow Transplant. 2003;9(5):320–9.

20. Childs R, Clave E, Contentin N, et al. Engraftment kinetics after nonmyeloablative allogeneic peripheral blood stem cell transplantation: full donor T-cell chimerism precedes alloimmune responses. Blood. 1999;94(9):3234–41.

21. Baron F, Baker JE, Storb R, et al. Kinetics of engraftment in patients with hematologic malignancies given allogeneic hematopoietic cell transplantation after nonmyeloablative conditioning. Blood. 2004;104(8):2254–62.

22. Bornhauser M, Thiede C, Platzbecker U, et al. Dose-reduced conditioning and allogeneic hematopoietic stem cell transplantation from unrelated donors in 42 patients. Clin Cancer Res. 2001;7(8):2254–62.

23. de Lima M, Anagnostopoulos A, Munsell M, et al. Nonablative versus reduced-intensity conditioning regimens in the treatment of acute myeloid leukemia and high-risk myelodysplastic syndrome: dose is relevant for long-term disease control after allogeneic hematopoietic stem cell transplantation. Blood. 2004;104(3):865–72.

24. Baron F, Sandmaier BM. Chimerism and outcomes after allogeneic hematopoietic cell transplantation following nonmyeloablative conditioning (review). Leukemia. 2006;20: 1690–700.

25. Maris MB, Sandmaier BM, Storer BE, et al. Unrelated donor granulocyte colony-stimulating factor-mobilized peripheral blood mononuclear cell transplantation after nonmyeloablative conditioning: the effect of postgrafting mycophenolate mofetil dosing. Biol Blood Marrow Transplant. 2006;12:454–65.
26. Carvallo C, Geller N, Kurlander R, et al. Prior chemotherapy and allograft CD34+ dose impact donor engraftment following nonmyeloablative allogeneic stem cell transplantation in patients with solid tumors. Blood. 2004;103(4):1560–3.
27. Maris MB, Niederwieser D, Sandmaier BM, et al. HLA-matched unrelated donor hematopoietic cell transplantation after nonmyeloablative conditioning for patients with hematologic malignancies. Blood. 2003;102(6):2021–30.
28. Baron F, Maris MB, Storer BE, et al. High doses of transplanted CD34$^+$ cells are associated with rapid T-cell engraftment and lessened risk of graft rejection, but not more graft-versus-host disease after nonmyeloablative conditioning and unrelated hematopoietic cell transplantation. Leukemia. 2005;19:822–8.
29. Mattsson J, Uzunel M, Brune M, et al. Mixed chimaerism is common at the time of acute graft-versus-host disease and disease response in patients receiving non-myeloablative conditioning and allogeneic stem cell transplantation. Br J Haematol. 2001;115(4):935–44.
30. Baron F, Petersdorf EW, Gooley T, et al. What is the role for donor NK cells after nonmyeloablative conditioning? Biol Blood Marrow Transplant. 2009;15(5):580–8.
31. Hogan WJ, Maris M, Storer B, et al. Hepatic injury after nonmyeloablative conditioning followed by allogeneic hematopoietic cell transplantation: a study of 193 patients. Blood. 2004; 103(1):78–84.
32. Fukuda T, Hackman RC, Guthrie KA, et al. Risks and outcomes of idiopathic pneumonia syndrome after nonmyeloablative and conventional conditioning regimens for allogeneic hematopoietic stem cell transplantation. Blood. 2003;102(8):2777–85.
33. Chien JW, Maris MB, Sandmaier BM, Maloney DG, Storb RF, Clark JG. Comparison of lung function after myeloablative and 2Gy of total body irradiation-based regimens for hematopoietic stem cell transplantation. Biol Blood Marrow Transplant. 2005;11:288–96.
34. Parikh CR, Schrier RW, Storer B, et al. Comparison of ARF after myeloablative and nonmyeloablative hematopoietic cell transplantation. Am J Kidney Dis. 2005;45(3):502–9.
35. Junghanss C, Marr KA, Carter RA, et al. Incidence and outcome of bacterial and fungal infections following nonmyeloablative compared with myeloablative allogeneic hematopoietic stem cell transplantation: a matched control study. Biol Blood Marrow Transplant. 2002;8:512–20.
36. Junghanss C, Boeckh M, Carter RA, et al. Incidence and outcome of cytomegalovirus infections following nonmyeloablative compared with myeloablative allogeneic stem cell transplantation, a matched control study. Blood. 2002;99(6):1978–85.
37. Nakamae H, Kirby KA, Sandmaier BM, et al. Effect of conditioning regimen intensity on CMV infection in allogeneic hematopoietic cell transplantation. Biol Blood Marrow Transplant. 2009;15:694–703.
38. Schiffer JT, Kirby K, Sandmaier B, Storb R, Corey L, Boeckh M. Timing and severity of community acquired respiratory virus infections after myeloablative versus non-myeloablative hematopoietic stem cell transplantation. Haematologica. 2009;94(8):1101–8.
39. Ruiz-Arguelles GJ, Lopez-Martinez B, Gomez-Rangel D, et al. Decreased transfusion requirements in patients given stem cell allografts using a non-myeloablative conditioning regimen: a single institution experience. Hematology. 2003;8(3):151–4.
40. Weissinger F, Sandmaier BM, Maloney DG, Bensinger WI, Gooley T, Storb R. Decreased transfusion requirements for patients receiving nonmyeloablative compared with conventional peripheral blood stem cell transplants from HLA-identical siblings. Blood. 2001;98(13): 3584–8.
41. Wang Z, Sorror ML, Leisenring W, et al. The impact of donor type and ABO incompatibility on transfusion requirements after nonmyeloablative hematopoietic cell transplantation. Br J Haematol. 2010;149:101–10.

42. Sorror ML, Maris MB, Storer B, et al. Comparing morbidity and mortality of HLA-matched unrelated donor hematopoietic cell transplantation after nonmyeloablative and myeloablative conditioning: influence of pretransplant comorbidities. Blood. 2004;104(4):961–8.

43. Charlson ME, Pompei P, Ales KL, MacKenzie CR. A new method of classifying prognostic comorbidity in longitudinal studies: development and validation. J Chronic Dis. 1987;40(5):373–83.

44. Diaconescu R, Flowers CR, Storer B, et al. Morbidity and mortality with nonmyeloablative compared to myeloablative conditioning before hematopoietic cell transplantation from HLA matched related donors. Blood. 2004;104(5):1550–8.

45. Sorror ML, Maris MB, Storb R, et al. Hematopoietic cell transplantation (HCT)-specific comorbidity index: a new tool for risk assessment before allogeneic HCT. Blood. 2005;106(8):2912–9.

46. Farina L, Bruno B, Patriarca F, et al. The hematopoietic cell transplantation comorbidity index (HCT-CI) predicts clinical outcomes in lymphoma and myeloma patients after reduced-intensity or non-myeloablative allogeneic stem cell transplantation. Leukemia. 2009;23(6): 1131–8.

47. Pollack SM, Steinberg SM, Odom J, Dean RM, Fowler DH, Bishop MR. Assessment of the hematopoietic cell transplantation comorbidity index in non-Hodgkin lymphoma patients receiving reduced-intensity allogeneic hematopoietic stem cell transplantation. Biol Blood Marrow Transplant. 2009;15(2):223–30.

48. Sorror ML, Giralt S, Sandmaier BM, et al. Hematopoietic cell transplantation-specific comorbidity index as an outcome predictor for patients with acute myeloid leukemia in first remission: combined FHCRC and MDACC experiences. Blood. 2007;110(13):4608–13.

49. Sorror ML, Sandmaier BM, Storer BE, et al. Comorbidity and disease status-based risk stratification of outcomes among patients with acute myeloid leukemia or myelodysplasia receiving allogeneic hematopoietic cell transplantation. J Clin Oncol. 2007;25(27):4246–54.

50. Deeg HJ. New strategies for prevention and treatment of graft-versus-host disease and for induction of graft-versus-leukemia effects. Int J Hematol. 2003;77:15–21.

51. Goker H, Haznedaroglu IC, Chao NJ. Acute graft-vs-host disease: pathobiology and management (Review) [erratum appears in Exp Hematol 2001 May;29(5):653]. Exp Hematol. 2001;29(3):259–77.

52. Shlomchik WD, Couzens MS, Tang CB, et al. Prevention of graft versus host disease by inactivation of host antigen-presenting cells. Science. 1999;285(5426):412–5.

53. Mielcarek M, Martin PJ, Leisenring W, et al. Graft-versus-host disease after nonmyeloablative versus conventional hematopoietic stem cell transplantation. Blood. 2003;102(2):756–62.

54. Levine JE, Uberti JP, Ayash L, et al. Lowered-intensity preparative regimen for allogeneic stem cell transplantation delays acute graft-versus-host disease but does not improve outcome for advanced hematologic malignancy. Biol Blood Marrow Transplant. 2003;9(3):189–97.

55. Filipovich AH, Weisdorf D, Pavletic S, et al. National institutes of health consensus development project on criteria for clinical trials in chronic graft-versus-host disease: I. Diagnosis and Staging Working Group report. Biol Blood Marrow Transplant. 2005;11(12):945–56.

56. Vigorito AC, Campregher PV, Storer BE, et al. Evaluation of NIH consensus criteria for classification of late acute and chronic GVHD. Blood. 2009;114(3):702–8.

57. Martino R, Caballero MD, Simón JA, et al. Evidence for a graft-versus-leukemia effect after allogeneic peripheral blood stem cell transplantation with reduced-intensity conditioning in acute myelogenous leukemia and myelodysplastic syndromes. Blood. 2002;100(6): 2243–5.

58. Kroger N, Perez-Simon JA, Myint H, et al. Relapse to prior autograft and chronic graft-versus-host disease are the strongest prognostic factors for outcome of melphalan/fludarabine-based dose-reduced allogeneic stem cell transplantation in patients with multiple myeloma. Biol Blood Marrow Transplant. 2004;10(10):698–708.

59. Crawley C, Lalancette M, Szydlo R, et al. Outcomes for reduced-intensity allogeneic trans-plantation for multiple myeloma: an analysis of prognostic factors from the Chronic Leukemia Working Party of the EBMT. Blood. 2005;105(11):4532–9.
60. Blaise DP, Boiron JM, Faucher C, et al. Reduced intensity conditioning prior to allogeneic stem cell transplantation for patients with acute myeloblastic leukemia as a first-line treat-ment. Cancer. 2005;104(9):1931–8.
61. Baron F, Maris MB, Sandmaier BM, et al. Graft-versus-tumor effects after allogeneic hematopoietic cell transplantation with nonmyeloablative conditioning. J Clin Oncol. 2005; 23(9):1993–2003.
62. Baron F, Sandmaier BM. Nonmyeloablative transplantation. In: Soiffer RJ, editor. Hematopoietic stem cell transplantation. Totowa: Humana Press; 2008. p. 349–74.
63. Avivi I, Montoto S, Canals C, et al. Matched unrelated donor stem cell transplant in 131 patients with follicular lymphoma: an analysis from the Lymphoma Working Party of the European Group for Blood and Marrow Transplantation. Br J Haematol. 2009;147(5):719–28.
64. Robinson SP, Sureda A, Canals C, et al. Reduced intensity conditioning allogeneic stem cell transplantation for Hodgkin's lymphoma: identification of prognostic factors predicting out-come. Haematologica. 2009;94(2):230–8.
65. Hari P, Carreras J, Zhang MJ, et al. Allogeneic transplants in follicular lymphoma: higher risk of disease progression after reduced-intensity compared to myeloablative conditioning. Biol Blood Marrow Transplant. 2008;14(2):236–45.
66. Sorror ML, Storer BE, Sandmaier BM, et al. Five-year follow-up of patients with advanced chronic lymphocytic leukemia treated with allogeneic hematopoietic cell transplantation after nonmyeloablative conditioning. J Clin Oncol. 2008;26(30):4912–20.
67. Rezvani AR, Norasetthada L, Gooley T, et al. Non-myeloablative allogeneic haematopoietic cell transplantation of relapsed diffuse large B-cell lymphoma: a multicentre experience. Br J Haematol. 2008;143:395–403.
68. Burroughs LM, O'Donnell PV, Sandmaier BM, et al. Comparison of outcomes of HLA-matched related, unrelated, or HLA-haploidentical related hematopoietic cell transplantation following nonmyeloablative conditioning for relapsed or refractory Hodgkin lymphoma. Biol Blood Marrow Transplant. 2008;14:1279–87.
69. Rezvani AR, Storer B, Maris M, et al. Nonmyeloablative allogeneic hematopoietic cell trans-plantation in relapsed, refractory, and transformed indolent non-Hodgkin lymphoma. J Clin Oncol. 2008;28(2):211–7.
70. Maris MB, Sandmaier BM, Storer BE, et al. Allogeneic hematopoietic cell transplantation after fludarabine and 2 Gy total body irradiation for relapsed and refractory mantle cell lym-phoma. Blood. 2004;104(12):3535–42.
71. Ram R, Storb RF, Maloney DG, Sandmaier BM, Maris M, Shizuru J, et al. Reduced intensity conditioning with allogeneic hematopoietic cell transplantation for the treatment of high-risk acute lymphoblastic leukemia. Blood. 2009;114(22):497–8, 497–498, #1210. 11-20-2009.
72. Rotta M, Storer BE, Sahebi F, et al. Long-term outcome of patients with multiple myeloma after autologous hematopoietic cell transplantation and nonmyeloablative allografting. Blood. 2009;113(14):3383–91.
73. Bruno B, Rotta M, Patriarca F, et al. Non-myeloablative allografting for newly diagnosed multiple myeloma: the experience of the Gruppo Italiano Trapianti di Midollo. Blood. 2009;113(14):3375–82.
74. Dreger P, Brand R, Hansz J, et al. Treatment-related mortality and graft-versus-leukemia activity after allogeneic stem cell transplantation for chronic lymphocytic leukemia using intensity-reduced conditioning (Review). Leukemia. 2003;17(5):841–8.
75. Robinson SP, Goldstone AH, Mackinnon S, et al. Chemoresistant or aggressive lymphoma predicts for a poor outcome following reduced-intensity allogeneic progenitor cell transplan-tation: an analysis from the Lymphoma Working Party of the European Group for Blood and Bone Marrow Transplantation. Blood. 2002;100(13):4310–6.
76. Mohty M, Labopin M, Tabrizzi R, et al. Reduced intensity conditioning allogeneic stem cell transplantation for adult patients with acute lymphoblastic leukemia: a retrospective study

from the European Group for Blood and Marrow Transplantation. Haematologica. 2008; 93(2):303–6.

77. Crawley C, Iacobelli S, Björkstrand B, Apperley JF, Niederwieser D, Gahrton G. Reduced-intensity conditioning for myeloma: lower nonrelapse mortality but higher relapse rates compared with myeloablative conditioning. Blood. 2007;109(8):3588–94.

78. Devetten MP, Hari PN, Carreras J, et al. Unrelated donor reduced-intensity allogeneic hematopoietic stem cell transplantation for relapsed and refractory Hodgkin lymphoma. Biol Blood Marrow Transplant. 2009;15(1):109–17.

79. Anderlini P, Saliba R, Acholonu S, et al. Fludarabine-melphalan as a preparative regimen for reduced-intensity conditioning allogeneic stem cell transplantation in relapsed and refractory Hodgkin's lymphoma: the updated M.D. Anderson cancer center experience. Haematologica. 2008;93(2):257–64.

80. Tam CS, Bassett R, Ledesma C, et al. Mature results of the M. D. Anderson Cancer Center risk-adapted transplantation strategy in mantle cell lymphoma. Blood. 2009;113(18): 4144–52.

81. Khouri IF, McLaughlin P, Saliba RM, et al. Eight-year experience with allogeneic stem cell transplantation for relapsed follicular lymphoma after nonmyeloablative conditioning with fludarabine, cyclophosphamide, and rituximab. Blood. 2008;111(12):5530–6.

82. Khouri IF, Saliba RM, Admirand J, et al. Graft-versus-leukaemia effect after non-myeloablative haematopoietic transplantation can overcome the unfavourable expression of ZAP-70 in refractory chronic lymphocytic leukaemia. Br J Haematol. 2007;137(4):355–63.

83. Laport GG, Sandmaier BM, Storer BE, et al. Reduced-intensity conditioning followed by allogeneic hematopoietic cell transplantation for adult patients with myelodysplastic syndrome and myeloproliferative disorders. Biol Blood Marrow Transplant. 2008;14: 246–55.

84. Hegenbart U, Niederwieser D, Sandmaier BM, et al. Treatment for acute myelogenous leukemia by low-dose, total-body, irradiation-based conditioning and hematopoietic cell transplantation from related and unrelated donors. J Clin Oncol. 2006;24(3):444–53.

85. Kerbauy FR, Storb R, Hegenbart U, et al. Hematopoietic cell transplantation from HLA-identical sibling donors after low-dose radiation-based conditioning for treatment of CML. Leukemia. 2005;19:990–7.

86. Crawley C, Szydlo R, Lalancette M, et al. Outcomes of reduced-intensity transplantation for chronic myeloid leukemia: an analysis of prognostic factors from the Chronic Leukemia Working Party of the EBMT. Blood. 2005;106(9):2969–76.

87. Lim Z, Brand R, Martino R, et al. Allogeneic hematopoietic stem-cell transplantation for patients 50 years or older with myelodysplastic syndromes or secondary acute myeloid leukemia. J Clin Oncol. 2010;28(3):405–11.

88. Aoudjhane M, Labopin M, Gorin NC, et al. Comparative outcome of reduced intensity and myeloablative conditioning regimen in HLA identical sibling allogeneic haematopoietic stem cell transplantation for patients older than 50 years of age with acute myeloblastic leukaemia: a retrospective survey from the Acute Leukemia Working Party (ALWP) of the European Group for Blood and Marrow Transplantation (EBMT). Leukemia. 2005;19: 2304–12.

89. Oran B, Giralt S, Saliba R, et al. Allogeneic hematopoietic stem cell transplantation for the treatment of high-risk acute myelogenous leukemia and myelodysplastic syndrome using reduced-intensity conditioning with fludarabine and melphalan. Biol Blood Marrow Transplant. 2007;13(4):454–62.

90. Kebriaei P, Detry MA, Giralt S, et al. Long-term follow-up of allogeneic hematopoietic stem-cell transplantation with reduced-intensity conditioning for patients with chronic myeloid leukemia. Blood. 2007;110(9):3456–62.

91. Kroger N, Holler E, Kobbe G, et al. Allogeneic stem cell transplantation after reduced-intensity conditioning in patients with myelofibrosis: a prospective, multicenter study of the Chronic Leukemia Working Party of the European Group for Blood and Marrow Transplantation. Blood. 2009;114(26):5264–70.

92. Kahl C, Storer BE, Sandmaier BM, et al. Relapse risk among patients with malignant diseases given allogeneic hematopoietic cell transplantation after nonmyeloablative conditioning. Blood. 2007;110(7):2744–8.
93. Radich JP, Gooley T, Sanders JE, Anasetti C, Chauncey T, Appelbaum FR. Second allogeneic transplantation after failure of first autologous transplantation. Biol Blood Marrow Transplant. 2000;6:272–9.
94. Nagler A, Or R, Naparstek E, Varadi G, Slavin S. Second allogeneic stem cell transplantation using nonmyeloablative conditioning for patients who relapsed or developed secondary malignancies following autologous transplantation. Exp Hematol. 2000;28:1096–104.
95. Dey BR, McAfee S, Sackstein R, et al. Successful allogeneic stem cell transplantation with nonmyeloablative conditioning in patients with relapsed hematologic malignancy following autologous stem cell transplantation. Biol Blood Marrow Transplant. 2001;7:604–12.
96. Fung HC, Cohen S, Rodriguez R, et al. Reduced-intensity allogeneic stem cell transplantation for patients whose prior autologous stem cell transplantation for hematologic malignancy failed. Biol Blood Marrow Transplant. 2003;9(10):649–56.
97. Baron F, Storb R, Storer BE, et al. Factors associated with outcomes in allogeneic hematopoietic cell transplantation with nonmyeloablative conditioning after failed myeloablative hematopoietic cell transplantation. J Clin Oncol. 2006;24(25):4150–7.
98. Shaw BE, Mufti GJ, Mackinnon S, et al. Outcome of second allogeneic transplants using reduced-intensity conditioning following relapse of haematological malignancy after an initial allogeneic transplant. Bone Marrow Transplant. 2008;42(12):783–9.
99. Gyurkocza B, Cao TM, Storb RF, et al. Salvage allogeneic hematopoietic cell transplantation with fludarabine and low-dose total body irradiation after rejection of first allografts. Biol Blood Marrow Transplant. 2009;15:1314–22.
100. Alyea EP, Kim HT, Ho V, et al. Impact of conditioning regimen intensity on outcome of allogeneic hematopoietic cell transplantation for advanced acute myelogenous leukemia and myelodysplastic syndrome. Biol Blood Marrow Transplant. 2006;12(10):1047–55.
101. Ringdén O, Labopin M, Ehninger G, et al. Reduced intensity conditioning compared with myeloablative conditioning using unrelated donor transplants in patients with acute myeloid leukemia. J Clin Oncol. 2009;27(27):4570–7.
102. Scott BL, Sandmaier BM, Storer B, et al. Myeloablative vs nonmyeloablative allogeneic transplantation for patients with myelodysplastic syndrome or acute myelogenous leukemia with multilineage dysplasia: a retrospective analysis. Leukemia. 2006;20:128–35.
103. Sorror ML, Storer BE, Maloney DG, Sandmaier BM, Martin PJ, Storb R. Outcomes after allogeneic hematopoietic cell transplantation with nonmyeloablative or myeloablative regimens for treatment of lymphoma and chronic lymphocytic leukemia. Blood. 2008;111(1):446–52.
104. Dreger P, Brand R, Milligan D, et al. Reduced-intensity conditioning lowers treatment-related mortality of allogeneic stem cell transplantation for chronic lymphocytic leukemia: a population-matched analysis. Leukemia. 2005;19(6):1029–33.
105. Sureda A, Robinson S, Canals C, et al. Reduced-intensity conditioning compared with conventional allogeneic stem-cell transplantation in relapsed or refractory Hodgkin's lymphoma: an analysis from the Lymphoma Working Party of the European Group for Blood and Marrow Transplantation. J Clin Oncol. 2008;26(3):455–62.
106. Carella AM, Cavaliere M, Lerma E, et al. Autografting followed by nonmyeloablative immunosuppressive chemotherapy and allogeneic peripheral-blood hematopoietic stem-cell transplantation as treatment of resistant Hodgkin's disease and non-Hodgkin's lymphoma. J Clin Oncol. 2000;18(23):3918–24.
107. Kroger N, Badbaran A, Lioznov M, et al. Post-transplant immunotherapy with donor-lymphocyte infusion and novel agents to upgrade partial into complete and molecular remission in allografted patients with multiple myeloma. Exp Hematol. 2009;37(7):791–8.
108. Koreth J, Alyea EP, Murphy WJ, Welniak LA. Proteasome inhibition and allogeneic hematopoietic stem cell transplantation: a review. Biol Blood Marrow Transplant. 2009;15(12):1502–12.

109. Luznik L, O'Donnell PV, Symons HJ, et al. HLA-haploidentical bone marrow transplantation for hematologic malignances using nonmyeloablative conditioning and high-dose, post-transplantation cyclophosphamide. Biol Blood Marrow Transplant. 2008;14:641–50.
110. Slattery JT, Clift RA, Buckner CD, et al. Marrow transplantation for chronic myeloid leukemia: the influence of plasma busulfan levels on the outcome of transplantation. Blood. 1997;89(8):3055–60.
111. Kashyap A, Wingard J, Cagnoni P, et al. Intravenous versus oral busulfan as part of a busulfan/cyclophosphamide preparative regimen for allogeneic hematopoietic stem cell transplantation: decreased incidence of hepatic venoocclusive disease (HVOD), HVOD-related mortality, and overall 100-day mortality. Biol Blood Marrow Transplant. 2002;8(9): 493–500.
112. Cutting R, Mirelman A, Vora A. Treosulphan as an alternative to busulphan for myeloablative conditioning in paediatric allogeneic transplantation. Br J Haematol. 2008;143(5):748–51.
113. Bacher U, Klyuchnikov E, Wiedemann B, Kroeger N, Zander AR. Safety of conditioning agents for allogeneic haematopoietic transplantation. Expert Opin Drug Saf. 2009; 8(3):305–15.
114. Kroger N, Shimoni A, Zabelina T, et al. Reduced-toxicity conditioning with treosulfan, fludarabine and ATG as preparative regimen for allogeneic stem cell transplantation (alloSCT) in elderly patients with secondary acute myeloid leukemia (sAML) or myelodysplastic syndrome (MDS). Bone Marrow Transplant. 2006;37(4):339–44.
115. Shimoni A, Hardan I, Shem-Tov N, Rand A, Yerushalmi R, Nagler A. Fludarabine and treosulfan: a novel modified myeloablative regimen for allogeneic hematopoietic stem-cell transplantation with effective antileukemia activity in patients with acute myeloid leukemia and myelodysplastic syndromes. Leuk Lymphoma. 2007;48(12):2352–9.
116. Carella AM, Champlin R, Slavin S, McSweeney P, Storb R. Mini-allografts: ongoing trials in humans (editorial). Bone Marrow Transplant. 2000;25:345–50.
117. Carella AM, Giralt S, Slavin S. Low intensity regimens with allogeneic hematopoietic stem cell transplantation as treatment of hematologic neoplasia (review). Haematologica. 2000; 85(3):304–13.
118. Champlin R, Khouri I, Kornblau S, et al. Allogeneic hematopoietic transplantation as adoptive immunotherapy. Induction of graft-versus-malignancy as primary therapy (review). Hematol Oncol Clin North Am. 1999;13(5):1041–57.
119. Scott BL, Sandmaier BM. Outcomes with myeloid malignancies. In: Berliner N, Linker C, Schiffer CA, editors. Hematology 2006: American society of hematology education program book. Washington, DC: American Society of Hematology; 2006. p. 381–9.
120. Shenoi J, Gopal AK, Press OW, Pagel JM. Recent advances in novel radioimmunotherapeutic approaches for allogeneic hematopoietic cell transplantation (review). Curr Opin Oncol. 2010;22(2):143–9.
121. Pagel JM, Gooley TA, Rajendran J, et al. Allogeneic hematopoietic cell transplantation after conditioning with ^{131}I-anti-CD45 antibody plus fludarabine and low-dose total body irradiation for elderly patients with advanced acute myeloid leukemia or high-risk myelodysplastic syndrome. Blood. 2009;114(27):5444–53.
122. Gopal AK, Rajendran JG, Pagel JM, Guthrie KA, Maloney DG, Appelbaum FR, et al. A phase II trial of 90Y-ibritumomab tiuxetan-based reduced intensity allogeneic peripheral blood stem cell (PBSC) transplantation for relapsed CD20+ B-cell non-Hodgkins lymphoma (NHL). Blood. 2006;108(Part 1 [11]):98a, #316. 11-16-2006. Ref Type: Abstract.
123. Gopal AK, Pagel JM, Rajendran JG, et al. Improving the efficacy of reduced intensity allogeneic transplantation for lymphoma using radiotherapy. Biol Blood Marrow Transplant. 2006;12:697–702.
124. de Lima M, Champlin RE, Thall PF, et al. Phase I/II study of gemtuzumab ozogamicin added to fludarabine, melphalan and allogeneic hematopoietic stem cell transplantation for high-risk CD33 positive myeloid leukemias and myelodysplastic syndrome. Leukemia. 2008; 22(2):258–64.

125. Green DJ, Pagel JM, Nemecek ER, et al. Pretargeting CD45 enhances the selective delivery of radiation to hematolymphoid tissues in nonhuman primates. Blood. 2009;114(6): 1226–35.
126. Nakamae H, Wilbur DS, Hamlin DK, et al. Biodistribution, myelosuppression, and toxicities in mice treated with an anti-CD45 antibody labeled with the a-emitting radionuclides bismuth-213 or astatine-211. Cancer Res. 2009;69(6):2408–15.
127. Pagel JM. Radioimmunotherapeutic approaches for leukemia: the past, present and future (review). Cytotherapy. 2008;10(1):13–20.
128. Walter RB, Boyle KM, Appelbaum FR, Bernstein ID, Pagel JM. Simultaneously targeting CD45 significantly increases cytotoxicity of the anti-CD33 immunoconjugate, gemtuzumab ozogamicin, against acute myeloid leukemia (AML) cells and improves survival of mice bearing human AML xenografts. Blood. 2008;111(9):4813–6.
129. Kantarjian HM, O'Brien S, Cortes JE, et al. Imatinib mesylate therapy for relapse after allogeneic stem cell transplantation for chronic myelogenous leukemia. Blood. 2002;100(5): 1590–5.
130. Olavarria E, Ottmann OG, Deininger M, et al. Response to imatinib in patients who relapse after allogeneic stem cell transplantation for chronic myeloid leukemia. Leukemia. 2003; 17(9):1707–12.
131. Hess G, Bunjes D, Siegert W, et al. Sustained complete molecular remissions after treatment with imatinib-mesylate in patients with failure after allogeneic stem cell transplantation for chronic myelogenous leukemia: results of a prospective phase II open-label multicenter study. J Clin Oncol. 2005;23(30):7583–93.
132. Olavarria E, Siddique S, Griffiths MJ, et al. Posttransplantation imatinib as a strategy to postpone the requirement for immunotherapy in patients undergoing reduced-intensity allografts for chronic myeloid leukemia. Blood. 2007;110(13):4614–7.
133. Metzelder S, Wang Y, Wollmer E, et al. Compassionate use of sorafenib in FLT3-ITD-positive acute myeloid leukemia: sustained regression before and after allogeneic stem cell transplantation. Blood. 2009;113(26):6567–71.
134. Verstovsek S, Odenike O, Scott B, Estrov Z, Cortes J, Thomas DA, et al. Phase I dose-escalation trial of SB1518, a novel JAK2/FLT3 inhibitor, in acute and chronic myeloid diseases, including primary or post-essential thrombocythemia/polycythemia vera myelofibrosis (abstract). Blood. 2009;114(22):1502.
135. Giles FJ, Cortes J, Jones D, Bergstrom D, Kantarjian H, Freedman SJ. MK-0457, a novel kinase inhibitor, is active in patients with chronic myeloid leukemia or acute lymphocytic leukemia with the T315I BCR-ABL mutation. Blood. 2007;109(2):500–2.
136. Barrett AJ, Le Blanc K. Prophylaxis of acute GVHD: manipulate the graft or the environment? (review). Bailliere's Best Pract Clin Haematol. 2008;21(2):165–76.
137. Goldman JM, Gale RP, Horowitz MM, et al. Bone marrow transplantation for chronic myelogenous leukemia in chronic phase: increased risk of relapse associated with T-cell depletion. Ann Intern Med. 1988;108:806–14.
138. Martin PJ, Hansen JA, Torok-Storb B, et al. Graft failure in patients receiving T cell-depleted HLA-identical allogeneic marrow transplants. Bone Marrow Transplant. 1988;3:445–56.
139. Chakrabarti S, Mackinnon S, Chopra R, et al. High incidence of cytomegalovirus infection after nonmyeloablative stem cell transplantation: potential role of Campath-1H in delaying immune reconstitution. Blood. 2002;99(12):4357–63.
140. Lan F, Zeng D, Higuchi M, Huie P, Higgins JP, Strober S. Predominance of NK1.1 + TCR alpha beta + or DX5 + TCR alpha beta + T cells in mice conditioned with fractionated lymphoid irradiation protects against graft-versus-host disease: "natural suppressor" cells. J Immunol. 2001;167(4):2087–96.
141. Kohrt HE, Turnbull BB, Heydari K, et al. TLI and ATG conditioning with low risk of graft-versus-host disease retains antitumor reactions after allogeneic hematopoietic cell transplantation from related and unrelated donors. Blood. 2009;114(5):1099–109.
142. Rezvani AR, Storb RF. Separation of graft-vs.-tumor effects from graft-vs.-host disease in allogeneic hematopoietic cell transplantation. J Autoimmun. 2008;30(3):172–9.

143. Armand P, Gannamaneni S, Kim HT, et al. Improved survival in lymphoma patients receiving sirolimus for graft-versus-host disease prophylaxis after allogeneic hematopoietic stem-cell transplantation with reduced-intensity conditioning. J Clin Oncol. 2008;26(35):5767–74.
144. Valmori D, Tosello V, Souleimanian NE, et al. Rapamycin-mediated enrichment of T cells with regulatory activity in stimulated CD4+ T cell cultures is not due to the selective expansion of naturally occurring regulatory T cells but to the induction of regulatory functions in conventional CD4+ T cells. J Immunol. 2006;177(2):944–9.
145. Sun K, Welniak LA, Panoskaltsis-Mortari A, et al. Inhibition of acute graft-versus-host disease with retention of graft-versus-tumor effects by the proteasome inhibitor bortezomib [erratum appears in Proc Natl Acad Sci U S A. 2004 Aug 24;101(34):12777]. PNAS. 2004;101(21):8120–5.
146. Reddy P, Maeda Y, Hotary K, et al. Histone deacetylase inhibitor suberoylanilide hydroxamic acid reduces acute graft-versus-host disease and preserves graft-versus-leukemia effect. Proc Natl Acad Sci USA. 2004;101(11):3921–6.
147. Koreth J, Stevenson KE, Kim HT, et al. Bortezomib, tacrolimus, and methotrexate for prophylaxis of graft-versus-host disease after reduced-intensity conditioning allogeneic stem cell transplantation from HLA-mismatched unrelated donors. Blood. 2009;114(18):3956–9.
148. Rotta M, Storer BE, Storb RF, et al. Donor statin treatment protects against severe acute graft-versus-host disease after related allogeneic hematopoietic cell transplantation. Blood. 2010;115(6):1288–95.

Chapter 8
Alternative Donor Hematopoietic Stem Cell Transplantation: A Role for Umbilical Cord Blood Transplantation for Hematologic Malignancies

Laura F. Newell, Jonathan A. Gutman, and Colleen Delaney

Abstract Hematopoietic stem cell transplantation (HSCT) is a widely accepted therapy with potentially curative benefit for patients with benign and malignant hematologic disorders. There are currently three possible sources of allogeneic hematopoietic stem cells (HSCs) – bone marrow, granulocyte colony-stimulating factor (G-CSF) mobilized peripheral blood (PBSC), and umbilical cord blood (CB). Donors can be either related or unrelated and must match recipients at human leukocyte antigens (HLA). Based on the average size of American families, and the 25% probability that a given sibling pair will be HLA-matched, it is estimated that approximately 35% of persons in the United States will have an HLA-matched sibling.

Keywords Alternative donor • Hematopoietic stem cell transplantation • Umbilical cord blood • Transplantation • Leukemia • Stem cells • Bone marrow • Granulocyte colony-stimulating factor • Mobilized peripheral blood

L.F. Newell, M.D.
Division of Hematology, University of Washington School of Medicine,
825 Eastlake Ave E, Seattle, WA 98109, USA
e-mail: lnewell@fhcrc.org; lnewell@u.washington.edu

J.A. Gutman, M.D.
Department of Medical Oncology, University of Colorado School of Medicine,
1665 Aurora Court, Room 2251A, Aurora, CO 80045, USA
e-mail: jonathan.gutman@ucdenver.edu

C. Delaney, M.D., M.Sc. (✉)
Department of Pediatrics, University of Washington School of Medicine,
Seattle, WA, USA

Clinical Research Division, Fred Hutchinson Cancer Research Center,
1100 Fairview Ave N, D2-100, Seattle, WA 98109, USA
e-mail: sdelaney@fhcrc.org

E.H. Estey and F.R. Appelbaum (eds.), *Leukemia and Related Disorders:*
Integrated Treatment Approaches, Contemporary Hematology,
DOI 10.1007/978-1-60761-565-1_8, © Springer Science+Business Media, LLC 2012

Introduction

Hematopoietic stem cell transplantation (HSCT) is a widely accepted therapy with potentially curative benefit for patients with benign and malignant hematologic disorders. There are currently three possible sources of allogeneic hematopoietic stem cells (HSCs) – bone marrow, granulocyte colony-stimulating factor (G-CSF) mobilized peripheral blood (PBSC), and umbilical cord blood (CB). Donors can be either related or unrelated and must match recipients at human leukocyte antigens (HLA). Based on the average size of American families, and the 25% probability that a given sibling pair will be HLA-matched, it is estimated that approximately 35% of persons in the United States will have an HLA-matched sibling. For those patients without a matched related donor (MRD), the overall chance of finding an unrelated matched donor (for HLA-A, B, DRB1, and DQB1) is approximately 60% [1]. For ethnic minorities, however, the chance of finding a high-resolution 8/8 matched unrelated donor (MURD) is significantly less than for Caucasians, and ranges from 10% to 40% [2]. Thus, these patients must rely on alternative donor sources, which include related HLA-haploidentical donors, mismatched unrelated donors (MMURDs), and CB. The prioritization of alternative donors remains largely institution dependent.

HLA matching requirements for using CB as the source of HSC are less stringent than for traditional donors; nearly all (>95%) patients are able to find at least one potential 4/6 HLA-matched CB unit, and the majority of patients are able to find a potential 5/6 match [3].

Furthermore, as a cryopreserved product, CB is rapidly available for use as soon as confirmatory typing is complete. This leads to patients receiving CB transplants at a median of 25–36 days earlier than patients receiving traditional URD transplants [4]. CB is collected after delivery of the infant without safety risks for mother and child. There is also lower risk of transmitting infections by latent viruses. In addition, current outcomes following cord blood transplantation (CBT) indicate a potentially lower incidence of chronic extensive graft-versus-host disease (GVHD), and possibly an enhanced graft-versus-leukemia (GVL) effect [5–7].

Despite the benefits noted for CBT, several concerns exist primarily related to the limited cell dose in CB units and the immunologic characteristics unique to a CB graft. Delayed hematopoietic recovery of both neutrophils and platelets remains problematic with most reports describing a median neutrophil recovery of 20–30 days following myeloablative conditioning [8], and only ~50% of patients achieving platelet recovery to $\geq 50,000/\mu L$ by day 100 [5–7]. Other concerns include an increased risk of primary or secondary graft failure and delayed immune reconstitution relative to other donor sources. Additionally, the potential for donor-lymphocyte infusion (DLI) does not currently exist after CBT.

This chapter will focus on issues relevant to CBT as an alternative donor source of hematopoietic stem cells for transplantation, as well as the unique potential benefits seen with CBT. In addition, areas of research and future directions to improve CBT outcomes will be discussed. Finally, data regarding haploidentical transplantation will be briefly reviewed.

History of Umbilical Cord Blood Transplantation

The first CBT was performed in 1988, on a 5-year-old boy with Fanconi's anemia using his HLA-identical sibling's CB [9]. The patient, now age 26, remains engrafted and clinically well [10]. The transplant demonstrated proof of principle that hematopoietic reconstitution could be achieved using CB stem cells, and reports of additional successful HLA-identical sibling donor CBTs soon followed [11–14].

In May 1990, the first related HLA-mismatched CBT was performed in a 30-month-old boy with ALL in second remission [15]. In 1996, the first series of URD CBTs was reported by Kurtzberg et al. [16] and Wagner et al. [17]. Collectively, the patients ranged in age from 0.1 to 23.5 years and were transplanted for both malignant and nonmalignant conditions [16, 17]. In their report of 25 consecutive transplants using unrelated single CB units from the New York Blood Center, Kurtzberg et al. described myeloid engraftment in 23 of the patients receiving units discordant for 0–3 HLA antigens (6/6 matched ($n=1$), 5/6 matched ($n=20$), 4/6 matched ($n=3$), 3/6 matched ($n=1$)). Similarly, Wagner et al. reported engraftment in 13 of 18 patients using units that were 3/6 to 6/6 matched (3/6 matched ($n=1$), 4/6 matched ($n=3$), 5/6 matched ($n=7$), and 6/6-matched ($n=7$)). These reports supported the feasibility of using unrelated, variably HLA-matched CB units as a source of HSC for pediatric patients, even at low total nucleated cell (TNC) doses, and established a role for CB banking.

The first adult CBT was performed in 1996 on a 26-year-old woman with chronic myelogenous leukemia (CML) [18]. Though the transplant was a success, subsequent studies demonstrated that the limited hematopoietic cell dose in a single CB unit negatively affected both hematopoietic recovery and overall survival among adults and large children [19–21].

Issues in Cord Blood Transplantation

During the last several decades, additional experience with CBT has resulted in significant improvements in the field. CB is being used increasingly as an alternative source of HSC, with more than 20,000 CB transplants performed in children and adults to date (Fig. 8.1) [22]. Analyses of transplant outcomes over the last two decades have identified several concerns critically relevant to the field of CBT and to the more widespread use of CB as a donor source. These issues include: graft rejection, engraftment and factors associated with delayed hematopoietic recovery of both platelets and neutrophils, infections and immune reconstitution posttransplantation, acute and chronic GVHD, and relapse after CBT. Currently, significant effort is ongoing to try to better understand these crucial issues, as well as to develop strategies to overcome these challenges.

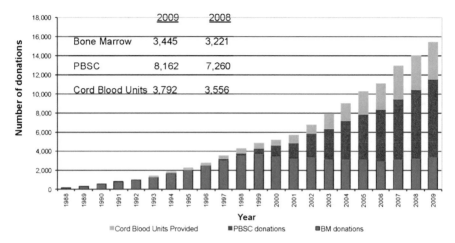

Fig. 8.1 Stem cell products provided for unrelated transplantation (With permission from LM Foeken, Working Group of the World Marrow Donor Association (WMDA) [139]))

Engraftment of Umbilical Cord Blood Hematopoietic Stem Cells

Major historical challenges with CBT include an increased incidence of graft failure relative to other donor sources and delayed time to engraftment following myeloablative conditioning. Recognition of cell dose and matching requirements as well as optimization of conditioning regimen have greatly reduced graft failures, but delayed engraftment remains an issue. Consistent with previous reports, a recent large retrospective study of myeloablative HSCT demonstrated a median time to neutrophil engraftment of approximately 24 days and platelet engraftment of 52 days following single CBT, in contrast to neutrophil engraftment 14 days after peripheral blood stem cell transplantation (PBSCT) and 19 days after BM, and platelet engraftment at 19 and 28 days, respectively [23]. Importantly, a portion of CBT patients will experience significantly prolonged time to engraftment of neutrophils (>40 days) and platelets (>100 days).

Importance of Cell Dose and HLA Match

Major factors found to be associated with engraftment include the TNC and CD34+ cells infused, as well as the number of HLA mismatches. There is also increasing evidence that cell dose and HLA matching interact [22]; two large series have investigated this issue [24, 25] Gluckman et al. [24] analyzed 550 patients undergoing single-unit CBT for hematologic malignancies and found that both the TNC

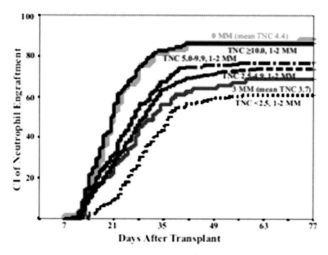

Fig. 8.2 Cumulative incidence (CI) of neutrophil engraftment by day 77 in patients given units with O-MM (mean TNC, 44) or 3-MM (mean TNC, 3.9), or according to the TNC×10⁷/kg in patients with 1- or 2-MM CB grafts (With permission from Barker et al. [25])

dose prefreeze and the number of HLA disparities had a significant influence on outcome. The 60-day cumulative incidence (CI) of neutrophil engraftment was 83% in the case of no HLA disparity, and 53.2% in the case of at least three HLA disparities $(HR=0.786, p=0.0010)$. TNC dose$\geq 4 \times 10^7$/kg at the time of freezing of the unit was also associated with occurrence of neutrophil recovery, with 60-day CI of 79.6%, versus CI of 69% with $<4 \times 10^7$ TNC/kg $(HR=1.004, p=0.00077)$. In addition, the hazard of neutrophil engraftment was log linearly related to both the number of HLA disparities and to the TNC at freezing.

In a more recent analysis, Barker et al. [25] retrospectively analyzed the outcomes of 1,061 patients receiving single-unit myeloablative CBT for leukemia or myelodysplasia (Fig. 8.2). Both TNC dose and HLA match affected transplant-related mortality (TRM) and survival. TNC dose was associated with neutrophil and platelet engraftment in a dose–response relationship. Improved HLA match was associated with improved neutrophil and platelet engraftment, though there was no difference between 1 and 2 level mismatch for myeloid recovery. Recipients of fully matched CB units had the lowest TRM regardless of cell dose, while the TRM for recipients of 1–2 mismatched units with TNC$\geq 5.0 \times 10^7$/kg was similar to single mismatched groups with TNC 2.5–4.9×10⁷/kg, despite the greater cell dose given. The highest TRM was seen in those receiving units with two mismatches and TNC$<2.5 \times 10^7$/kg. Similar results were seen for overall mortality, treatment failure, and disease-free survival (DFS). These findings supported the author's hypothesis that in certain situations, an improved HLA match could compensate for a lower TNC dose.

Transplantation of Multiple Cord Blood Units: Rationale for Double Cord Blood Transplantation

In order to overcome the limited cell dose from a single CB unit and to ensure adequate stem cell dose for hematopoietic reconstitution of adolescent and adult patients with hematologic malignancies, investigators have examined the coinfusion of more than one CB unit at the time of transplantation. While there were early case reports in which patients received more than one unit of CB for transplantation [26–28], it was the concentrated efforts of the Minnesota group that firmly established the safety of this approach. In 2005, Barker et al. [25] reported results of the first series of double-unit CBT (dCBT) patients. Patients without a single unit containing a cryopreserved TNC dose of at least 2.5×10^7 nucleated cells/kg were eligible for double-unit transplant (the threshold for single-unit cord was raised to 3.5×10^7 nucleated cells/kg in 2002). Units were 4–6/6 HLA-A, B, DRB1 matched to the recipient and each other. Between January 2000 and October 2003, 23 patients with acute myeloid leukemia (AML), acute lymphoblastic leukemia (ALL), and chronic myeloid leukemia (CML) were transplanted with two units. The majority of patients received conditioning with cyclophosphamide (CY), fludarabine (FLU), and 1,320 cGy total body irradiation (TBI); for GVHD prophylaxis, most patients received cyclosporine (CSP) and mycophenolate mofetil (MMF). The median cryopreserved TNC was 4.8×10^7/kg (range $1.6–7.0 \times 10^7$ TNC/kg); median infused TNC was 3.5×10^7/kg (range $1.1–6.3 \times 10^7$/kg). The median infused CD34+ cell dose was 4.9×10^5/kg (range $1.2–14.5 \times 10^5$/kg). Of the 21 evaluable patients, 100% engrafted, with neutrophil engraftment occurring at a median of 23 days. Six-month TRM was 22%; disease-free survival (DFS) was 57% at 1 year, and in patients transplanted in remission the DFS was 72%. In the majority of cases, one unit emerged as the sole source of long-term hematopoiesis.

Importantly, although the TNC dose of the individual units infused in the dCBT setting did not differ significantly from the cell doses infused in historical single-unit CBTs, the incidence of sustained donor engraftment and survival were both improved with dCBT. Prior results in adult patients receiving single-unit CBT at the University of Minnesota showed that only 72% engrafted at a median of 34 days (range 17–54 days) when the infused cell dose was less than 1.7×10^5 CD34/kg [29]. This suggests that the "losing" unit could potentially be facilitating the engraftment of the "winning" unit by a yet to be determined mechanism.

Subsequent investigation has confirmed improved engraftment rates following double CBT and has also demonstrated that in the vast majority of dCBTs, a "winning" unit emerges. Of particular interest, as discussed later, evidence suggests that double-unit CBT may be associated with decreased rates of relapse.

Single-Donor Dominance After Double Cord Blood Transplant

No studies to date have established a reliable mechanism of predicting which unit will predominate in the double-CBT setting; descriptive analyses have examined numerous potential factors, including TNC dose, CD34+ cell dose, CD3+ cell dose, degree of HLA matching, ABO typing, gender match, and order of unit infusion. Limited data do suggest that a unit with very low CD34+ viability is unlikely to engraft in the double-unit setting. In a small series by Scaradavou et al. [30], 46 dCBT patients were evaluated for CD34+ viability and the emergence of single-donor dominance. Of the 46, 44 engrafted with a single CB unit. When both units had a high CD34+ viability (≥75%), the winning unit could not be predicted. In contrast, of the 16 patients receiving a dCBT with high CD34+ viability in only one unit, that CB unit became the single engrafting donor in all but one case. Notably, the single patient without engraftment received two low viability units.

Additional biology underlying the emergence of the winning unit is also not clear, but evidence suggests that an immunologic interaction is important. In a recent study conducted at the Fred Hutchinson Cancer Research Center (FHCRC), Gutman et al. [31] demonstrated that among patients in whom single-donor dominance was established by day 28 posttransplant, effector CD8+ T cells derived from the winning unit were present and targeted against the nondominant unit, producing interferon-gamma (IFN-γ) in response to the nonengrafting unit. Neither the engrafting unit nor HLA-mismatched third-party donors stimulated this IFN-γ response. In contrast, in those patients maintaining mixed chimerism, these T cells were not detectable. There was 1 patient with primary graft failure; in this patient, there was a significant frequency of IFN-γ secreting CD8+ T cells to each CB unit. These findings are the first to demonstrate that immune recognition by the T cells from the dominant CB unit likely contributes to the failure of the second unit to engraft, and leads to the question of whether this immune interaction between units could contribute to an enhanced GVL effect in the dCBT setting.

Importance of Conditioning Regimen and GVHD Prophylaxis

In addition to cell dose and HLA matching, preparative regimen and GVHD prophylaxis play a critical role in achieving CB engraftment. Conditioning regimens must be sufficiently immunosuppressive to allow the small inoculum of CB to establish in the bone marrow niche and not be rejected by the patient. The majority of experience with CB as a stem cell source for transplantation has been with TBI-based myeloablative regimens, initially with the addition of antithymocyte globulin (ATG) to intensify immunosuppression [29, 32], but now more commonly with FLU [7, 33, 34]. With better donor selection and cell dose threshold criteria more firmly established, however, the importance of FLU as part of the regimen is not certain. More limited data are available regarding non-TBI-based intensive conditioning regimens. Traditional busulfan (BU)-based conditioning regimens have yielded disappointing engraftment rates [35, 36]. The Spanish, however, have reported high rates of engraftment following the addition of thiotepa and ATG to BU, CY or BU, FLU [37, 38]. Optimal reduced-intensity conditioning regimens remain under investigation, as discussed in a subsequent section, but securing engraftment for patients without extensive prior treatment (CML, myelodysplastic syndrome (MDS), nonmalignant disease, etc.) remains a significant challenge [39].

Optimized posttransplantation immunosuppressive regimens may also improve engraftment. Calcineurin inhibitors are central to most regimens. While the Japanese have published data supporting short-course methotrexate (MTX) as additional GVHD prophylaxis [40], European data raise questions about potential delayed or decreased engraftment when MTX is used following CBT [41, 42]. Prednisone was combined with cyclosporine in several early trials [10, 21, 29], but MMF has replaced prednisone in most recent studies [7, 34]. Optimal dose and duration of MMF remain under investigation. More recently, the Boston group has reported high engraftment following tacrolimus combined with sirolimus [43].

Improving Time to Engraftment with CBT

Due to the morbidity and mortality associated with delayed engraftment of neutrophils and platelets, different strategies for improving engraftment with CBT are being investigated including ex vivo expansion of CB stem cells, coinfusion of third-party donor cells, techniques to improve CB homing to the marrow, and reduced-intensity conditioning (RIC) regimens.

Ex Vivo Expansion of Cord Blood Hematopoietic Stem Cells

One potential solution to overcome the problem of low stem cell numbers is ex vivo proliferation of the cells prior to transplantation. Extensive research has been done to define the optimal conditions necessary for ex vivo expansion of HSC, with various expansion methodologies developed for this purpose [44–50], including cytokine-mediated expansion systems, co-culture of unmanipulated CB cells with mesenchymal stem cell monolayers, and automated continuous perfusion systems.

In addition, substantial effort has focused on the exogenous signals that may be used to favor stem cell self-renewal versus differentiation in order to develop optimal conditions for the ex vivo expansion of stem and progenitor cells for clinical application. The effect of cytokines that support hematopoietic cell survival, proliferation, and differentiation has been extensively studied in vitro, but a significant role for these cytokines in enhancing self-renewal has not been shown. Clinical trials, which have also mainly evaluated cytokine-driven expansion systems, have not yet provided evidence for stem cell expansion but have demonstrated the feasibility and safety of ex vivo culturing of stem cells.

More recent studies are aimed at identifying intrinsic and extrinsic factors that regulate HSC fate. The specific interactions between stem and other cells within a particular microenvironment or "stem cell niche" are likely to play a key role in vivo in maintaining numbers of HSC by regulating their self-renewal and differentiation, as has been demonstrated by the work of several groups [51–53]. Newer generations of clinical trials are now underway evaluating the use of extrinsic regulators of stem cell fate (such as Notch, copper chelators) and co-culture systems utilizing nonhematopoietic components (mesenchymal stromal cells, (MSCs)) of the stem cell niche.

De Lima et al. at MD Anderson reported their results with MSC-mediated expansion at the 2010 American Society of Hematology (ASH) meeting [54]. Patients undergoing double CBT with myeloablative conditioning had the smaller of their two CB units ex vivo expanded on confluent MSC layers generated from either commercially available versus family donor MSC sources. After the 14-day culture period, patients were transplanted with the unmanipulated unit as well as the expansion fractions. This technique resulted in a 14-fold expansion of TNCs (range 1–30) and a 40-fold expansion of CD34+ cells (range 4–140); clinically, this translated into a median time to neutrophil and platelet engraftment of 15 days (range 9–42) and 40 days (range 13–62).

Additionally, the MD Anderson group has also incorporated the copper chelator tetraethylenepentamine (TEPA; StemEx) as a differentiation inhibitor into their expansion cultures, in order to augment the expansion potential of CB progenitor cells [55]. Ten patients were transplanted with a single CB unit that had been originally frozen into two fractions; for expansion, purified CD133+ cells from the smaller CB fraction were ex vivo cultured for 21 days with thrombopoietin, IL-6, Flt-3 ligand, and stem cell factor, prior to infusion following the unmanipulated fraction [56]. The average TNC expansion was 219 (range 2–620), with a mean increase in CD34+ cell count of six over the CD34+ cell count of the entire unit. Of ten patients, nine were engrafted, despite a low infused TNC/kg (1.8×10^7/kg median); the median time to neutrophil and platelet engraftment was 30 days (range 16–46) and 48 days (range 35–105), respectively. Further efforts are ongoing to optimize both the cell type(s) used for culture initiation (i.e., CD34+ or CD133+ selection, versus CD3+, CD14+ depletion), as well as the culture conditions for ex vivo expansion including the cytokine cocktail, incorporation of cell fate regulators, and the use of MSC monolayers.

Notch-Mediated Expansion of Human Cord Blood Progenitor Cells

At our center, we have developed a Notch-ligand-mediated ex vivo culture and expansion system able to generate large-scale expansion of CD34+ CB stem and progenitor cells with rapid myeloid reconstituting potential in a clinical setting. Initial work demonstrated the role of Notch in hematopoiesis, and the ability to ex vivo expand mouse marrow progenitor cells by activation of endogenous Notch receptors by immobilized Notch ligand that were capable of short-term lymphoid and myeloid repopulating ability [57–59]. Subsequently, the incubation of human CB progenitor cells in the presence of immobilized Notch ligand was shown to generate an approximate 100-fold increase in the number of CD34+ cells with enhanced repopulating ability in immunodeficient mice [60, 61].

Fig. 8.3 Time to neutrophil recovery to ≥500/μL for patients receiving dCBT with two unmanipulated CB units (conventional) versus one unmanipulated and one ex vivo expanded unit (expanded) (Unpublished data)

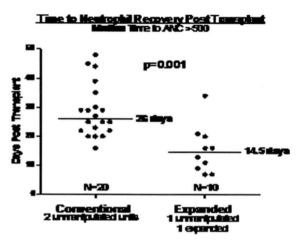

Most recently, the ex vivo culture of CD34+ CB stem/progenitor cells in the presence of Notch ligand has been shown to increase CD34+ cells by greater than 100-fold, and in the preliminary results of a phase I clinical trial has shown to provide more rapid myeloid engraftment [62]. Using the double-unit CBT platform pioneered by Wagner et al. 11 patients with high-risk leukemia were conditioned with 1,320 cGy of TBI, 120 mg/kg CY, and 75 mg/m^2 FLU prior to double-unit CBT with one unmanipulated unit plus one ex vivo expanded CB unit. Sixteen days prior to transplantation, the unit for expansion was thawed, CD34+ selected, and ex vivo expanded on Notch ligand and in serum-free medium supplemented with recombinant human IL-3, IL-6, thrombopoietin, Flt-3 ligand, and stem cell factor. At the time of harvest of the cultured cells, there was a 164-fold average expansion of CD34+ cells, and an average total nucleated cell fold expansion of 562. The average infused CD34+ cell dose was 6×10^6 CD34+ cells/kg from the expanded unit, versus 0.24×10^6 CD34+ cell/kg from the unmanipulated CB graft. The time to an absolute neutrophil count of ≥500 cells/uL, in the nine of ten evaluable patients, was significantly shortened as compared to a concurrent cohort of patients undergoing myeloablative double unexpanded unit CBT transplant. Median time to ANC of ≥500 cells/uL was 14.5 days, compared to 26 days in the double unexpanded unit setting ($p=0.002$), (Fig. 8.3). The median time to an ANC of >100 cells was 9 days, versus 19 days in the unmanipulated dCBT setting. There was one patient with primary graft failure.

Notably, while early myeloid recovery at day 7 posttransplantation was predominately from the expanded unit, the expanded graft in general did not persist beyond day 21 posttransplantation. The observation that the overall time to engraftment was shortened despite the absence of the second expanded unit suggests that there was facilitation of hematopoietic recovery and engraftment of the unmanipulated graft by the ex vivo expanded unit. Additionally, this study was the first to demonstrate that ex vivo expanded CB hematopoietic stem/progenitor cells can be manufactured and used to improve engraftment in a clinical setting.

Coinfusion of Third-Party Donor Cells

An additional strategy for increasing TNC and CD34+ cell counts, pioneered by the Madrid group, is coinfusion of third-party donor HSC. Different third-party donor sources have been described, including infusion of haploidentical peripheral blood CD34+ cells with a CB graft [63] coinfusion of CB with third-party donor mobilized CD34+ cells [64, 65], and coinfusion of third-party bone marrow MSCs along with same donor mobilized CD34+ cells [66]. Third-party HSCs rapidly engraft neutrophils, providing a bridge until the CB unit engrafts, and may also facilitate CB engraftment. In the most recent update of their work, median time to engraftment following myeloablative conditioning and coinfusion with third-party HSC was 10 days, while median time to CB engraftment was 21 days. Using third-party HSC, single CB units with infused TNC from 1.14×10^7/kg to 4.5×10^7/kg (median 2.39×10^7/kg) reliably engrafted (cumulative incidence of engraftment 91%) [65]. Other groups are now investigating this strategy.

Improved Homing Strategies

Methods to improve the establishment of CB HSC in the marrow niche are also under investigation. Strategies to bypass homing have included intrabone infusion of CB into the superior-posterior iliac crest of patients [67]. While results have been mixed, a recent report describes the outcomes of 75 patients receiving a median TNC from single CB units of 2.6×10^7/kg (range $1.35-5.4 \times 10^7$/kg) transplanted via intrabone injection. Ninety-six percent of patients engrafted, with a median ANC recovery to $>500 \times 10^9$/L by day 23 (range 14–44 days) and median platelet recovery to $>20,000 \times 10^9$/L by day 35 (range 16–70 days) [68]. While logistical challenges associated with the procedure remain an important consideration and obstacle, further investigation is warranted [69, 70].

Alternative strategies include manipulation of the stromal cell-derived factor-1 (SDF-1) and its chemokine receptor CXCR4 axis, which is important in the homing of hematopoietic stem and progenitor cells to the marrow microenvironment. The inhibition of CD26/dipeptidyl peptidase IV, which prevents enzymatic cleavage of SDF-1, has been demonstrated to improve engraftment in murine models [71, 72]; C3a priming, as a means to enhance CB HSC responsiveness to SDF-1, is also being evaluated [73]. Preliminary data also suggest that ex vivo fucosylation of CB ligands, necessary for extravasation of HSCs from the vasculature, as well as exposure to prostaglandin E2, postulated to increase CXCR4 expression may improve homing [74, 75].

Reduced-Intensity Conditioning Regimens

An additional strategy to overcome the cell dose limitation and the delay in engraftment seen with adult CBT is the use of RIC regimens. By decreasing the degree of marrow suppression from conditioning, temporary autologous hematopoietic recovery is permitted, thus potentially minimizing the duration of pancytopenia and specifically neutropenia. The regimen of CY 50 mg/kg, FLU 200 mg/m^2, and 200 cGy of TBI pioneered at the University of Minnesota has resulted in a median time to neutrophil engraftment of 12 days and produces reliable engraftment in patients who have received significant prior treatment [39]. Further review of RIC regimens and outcomes is provided later in this chapter.

Infectious Complications and Immune Reconstitution After Cord Blood Transplantation

Infectious complications and immune reconstitution remain significant challenges following CBT. The prolonged neutropenia following myeloablative conditioning increases patients' vulnerability to fungal and bacterial infections, while the unique immunologic properties of cord blood T cells raise concerns about delays in T cell immune reconstitution and consequent increased risk of clinical infections.

Clinical literature regarding infectious outcomes following CBT is difficult to interpret due to heterogeneity in patient populations, conditioning regimens, evolving standards for matching and size criteria for CB units, etc. Most large series suggest an increased risk of infectious complications following CBT as compared to other donor sources [5, 76, 77]. Two recent large retrospective analyses comparing outcomes in adult patients following transplantation with various donor sources demonstrated an increased incidence of infection-related early TRM following CBT [6, 23]. A similar comparative analysis of pediatric patients did not demonstrate increased early infection-related TRM among well-matched CBT patients but did suggest increased infection-related TRM following CBT with a 4/6 matched unit. Data are more limited regarding late infectious complications of CBT, but available evidence suggests comparable long-term infectious mortality regardless of donor source [23, 78]. As supportive care improves, infectious complications after HCT are equalizing among donor source; however, viral infections remain of particular concern among CBT patients.

Numerous studies have reported the viral complications of CBT with a specific emphasis on cytomegalovirus (CMV) [79–84]. While heterogeneity of patients and treatment strategies again make analysis difficult, a recent large study from the University of Minnesota suggests comparable rates of CMV reactivation and disease following CBT as compared to transplantation with other donor sources [85]. Optimal preemptive therapies to treat CMV in CBT patients remain under investigation, and numerous strategies have been described [81, 84, 86]. In a recent single center analysis at the FHCRC, Milano et al. compared the outcomes of CBT patients receiving CMV prophylaxis with either standard-dose acyclovir/valacyclovir versus an intensified regimen consisting of pretransplant ganciclovir with high-dose acyclovir posttransplant and preemptive biweekly CMV DNA monitoring [87]. Patients receiving the intensified strategy had a significantly lower cumulative incidence of CMV reactivation in the multivariate analysis (HR 0.31, 95% CI 0.16–0.58,

$p < 0.001$), with a trend toward fewer episodes of invasive CMV disease (3% versus 16%, $p = 0.09$). Several reports do describe increased incidence of other viral complications, particularly Epstein-Barr virus (EBV) – posttransplant lymphoproliferative disorder (PTLD) and human herpesvirus 6 (HHV6), in selected CBT patient populations [88–92].

Several descriptive analyses have characterized delayed immune reconstitution following CBT [93–95]. In the most comprehensive prospective study to date, Komanduri et al. assessed T cell immune reconstitution in 32 heavily pretreated CB transplant recipients using immunophenotyping, cytokine flow cytometry analysis of superantigen-stimulated and virus-specific T cells, and analysis of T cell receptor excision circles (TREC) to assess thymopoiesis [96]. Findings demonstrated inadequate thymic regeneration associated with lymphopenia and compensatory expansion of NK and B cells, delayed functional immune recovery, and skewing of the T cell compartment away from naïve and early memory T cells [96]. In contrast to this study, others have demonstrated that early viral-specific T cell responses do develop in a portion of CBT patients, and have correlated improved survival with effective thymopoiesis [56, 97]. Strategies to improve immune reconstitution through ex vivo manipulation of CB and adoptive immunotherapy remain investigational [98, 99].

Studies have also shown that T regulatory cells (Tregs) from CB possess more potent suppressor function than Tregs isolated from peripheral blood [100]. It is unknown whether these highly suppressive CB Tregs may be able to inhibit responses of effector cells in the recipients of CB [101].

Graft-Versus-Host Disease (GVHD) After Cord Blood Transplantations

A greater degree of HLA mismatching appears to be tolerable in CBT. Activated T cells from CB have been shown in vitro to produce lower amounts of Th1 and Th2 cytokines compared with adult T cells after stimulation, including cytokines known to contribute to GVHD such as tumor necrosis factor-α (TNF-α) and INF-γ [102, 103]. Kleen et al. analyzed circulating lymphocytes collected 3 months post-CB transplant [104]. The circulating peripheral blood CB-derived lymphocytes produced normal levels of INF-γ, and proliferated normally after stimulation with mitogen or third-party alloantigen. However, after stimulation with recipient antigen, the circulating CB-derived lymphocytes did not proliferate or produce INF-γ, suggesting recipient immune tolerance induction. Other proposed differences with cord blood grafts include the presence of increased regulatory T cells, altered cytokine profiles, decreased HLA expression, and functional immaturity with decreased cytotoxicity of the infused lymphocytes [105].

Clinically, despite the often greater degree of HLA mismatch seen in the CBT setting, the incidence of acute and chronic GVHD has been lower than expected. Several older registry analyses have demonstrated lower or comparable rates of acute GVHD among CBT patients as compared to bone marrow and peripheral blood HSCT patients, with well-matched CB units associated with the lowest rates of GVHD of any URD source [5, 77]. Two recent large analyses confirm the decreased incidence of GVHD among CBT patients [7, 23]. A Japanese series describing 1,072 patients demonstrated a 28% 2-year cumulative incidence of cGVHD [106], and several reports suggest a low incidence of clinically significant cGVHD following CBT [107, 108]. Notably, the incidence of mild to moderate aGVHD appears higher following double-unit CBT versus single-unit CBT [109].

In addition, a recent analysis suggests that GVHD following CBT may be more treatment responsive versus conventional transplant recipients. Arora et al. compared the clinical presentation and response to treatment in 170 patients with chronic GVHD, of which 123 patients had undergone URD, predominately HLA-matched bone marrow, and 47 CB donor transplants [110]. At 2 months, URD response rates were 48% versus 74% among CB patients ($p=0.005$). Six-month response rates were 49% versus 78% ($p=0.001$); 1-year responses were 51% versus 72% ($p=0.03$); and at 2 years, the responses were 47% versus 70% ($p=0.05$) for URD compared with CB patients, respectively. Despite higher response rates in the CB recipients, the incidence and timing of discontinuation of immunosuppression was similar in the two cohorts, though there was a trend toward better survival seen with CBT.

Relapse Risk After Cord Blood Transplantation

Possibility of Enhanced Graft-Versus-Leukemia Effect After Double-Unit CBT

A growing body of evidence suggests that double cord transplant may be associated with a lower risk of relapse than transplant with other donor sources [7, 34, 111, 112]. A recent single center analysis of 177 patients with acute leukemia at the University of Minnesota assessed risk factors associated with leukemia relapse following myeloablative CB transplantation [111]. Eighty-eight patients with ALL and 89 with AML were included, with a median age of 17. While the overall incidence of relapse was 26%, in the multivariate analysis, a trend toward less relapse was seen in recipients of 2 CB units ($RR=0.6$, $p=0.07$); relapse was significantly lower for patients transplanted in first or second complete remission with 2 CB units ($RR=0.5$, $p<0.03$). In another recent analysis from the University of Minnesota and FHCRC comparing outcomes among 536 patients following double-unit CBT or transplantation with other donor sources [5], relapse rates were significantly lower following dCBT (15%, 95% CI 9–22%) compared to MRD (43%, 95% CI 35–52%), MUD (37%, 95% CI 29–46%) and MMUD (35%, 95% CI 21–48%), though early TRM was highest following dCBT (34%, 95% CI 25–42%) versus MRD (24%, 95% CI 17–39%) and MUD (14%, 95% CI 9–20%). Immunologic interactions between the two units have been speculated as a possible mechanism for lower relapse following double-unit CBT, and ongoing investigation is examining this issue. The Bone Marrow Transplant Clinical Trials Network (BMT CTN) is currently investigating this question in pediatric patients with high-risk leukemia and myelodysplasia, in a multicenter, open-label, randomized clinical trial comparing single versus double CB transplantation.

Importance of HLA Match

The role of HLA match is also of possible importance in the risk of relapse after CBT. The Eurocord group analyzed outcomes after single-unit CBT for both malignant disease ($n = 925$ patients) and nonmalignant disease ($n = 279$). In patients with malignant disease, increasing the number of HLA disparities decreased the incidence of relapse. However, the number HLA incompatible did not influence overall survival or disease-free survival. This observation was thought to be explained by the positive impact of HLA mismatches on relapse and the negative impact of mismatches on engraftment [113].

In contrast, the analysis of Barker et al. [25] found no association between HLA match and relapse. They analyzed the outcomes of 1,061 patients receiving single CB unit myeloablative transplant for leukemia or myelodysplasia. While HLA match affected survival, this was because of its effect on TRM; HLA match was not associated with relapse.

Outcomes After Cord Blood Transplantation

Pediatric Malignant Disease

Two large series have examined outcomes in pediatric patients undergoing CBT. Eapen et al. compared outcomes of CBT with those after bone marrow transplants (BMT) [78], in 503 children with acute leukemia aged <16 years (Fig. 8.4). Compared with matched BMT, early TRM was higher after two antigen-mismatched CBT (relative risk 2.31, $p = 0.0003$) and potentially also higher after one antigen-mismatched CBT with low cell dose defined as TNC $\leq 0.3 \times 10^8$/kg (*relative risk* 1.88, $p = 0.0455$). TRM was similar after matched CBT and one antigen-mismatched CBT with high cell dose. The probability of 5-year leukemia-free survival was 38% and 37%, respectively, after matched and mismatched BMT. After one antigen-mismatched CBT with a low cell dose, the probability was 36%; after one antigen-mismatched CBT with high cell dose, it was 45%; and after HLA-matched CBT, the probability of 5-year leukemia-free survival was 60%. Patients receiving 6/6 matched CBT had a nonstatistically significant trend toward improved survival over patients receiving matched BMT.

Kurtzberg et al. recently reported outcomes of the Cord Blood Transplantation Study (COBLT), a phase II multicenter trial of 191 pediatric patients undergoing unrelated single-unit CBT for hematologic malignancies. Patients were conditioned

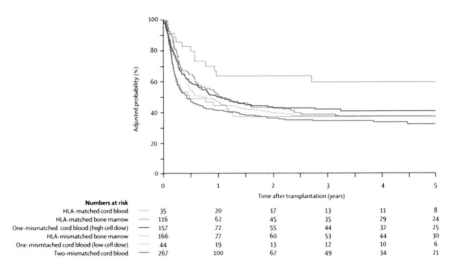

Numbers at risk

		0	1	2	3	4	5
HLA-matched cord blood	——	35	20	17	13	11	8
HLA-matched bone marrow	······	116	62	45	35	29	24
One-mismatched cord blood (high cell dose)	——	157	72	55	44	32	25
HLA-mismatched bone marrow	······	166	77	60	53	44	30
One-mismtached cord blood (low cell dose)	——	44	19	13	12	10	6
Two-mismatched cord blood	——	267	100	67	49	34	21

Fig. 8.4 Probability of leukemia-free survival after bone marrow and cord blood transplantation adjusted for disease status at transplantation (With permission from Eapen et al. [78])

with CY, TBI, and ATG, and received methylprednisolone and CSP for GVHD prophylaxis. The overall survival in the study at day 180 was 67.4%, at 1 year was 57.3%, and was 49.5% at 2 years. CMV seropositivity, female gender, ABO mismatch, and $TNC \leq 2.5 \times 10^7/kg$ were unfavorable factors significantly associated with survival in the multivariate analysis [32].

Together, these studies support the safety and efficacy of CBT for hematologic malignancies in the pediatric population. In addition, given the comparable results for matched BMT and mismatched CBT, and trend toward superior survival for matched CBT in the Eapen et al. study, these results suggest investigation of CB as the first choice of donor source for pediatric patients lacking a MRD.

Adult Malignant Disease

Myeloablative Conditioning

Outcomes after transplantation have also been evaluated in the adult population (Table 8.1). Two landmark series established the efficacy of CBT in adults. Laughlin et al. analyzed adult patients with leukemia receiving single-unit CB ($n = 150$ patients), HLA-matched BM ($n = 367$ patients), and 1 HLA-mismatched BM ($n = 83$ patients) [5]. The overall mortality rates were lowest after HLA-matched BMT, but similar after mismatched marrow and CB. Rocha et al. compared CBT ($n = 98$) and matched unrelated BMT ($n = 584$) outcomes in adult patients with acute leukemia [114]. CBT was associated with comparable leukemia-free survival.

Table 8.1 Summary of recent myeloablative cord blood transplant studies

Reference	Stem cell source	Sample size	Median age (years)	# CB units	Median TNC/ kg×10^8	Median CD34/ kg×10^6	Median time to ANC >500/μL (days)	Median time to platelets >20,000/μL (days)	aGVHD II-IV (%)	cGVHD (%)	TRM day-100 (%)	Relapse (%)	DFS (%)	Survival 1-year (%)
Laughlin 2004 [5]	CB	150	16–60[a]	1	0.22	NS	27	60	41	51	63	17	19	26
	MUD BM	367	16–60[a]	–	2.4	NS	18	29	48	35	46	23	31	35
	MMUD BM	83	16–60[a]	–	2.2	NS	20	29	52	40	65	14	20	20
Rocha 2004 [114]	CB	98	25	1	0.23	0.11	26	NS	26	30	44	23	33	36
	MUD BM	584	32	1	2.9	NS	19	NS	39	46	38	23	38	42
Takahashi 2007 [115]	CB	100	38	1	NS	0.093	22	40	60	89	8	17	70	NS
	REL BM,PB	71	40		NS	NS	17	22.5	55	89	4	26	60	NS
Atsuta 2009 [76]	CB AML	173	38	1	0.244	NS	NS	NS	32	28	30[b]	31	36	43
	MUD BM AML	311	38	–	2.63	NS	NS	NS	35	32	19[b]	24	54	60
	CB ALL	114	34	1	0.248	NS	NS	NS	28	27	21[b]	31	45	49
	MUD BM ALL	222	32	–	2.82	NS	NS	NS	42	30	23[b]	24	51	57
Verneris 2009 [111]	CB	177	8	1	0.33	0.35	22	NS	29	10	26[b]	34	40	NS
			24	2	0.36	0.45	25	NS	48	18	29[b]	19	51	NS
Brunstein 2010 [7]	CB	128	25	2	0.4	NS	26	53[c]	60	26	NS	15	51	NS
	MRD PB>BM	204	40	–	8.6	NS	16	20[c]	65	47	NS	43	33	NS
	MUD PB, BM	152	31	–	2.0	NS	19	21[c]	80	43	NS	37	48	NS
	MMUD PB, BM	52	31	–	1.7	NS	18.5	21[c]	85	48	NS	39	38	NS

(continued)

Table 8.1 (continued)

Reference	Stem cell source	Sample size	Median age (years)	# CB units	Median TNC/ kg×10^8	Median CD34/ kg×10^6	Median time to ANC >500/μL (days)	Median time to platelets >20,000/μL (days)	aGVHD II-IV (%)	cGVHD (%)	TRM day-100 (%)	Relapse (%)	DFS (%)	Survival 1-year (%)
Eapen 2010 [23]	CB	165	28	1	0.26	NS	24	52	30	24	33	26	59	NS
	URD PB	888	33	–	NS	NS	14	19	49	50	27	32	59	NS
	URD BM	472	39	–	NS	NS	19	28	41	39	26	33	57	NS
Yoo 2010 [135]	CB	236[d]	7	1 (91%) 2 (9%)	0.484	0.2	18	45	41	36.1	19	NS	NS	47.5[e]

Abbreviations: *CB* cord blood, *TNC* total nucleated cell, *ANC* absolute neutrophil count, *aGVHD* acute graft-versus-host disease, *cGVHD* chronic graft-versus-host-disease, *TRM* transplant-related mortality, *DFS* disease-free survival, *BM* bone marrow, *PB* peripheral blood, *REL* related, *dCB* double cord blood, *MRD* matched related donor, *MUD* matched unrelated donor, *MMUD* mismatched unrelated donor, *NS* not specified

[a]Median age not reported

[b]1-year TRM

[c]Platelet recovery to ≥50,000/μL

[d]Includes 21 patients receiving reduced-intensity transplants

[e]5-year survival

Similarly, in an analysis of 171 adults with hematologic malignancies, Takahashi et al. reported on a pilot study using CBT as a primary unrelated stem cell source ($n = 100$), compared with related bone marrow ($n = 55$) or peripheral blood ($n = 16$) stem cell transplants [76, 115]. In the multivariate analysis, there was no significant difference in TRM, relapse rate, or DFS between the CBT and BM/PBSCT groups.

Two recent large retrospective analyses have further confirmed the efficacy of CBT in adults. Eapen et al. compared transplant outcomes among different stem cell sources – unrelated bone marrow ($n = 472$), peripheral blood ($n = 888$), and CB ($n = 165$) – using registry data from the United States and Europe [23]. Leukemia-free survival was comparable between CB and 8/8 and 7/8 PBSC or BM transplant. TRM was higher after CB transplantation than after 8/8 PBSC or BM transplant.

Using combined datasets at the University of Minnesota and the FHCRC, Brunstein et al. retrospectively analyzed 536 patients with leukemia transplanted between 2001 and 2008 [7]. Patients were transplanted with grafts from either matched sibling ($n = 204$), 8/8 MURD ($n = 152$), 7/8 MMURD ($n = 52$), or dCBT ($n = 128$). Progression-free survival at 5 years was similar among the four groups – and while a higher TRM was seen with the dCBT, the risk of relapse at 5 years was lowest following CBT.

These results confirm a role for CBT in adults lacking an MRD or readily available MURD. The reduced risk of relapse seen in the dCBT setting is especially encouraging; if new strategies could be developed to improve hematopoietic recovery and to reduce TRM, then potentially improved progression-free survival (PFS) and overall survival could be seen after CBT.

Reduced-Intensity Conditioning

Several small series have described CBT outcomes following heterogeneous RIC regimens (Table 8.2) [112, 116–119]. The University of Minnesota has reported the largest series of adult patients ($n = 110$), undergoing RIC CBT following a uniform conditioning regimen. Patients were conditioned with CY/FLU/TBI as described earlier in this chapter (engraftment section). Neutrophil recovery occurred in 92% of patients, at a median of 12 days, and was similar for those receiving one versus two units. Primary graft failure occurred in seven patients; secondary graft failure occurred in eight. While chimerisms were mixed at early time points, the vast majority of patients had single-donor bone marrow engraftment by day 100. TRM was 19% at day 180 and 26% at 3 years, with a 3-year survival of 45%. There was as trend toward lower relapse rate and higher event-free survival in recipients of 2 CB units [39]. In a follow-up study, the Minnesota group retrospectively compared the outcomes of the subset of patients aged greater than 55 years undergoing RIC CBT ($n = 43$) to comparable patients undergoing MRD ($n = 47$) transplants. Three-year progression-free survival was 30% versus 34% for MRD and CB, respectively [120].

The Dana-Farber Cancer Center and Massachusetts General Hospital have reported the largest series following a uniform non-TBI-based RIC regimen [121, 122].

Table 8.2 Summary of recent reduced-intensity conditioning cord blood transplant studies

Reference	Sample size	Conditioning regimen	GVHD prophylaxis	Median age (years)	# CB units	Median TNC/ kg×10^8	Median CD34/ kg×10^6	Median time to ANC >500/μL (days)	Median time to platelets >20,000/μL (days)	aGVHD II–IV (%)	cGVHD (%)	TRM day 100 (%)	Relapse (%)	DFS 1-year (%)	Survival (%)
Barker 2003 [33]	21	BU/FLU/TBI	CSA/MMF	49.5	2 (43%)	0.26	0.37	26	NS	44	21	48	NS	31	39 1-year
	22	CY/FLU/TBI[a]			2 (68%)	0.32	0.43	9.5	NS			28			1-year
Kishi 2005 [136]	57	FLU 125 mg/m² MEL or BU TBI 400–800 cGy	CSA	56	1	NS	0.29	19	NS	66	NS	62[b]	15 Day 180	NS	NS
Ballen 2007 [121]	21	FLU 180 mg/m² MEL 100 mg/m² ATG	CSA/MMF	49	2	0.4	0.19	20	41	40	31	14	NS	67	71 1-year
Brunstein 2007 [39]	110	CY 50 mg/kg FLU 200 mg/m² TBI 200 cGy +/– ATG	CSA/MMF	51	2 (85%) 1 (15%)	0.37 0.33	0.49 0.38	12	49[c]	59	23	19[b]	31 3-years	NS	45 3-year
Miyakoshi 2007 [137]	34	FLU 125 mg/m² MEL 80 mg/m² TBI 400 cGy	Tacrolimus	56.5	1	0.24	NS	20	38	45	27	12	5 patients	NS	70 1-year
Majhail 2008 [120]	43 CB	CY/FLU/TBI (84%) + ATG (40%)	CSA/MMF	59	2 (88%)	0.4	0.4	NS	NS	49	17	28[b]	NS	NS	34
	47 MRD	CY/FLU/TBI (70%) + ATG (13%)		58	–	9.2	5.3	NS	NS	42	40	23[b]	NS	NS	43 3-year

Study	n	Conditioning	GVHD prophylaxis	TNC											
Uchida 2008[d] [138]	70	[e]MEL 80 mg/m² FLU 125–180 mg/m² TBI 200–400 cGy	CSA (n=37) or Tacrolimus (n=33)	61	1	0.28	0.084	18	35	61	40	43	26[f]	NS	23	2-year
Rocha 2009 [116]	176	FLU-based (95%) BU-based (16%) Other (29%) +/− ATG	CSA/MMF (72%)	45	1	0.27	NS	20	35	30	30	38	41	31–42[g]	NS	1-year
Rocha 2009 [116]	155	CY 50 mg/kg FLU 200 mg/m² TBI 200 cGy	CSA/MMF	47	1 (62%) 2 (38%)	0.28 0.36	0.14 0.16	20	NS	37	39	18[b]	NS	51[h]	NS	2-years
Cutler 2010 [43]	32	FLU 180 mg/m² MEL 100 mg/m² ATG	Sirolimus + Tacrolimus	53	2	0.516	0.016	21	42	9.4	12.5	12	34	NS	53	2-year

Abbreviations: *CB* cord blood, *TNC* total nucleated cell, *ANC* absolute neutrophil count, *aGVHD* acute graft-versus-host-disease, *cGVHD* chronic graft-versus-host disease, *TRM* transplant-related mortality, *DFS* disease-free survival, *BU* busulfan, *FLU* fludarabine, *TBI* total body irradiation, *CY* cyclophosphamide, *CSA* cyclosporine, *MMF* mycophenolate mofetil, *NS* not specified, *MEL* melphalan, *ATG* antithymocyte globulin, *MRD* matched related donor

[a]One patient received CY/FLU/TBI with ATG
[b]Day-180
[c]Platelet recovery to ≥50,000/μL
[d]Includes patients from the study of Kishi et al.
[e]Four patients received busulfan instead of melphalan; 1 patient received thiotepa with FLU/MEL
[f]Disease progression occurred at a median of 134 days (range 13–785)
[g]31% for myelodysplastic syndromes/CML; 41% for acute leukemias; 42% lymphoid/plasmocytic diseases
[h]At 18-months

As part of two phase I–II studies, 53 patients were transplanted using FLU 180 mg/m^2, melphalan 100 mg/m^2, and ATG 6 mg/kg, followed by 2 CB units that were at least 4/6 HLA-matched. In this series, the 100-day TRM was only 12%, with long-term relapse-free and overall survival of 24.6% and 33.1%, respectively [122].

These analyses have demonstrated that nonmyeloablative conditioning is sufficient to promote engraftment with CBT; importantly, these regimens extend the potential benefit of transplantation to patients ineligible for conventional myeloablative therapy. Additional studies are ongoing to further optimize reduced-intensity conditioning regimens.

Nonmalignant Disease

In addition to the potential benefit of HSCT for hematologic malignancies, transplant can also offer the potential for cure in the nonmalignant setting. Given there is no need for the GVL effect, minimizing GVHD is desired, and the possibility of lower GVHD with CBT is appealing [123]. However, given the minimal immunosuppressive treatment many patients with nonmalignant diseases have experienced, as well as the unfavorable bone marrow environment associated with bone marrow failure syndromes, ensuring engraftment of CB is a challenge, and optimization of conditioning regimens and posttransplantation immunosuppression is necessary. Nonmalignant diseases for which CBT is being explored include hemoglobinopathies such as thalassemia and sickle cell disease [42, 124], and bone marrow failure syndromes including Fanconi anemia [124], primary immune deficiencies [125], and inborn errors of metabolism [126, 127].

Alternative Donors for Hematopoietic Stem Cell Transplant: Haploidentical Stem Cell Transplant

As an alternative to CBT for patients lacking a MRD or appropriate URD, several investigators have explored haploidentical transplantation. The possibility of using a related donor sharing at least one haplotype (the maternal or paternal #6 chromosome) with the patient has several advantages. Nearly all patients will have a family member – parent, child, sibling, or other relative – with whom they share a haplotype, and such a donor does not require expensive searching to identify and is typically immediately available. For patients with hematologic malignancies, the high degree of HLA mismatching might promote a more potent GVL effect. Nevertheless, the high degree of HLA mismatching associated with haploidentical transplantation creates significant immunologic challenges including potential graft rejection, GVHD, and poor immune reconstitution.

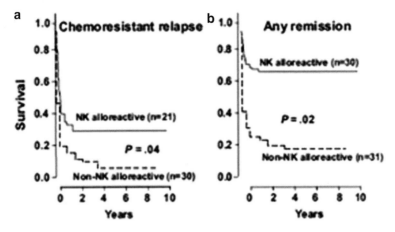

Fig. 8.5 Transplantation from haploidentical NK alloreactive donors improves EFS. (**a**) EFS in patients transplanted in relapse from NK-alloreactive versus non-NK alloreactive donors. (**b**) EFS in patients transplanted in CR from NK alloreactive versus non-NK alloreactive donors (With permission from Ruggeri et al. [130])

Haploidentical transplantation has been investigated over the last several decades. Initial attempts at myeloablative HSCT utilizing T cell replete bone marrow donors resulted in high rates of early TRM due to graft failure, severe GVHD, and infection [128]. Initial outcomes utilizing T cell–depleted haploidentical donors were also unsatisfactory due to high rates of graft failure, infectious complications, and recurrent malignancies [129].

More recently, however, novel approaches to haploidentical transplantation have offered more encouraging results. One newer strategy utilizes myeloablative conditioning followed by megadose CD34+ infusions versus a variety of reduced-intensity conditioning approaches using various in vivo manipulations to avoid overwhelming T cell responses.

The strategy of mega dose CD34+ haploidentical transplant, pioneered by the Perugia group, has demonstrated significant efficacy in the treatment of AML (Fig. 8.5) [130]. Its proponents suggest that alloreactive natural killer (NK) cells mediate GVL, destroy recipient T cells that might mediate graft failure, and destroy recipient dendritic cells that might trigger GVHD. This approach has been less successful in ALL, presumably due to lack of NK alloreactivity against ALL cells.

Following myeloablative conditioning with 8 Gy TBI, 10 mg/kg thiotepa, 200 mg/m^2 FLU, and 20 mg/kg rabbit ATG, patients receive large doses of G-CSF mobilized, CD34+ selected haploidentical cells (17.5 ± 5 × 10^6 CD34+ and 3.5 ± 2 × 10^4 CD3+ cells/kg in the most recently reported series). The highly immunosuppressive regimen combined with high CD34+ doses promotes reliable engraftment – in the largest series to date, 103 of 112 patients experienced primary engraftment. Grade II–IV GVHD developed in 10% of patients. Forty-eight (43%) patients experienced TRM with 42 of 48 deaths due to infection.

Transplantation using NK alloreactive donors, as predicted by the authors' "missing ligand" model, resulted in improved event-free survival as compared to patients with no predicted NK alloreactivity (67% versus 18%, $p = 0.02$ for patients transplanted in remission and 34% versus 6%, $p = 0.04$ for patients transplanted in relapse) [130]. In a more recent analysis, the Perugia group has suggested that maternal rather than paternal donors may result in better outcomes (overall survival hazard ratio, father versus mother $= 2.36$; $p = 0.003$) [131]. The authors suggest that maternal exposure to fetal antigens during pregnancy may contribute to these findings.

As an alternative to the approach discussed above, several reduced-intensity regimens have been investigated in an effort to reduce toxicity and extend haploidentical transplant to older and comorbid patients. The majority of experience is in patients with hematologic malignancies, but limited data have demonstrated potential efficacy of haploidentical transplantation in patients with nonmalignant diseases. Reported regimens have incorporated a variety of strategies to promote engraftment and avoid overwhelming GVHD. The Duke group has reported 31% 1-year survival (63% 1 year survival among standard risk patients) in 49 patients with hematologic malignancies or marrow failure conditioned with FLU, CY, and alemtuzumab followed by MMF +/– CSP as GVHD prophylaxis [132]. Ogawa et al. described 55% 3-year event-free survival in 26 hematologic malignancy patients receiving FLU, BU, and ATG conditioning followed by tacrolimus and methylprednisolone GVHD prophylaxis [133]. The Johns Hopkins and FHCRC groups have reported the largest reduced-intensity haploidentical experience (185 hematologic malignancy patients). Following conditioning with FLU, CY, and 2 Gy TBI, 50 mg/kg of CY is administered on day 3 ± 4 posttransplantation to eliminate nascent proliferation of activated T cells. TAC is administered as additional GVHD prophylaxis. One-year event-free survival was 35%, cumulative incidence of 1 year TRM was 15%, grade II–IV aGVHD was 31%, and cGVHD was 15%. Graft failure occurred in 29 of 177 (16%) evaluable patients [134]. This approach is currently under investigation in a multicenter BMT CTN trial.

Future Strategies for Haploidentical Transplant

Efforts to optimize donor selection, including investigation of the potential role of selection based on noninherited maternal antigens as well as developing techniques to better optimize NK cell alloreactivity, are important areas of research in haploidentical transplantation. As in all areas of allogeneic stem cell transplantation, graft engineering, including selective depletion of cells capable of causing GVHD as well as ex vivo manipulation and add back of leukemia-specific, GVHD-suppressive, and/or immune-reconstituting cells, is under investigation. Ongoing efforts are also underway to optimize conditioning regimens; at the FHCRC a trial has recently been initiated using a CD45 radioimmunotherapy-based conditioning regimen with the intention of decreasing relapse without increasing toxicity.

Conclusions

With over 20,000 transplants having been performed worldwide in adults and children, CBT is now an accepted alternative donor source for HSCT. CB banks have since been established (more than 50) with more than 400,000 units available [3], extending the donor pool and the potential benefit of hematopoietic stem cell transplant to patients without a conventional matched donor.

Recent data suggest that outcomes of adult patients, in addition to pediatric patients, after CBT are no longer inferior to matched unrelated marrow transplants. In addition, there is the possibility of improved graft-versus-leukemia effect seen with dCBT. Further research to improve CB stem cell homing, engraftment, immune reconstitution, and optimization of conditioning regimens, GVHD prophylaxis, and outcomes after transplantation is ongoing. With continued efforts to further decrease transplant-related mortality, there is hope that the suggested enhanced GVL effect seen with CBT will translate into improved overall survival after transplantation for adult and pediatric patients with hematologic malignancies.

References

1. Appelbaum FR. The current status of hematopoietic cell transplantation. Annu Rev Med. 2003;54:491–512.
2. Gragert L. Estimating match rates with adult donors and umbilical cord blood units in the NMDP Be the Match registry. In: 8th annual international umbilical cord blood transplantation symposium, San Francisco, 2010
3. NMDP. Likelihood of finding and unrelated donor or cord blood unit. 2010. Available from: http://www.marrow.org/PHYSICIAN/URD_Search_and_Tx/Likelihood_of_Finding_an_URD_o/index.html. Accessed on 01/24/11.
4. Barker JN, et al. Searching for unrelated donor hematopoietic stem cells: availability and speed of umbilical cord blood versus bone marrow. Biol Blood Marrow Transplant. 2002;8(5):257–60.
5. Laughlin MJ, et al. Outcomes after transplantation of cord blood or bone marrow from unrelated donors in adults with leukemia. N Engl J Med. 2004;351(22):2265–75.
6. Brunstein CG, Laughlin MJ. Extending cord blood transplant to adults: dealing with problems and results overall. Semin Hematol. 2010;47(1):86–96.
7. Brunstein CG, et al. Allogeneic hematopoietic cell transplantation for hematological malignancy: relative risks and benefits of double umbilical cord blood. Blood. 2010;116(22): 4693–9. Epub 2010 Aug 4.
8. Smith AR, Wagner JE. Alternative haematopoietic stem cell sources for transplantation: place of umbilical cord blood. Br J Haematol. 2009;147(2):246–61.
9. Gluckman E, et al. Hematopoietic reconstitution in a patient with Fanconi's anemia by means of umbilical-cord blood from an HLA-identical sibling. N Engl J Med. 1989;321(17):1174–8.
10. Kurtzberg J. Update on umbilical cord blood transplantation. Curr Opin Pediatr. 2009;21(1):22–9.
11. Wagner JE, et al. Transplantation of umbilical cord blood after myeloablative therapy: analysis of engraftment. Blood. 1992;79(7):1874–81.
12. Bogdanic V, et al. Umbilical cord blood transplantation in a patient with Philadelphia chromosome-positive chronic myeloid leukemia. Transplantation. 1993;56(2):477–9.

13. Issaragrisil S, et al. Brief report: transplantation of cord-blood stem cells into a patient with severe thalassemia. N Engl J Med. 1995;332(6):367–9.
14. Broxmeyer HE, et al. Umbilical cord blood hematopoietic stem and repopulating cells in human clinical transplantation. Blood Cells. 1991;17(2):313–29.
15. Vilmer E, et al. HLA-mismatched cord-blood transplantation in a patient with advanced leukemia. Transplantation. 1992;53(5):1155–7.
16. Kurtzberg J, et al. Placental blood as a source of hematopoietic stem cells for transplantation into unrelated recipients. N Engl J Med. 1996;335(3):157–66.
17. Wagner JE, et al. Successful transplantation of HLA-matched and HLA-mismatched umbilical cord blood from unrelated donors: analysis of engraftment and acute graft-versus-host disease. Blood. 1996;88(3):795–802.
18. Laporte JP, et al. Cord-blood transplantation from an unrelated donor in an adult with chronic myelogenous leukemia. N Engl J Med. 1996;335(3):167–70.
19. Gluckman E, et al. Outcome of cord-blood transplantation from related and unrelated donors. Eurocord Transplant Group and the European Blood and Marrow Transplantation Group. N Engl J Med. 1997;337(6):373–81.
20. Rubinstein P, et al. Outcomes among 562 recipients of placental-blood transplants from unrelated donors. N Engl J Med. 1998;339(22):1565–77.
21. Cornetta K, et al. Umbilical cord blood transplantation in adults: results of the prospective cord blood transplantation (COBLT). Biol Blood Marrow Transplant. 2005;11(2):149–60.
22. Gluckman E, Rocha V. Cord blood transplantation: state of the art. Haematologica. 2009;94(4):451–4.
23. Eapen M, et al. Effect of graft source on unrelated donor haemopoietic stem-cell transplantation in adults with acute leukaemia: a retrospective analysis. Lancet Oncol. 2010; 11(7):653–60.
24. Gluckman E, et al. Factors associated with outcomes of unrelated cord blood transplant: guidelines for donor choice. Exp Hematol. 2004;32(4):397–407.
25. Barker JN, Scaradavou A, Stevens CE. Combined effect of total nucleated cell dose and HLA match on transplantation outcome in 1061 cord blood recipients with hematologic malignancies. Blood. 2010;115(9):1843–9.
26. Shen BJ, et al. Unrelated, HLA-mismatched multiple human umbilical cord blood transfusion in four cases with advanced solid tumors: initial studies. Blood Cells. 1994; 20(2–3):285–92.
27. Weinreb S, et al. Transplantation of unrelated cord blood cells. Bone Marrow Transplant. 1998;22(2):193–6.
28. De Lima M, et al. Double-chimaerism after transplantation of two human leucocyte antigen mismatched, unrelated cord blood units. Br J Haematol. 2002;119(3):773–6.
29. Wagner JE, et al. Transplantation of unrelated donor umbilical cord blood in 102 patients with malignant and nonmalignant diseases: influence of CD34 cell dose and HLA disparity on treatment-related mortality and survival. Blood. 2002;100(5):1611–18.
30. Scaradavou A, et al. Cord blood units with low CD34+ cell viability have a low probability of engraftment after double unit transplantation. Biol Blood Marrow Transplant. 2010; 16(4):500–8.
31. Gutman JA, et al. Single-unit dominance after double-unit umbilical cord blood transplantation coincides with a specific CD8+ T-cell response against the nonengrafted unit. Blood. 2010;115(4):757–65.
32. Kurtzberg J, et al. Results of the cord blood transplantation study (COBLT): clinical outcomes of unrelated donor umbilical cord blood transplantation in pediatric patients with hematologic malignancies. Blood. 2008;112(10):4318–27.
33. Barker JN, et al. Rapid and complete donor chimerism in adult recipients of unrelated donor umbilical cord blood transplantation after reduced-intensity conditioning. Blood. 2003;102(5): 1915–19.
34. Gutman JA, et al. Low relapse without excessive transplant-related mortality following myeloablative cord blood transplantation for acute leukemia in complete remission: a matched cohort analysis. Biol Blood Marrow Transplant. 2009;15(9):1122–9.

35. Horwitz ME, et al. Myeloablative intravenous busulfan/fludarabine conditioning does not facilitate reliable engraftment of dual umbilical cord blood grafts in adult recipients. Biol Blood Marrow Transplant. 2008;14(5):591–4.
36. Ciurea SO, Andersson BS. Busulfan in hematopoietic stem cell transplantation. Biol Blood Marrow Transplant. 2009;15(5):523–36.
37. Sanz J, et al. Single-unit umbilical cord blood transplantation from unrelated donors in adult patients with chronic myeloid leukemia. Biol Blood Marrow Transplant. 2010;16(11):1589–95. Epub 2010 May 27.
38. Sanz J, et al. Cord blood transplantation from unrelated donors in adults with high-risk acute myeloid leukemia. Biol Blood Marrow Transplant. 2010;16(1):86–94.
39. Brunstein CG, et al. Umbilical cord blood transplantation after nonmyeloablative conditioning: impact on transplantation outcomes in 110 adults with hematologic disease. Blood. 2007;110(8):3064–70.
40. Yamada MF, et al. Myeloablative cord blood transplantation for adults with hematological malignancies using tacrolimus and short-term methotrexate for graft-versus-host disease prophylaxis: single-institution analysis. Transplant Proc. 2008;40(10):3637–42.
41. Locatelli F, et al. Factors associated with outcome after cord blood transplantation in children with acute leukemia. Eurocord-Cord Blood Transplant Group. Blood. 1999;93(11):3662–71.
42. Locatelli F, et al. Related umbilical cord blood transplantation in patients with thalassemia and sickle cell disease. Blood. 2003;101(6):2137–43.
43. Cutler C, et al. Double umbilical cord blood transplantation with reduced intensity conditioning and sirolimus-based GVHD prophylaxis. Bone Marrow Transplant. 2011;46:659–67.
44. Attar EC, Scadden DT. Regulation of hematopoietic stem cell growth. Leukemia. 2004;18(11):1760–8.
45. Hofmeister CC, et al. Ex vivo expansion of umbilical cord blood stem cells for transplantation: growing knowledge from the hematopoietic niche. Bone Marrow Transplant. 2007;39(1):11–23.
46. McNiece I, Briddell R. Ex vivo expansion of hematopoietic progenitor cells and mature cells. Exp Hematol. 2001;29(1):3–11.
47. Robinson SN, et al. Superior ex vivo cord blood expansion following co-culture with bone marrow-derived mesenchymal stem cells. Bone Marrow Transplant. 2006;37(4):359–66.
48. Sauvageau G, Iscove NN, Humphries RK. In vitro and in vivo expansion of hematopoietic stem cells. Oncogene. 2004;23(43):7223–32.
49. Verfaillie C. Ex vivo expansion of hematopoeitic stem cells. In: Zon L, editor. Hematopoiesis: a developmental approach. New York: Oxford University Press; 2001. p. 119–29.
50. Sorrentino BP. Clinical strategies for expansion of haematopoietic stem cells. Nat Rev Immunol. 2004;4(11):878–88.
51. Yin T, Li L. The stem cell niches in bone. J Clin Invest. 2006;116:1195–201.
52. Wilson A, Trumpp A. Bone-marrow haematopoietic-stem-cell niches. Nat Rev Immunol. 2006;6(2):93–106.
53. Adams GB, Scadden DT. The hematopoietic stem cell in its place. Nat Immunol. 2006;7:333–7.
54. De Lima M, et al. Mesenchymal stem cell based cord blood expansion leads to rapid engraftment of platelets and neutrophils. Orlando: American Society of Hematology; 2010.
55. de Lima M, et al. Transplantation of ex vivo expanded cord blood cells using the copper chelator tetraethylenepentamine: a phase I/II clinical trial. Bone Marrow Transplant. 2008;41(9):771–8.
56. Brown JA, et al. Clearance of CMV viremia and survival after double umbilical cord blood transplantation in adults depends on reconstitution of thymopoiesis. Blood. 2010;115(20):4111–19.
57. Milner LA, et al. A human homologue of the *Drosophila* developmental gene, Notch, is expressed in CD34+ hematopoietic precursors. Blood. 1994;83(8):2057–62.
58. Varnum-Finney B, et al. Pluripotent, cytokine-dependent, hematopoietic stem cells are immortalized by constitutive Notch1 signaling. Nat Med. 2000;6(11):1278–81.

59. Varnum-Finney B, Brashem-Stein C, Bernstein ID. Combined effects of Notch signaling and cytokines induce a multiple log increase in precursors with lymphoid and myeloid reconstituting ability. Blood. 2003;101(5):1784–9.

60. Delaney C, et al. Dose-dependent effects of the Notch ligand Delta1 on ex vivo differentiation and in vivo marrow repopulating ability of cord blood cells. Blood. 2005;106(8):2693–9.

61. Ohishi K, Varnum-Finney B, Bernstein ID. Delta-1 enhances marrow and thymus repopulating ability of human CD34(+)CD38(−) cord blood cells. J Clin Invest. 2002;110(8):1165–74.

62. Delaney C, et al. Notch-mediated expansion of human cord blood progenitor cells capable of rapid myeloid reconstitution. Nat Med. 2010;16(2):232–6.

63. Fernandez MN, et al. Unrelated umbilical cord blood transplants in adults: early recovery of neutrophils by supportive co-transplantation of a low number of highly purified peripheral blood CD34+ cells from an HLA-haploidentical donor. Exp Hematol. 2003;31(6):535–44.

64. Magro E, et al. Early hematopoietic recovery after single unit unrelated cord blood transplantation in adults supported by co-infusion of mobilized stem cells from a third party donor. Haematologica. 2006;91(5):640–8.

65. Bautista G, et al. Cord blood transplants supported by co-infusion of mobilized hematopoietic stem cells from a third-party donor. Bone Marrow Transplant. 2009;43(5):365–73.

66. Gonzalo-Daganzo R, et al. Results of a pilot study on the use of third-party donor mesenchymal stromal cells in cord blood transplantation in adults. Cytotherapy. 2009;11(3):278–88.

67. Frassoni F, et al. Direct intrabone transplant of unrelated cord-blood cells in acute leukaemia: a phase I/II study. Lancet Oncol. 2008;9(9):831–9.

68. Frassoni F, et al. The intra-bone marrow injection of cord blood cells extends the possibility of transplantation to the majority of patients with malignant hematopoietic diseases. Best Pract Res Clin Haematol. 2010;23(2):237–44.

69. Ramirez PA, Wagner JE, Brunstein CG. Going straight to the point: intra-BM injection of hematopoietic progenitors. Bone Marrow Transplant. 2010;45(7):1127–33.

70. Brunstein CG, et al. Intra-BM injection to enhance engraftment after myeloablative umbilical cord blood transplantation with two partially HLA-matched units. Bone Marrow Transplant. 2009;43(12):935–40.

71. Christopherson II KW, et al. CD26 inhibition on CD34+ or lineage- human umbilical cord blood donor hematopoietic stem cells/hematopoietic progenitor cells improves long-term engraftment into NOD/SCID/Beta2null immunodeficient mice. Stem Cells Dev. 2007;16(3):355–60.

72. Christopherson II KW, et al. Modulation of hematopoietic stem cell homing and engraftment by CD26. Science. 2004;305(5686):1000–3.

73. Wysoczynski M, et al. Cleavage fragments of the third complement component (C3) enhance stromal derived factor-1 (SDF-1)-mediated platelet production during reactive postbleeding thrombocytosis. Leukemia. 2007;21(5):973–82.

74. Taupin P. Ex vivo fucosylation of stem cells to improve engraftment: WO2004094619. Expert Opin Ther Pat. 2010;20(9):1265–9.

75. Hoggatt J, et al. Prostaglandin E2 enhances hematopoietic stem cell homing, survival, and proliferation. Blood. 2009;113(22):5444–55.

76. Atsuta Y, et al. Disease-specific analyses of unrelated cord blood transplantation compared with unrelated bone marrow transplantation in adult patients with acute leukemia. Blood. 2009;113(8):1631–8.

77. Rocha V, et al. Comparison of outcomes of unrelated bone marrow and umbilical cord blood transplants in children with acute leukemia. Blood. 2001;97(10):2962–71.

78. Eapen M, et al. Outcomes of transplantation of unrelated donor umbilical cord blood and bone marrow in children with acute leukaemia: a comparison study. Lancet. 2007;369(9577):1947–54.

79. Montesinos P, et al. Incidence, risk factors, and outcome of cytomegalovirus infection and disease in patients receiving prophylaxis with oral valganciclovir or intravenous ganciclovir after umbilical cord blood transplantation. Biol Blood Marrow Transplant. 2009;15(6):730–40.

80. Matsumura T, et al. Cytomegalovirus infections following umbilical cord blood transplantation using reduced intensity conditioning regimens for adult patients. Biol Blood Marrow Transplant. 2007;13(5):577–83.

81. Narimatsu H, et al. Reduced dose of foscarnet as preemptive therapy for cytomegalovirus infection following reduced-intensity cord blood transplantation. Transpl Infect Dis. 2007;9(1):11–5.

82. Takami A, et al. High incidence of cytomegalovirus reactivation in adult recipients of an unrelated cord blood transplant. Haematologica. 2005;90(9):1290–2.

83. Tomonari A, et al. Impact of cytomegalovirus serostatus on outcome of unrelated cord blood transplantation for adults: a single-institute experience in Japan. Eur J Haematol. 2008; 80(3):251–7.

84. Tomonari A, et al. Preemptive therapy with ganciclovir 5 mg/kg once daily for cytomegalovirus infection after unrelated cord blood transplantation. Bone Marrow Transplant. 2008;41(4):371–6.

85. Walker CM, et al. Cytomegalovirus infection after allogeneic transplantation: comparison of cord blood with peripheral blood and marrow graft sources. Biol Blood Marrow Transplant. 2007;13(9):1106–15.

86. Shereck EB, et al. A pilot phase II study of alternate day ganciclovir and foscarnet in preventing cytomegalovirus (CMV) infections in at-risk pediatric and adolescent allogeneic stem cell transplant recipients. Pediatr Blood Cancer. 2007;49(3):306–12.

87. Milano F, et al. Pre-transplant ganciclovir and high-dose valacyclovir prophylaxis decrease incidence of CMV reactivation in high-risk seropositive UCBT recipients. Orlando: American Society of Hematology; 2010.

88. Brunstein CG, et al. Marked increased risk of Epstein-Barr virus-related complications with the addition of antithymocyte globulin to a nonmyeloablative conditioning prior to unrelated umbilical cord blood transplantation. Blood. 2006;108(8):2874–80.

89. Ballen KK, et al. Donor-derived second hematologic malignancies after cord blood transplantation. Biol Blood Marrow Transplant. 2010;16(7):1025–31.

90. Mori Y, Miyamoto T, Nagafuji K, Kamezaki K, Yamamoto A, Saito N, Kato K, Takenaka K, Iwasaki H, Harada N, Abe Y, Teshima T, Akashi K. High incidence of human herpes virus 6-associated encephalitis/myelitis following a second unrelated cord blood transplantation. Biol Blood Marrow Transplant. 2010;16(11):1596–602. Epub 2010 May 26.

91. Chevallier P, et al. Human herpes virus 6 infection is a hallmark of cord blood transplant in adults and may participate to delayed engraftment: a comparison with matched unrelated donors as stem cell source. Bone Marrow Transplant. 2010;45(7):1204–11.

92. Sashihara J, et al. High incidence of human herpesvirus 6 infection with a high viral load in cord blood stem cell transplant recipients. Blood. 2002;100(6):2005–11.

93. Klein AK, et al. T-cell recovery in adults and children following umbilical cord blood transplantation. Biol Blood Marrow Transplant. 2001;7(8):454–66.

94. Inoue H, et al. The kinetics of immune reconstitution after cord blood transplantation and selected CD34+ stem cell transplantation in children: comparison with bone marrow transplantation. Int J Hematol. 2003;77(4):399–407.

95. Szabolcs P, Niedzwiecki D. Immune reconstitution after unrelated cord blood transplantation. Cytotherapy. 2007;9(2):111–22.

96. Komanduri KV, et al. Delayed immune reconstitution after cord blood transplantation is characterized by impaired thymopoiesis and late memory T-cell skewing. Blood. 2007;110(13): 4543–51.

97. Cohen G, et al. Antigen-specific T-lymphocyte function after cord blood transplantation. Biol Blood Marrow Transplant. 2006;12(12):1335–42.

98. Davis CC, et al. Interleukin-7 permits Th1/Tc1 maturation and promotes ex vivo expansion of cord blood T cells: a critical step toward adoptive immunotherapy after cord blood transplantation. Cancer Res. 2010;70(13):5249–58.

99. Micklethwaite KP, et al. Derivation of human T lymphocytes from cord blood and peripheral blood with antiviral and antileukemic specificity from a single culture as protection against infection and relapse after stem cell transplantation. Blood. 2010;115(13):2695–703.

100. Godfrey WR, et al. Cord blood CD4(+)CD25(+)-derived T regulatory cell lines express FoxP3 protein and manifest potent suppressor function. Blood. 2005;105(2):750–8.
101. Brown JA, Boussiotis VA. Umbilical cord blood transplantation: basic biology and clinical challenges to immune reconstitution. Clin Immunol. 2008;127(3):286–97.
102. Kadereit S, et al. Cyclosporin A effects during primary and secondary activation of human umbilical cord blood T lymphocytes. Exp Hematol. 2001;29(7):903–9.
103. Kaminski BA, et al. Reduced expression of NFAT-associated genes in UCB versus adult CD4+ T lymphocytes during primary stimulation. Blood. 2003;102(13):4608–17.
104. Kleen TO, et al. Recipient-specific tolerance after HLA-mismatched umbilical cord blood stem cell transplantation. Transplantation. 2005;80(9):1316–22.
105. Sauter C, Barker JN. Unrelated donor umbilical cord blood transplantation for the treatment of hematologic malignancies. Curr Opin Hematol. 2008;15(6):568–75.
106. Narimatsu H, et al. Chronic graft-versus-host disease following umbilical cord blood transplantation: retrospective survey involving 1072 patients in Japan. Blood. 2008; 112(6):2579–82.
107. Sugimoto K, et al. Clinical characteristics of chronic graft-versus-host disease following umbilical cord blood transplantation for adults. Bone Marrow Transplant. 2008;41(8): 729–36.
108. Alsultan A, Giller RH, Gao D, Bathurst J, Hild E, Gore L, Foreman NK, Keating A, Quinones RR. GVHD after unrelated cord blood transplant in children: characteristics, severity, risk factors and influence on outcome. Bone Marrow Transplant. 2011;46(5):668–75. Epub 2010 Aug 2.
109. MacMillan ML, et al. Acute graft-versus-host disease after unrelated donor umbilical cord blood transplantation: analysis of risk factors. Blood. 2009;113(11):2410–15.
110. Arora M, et al. Chronic graft-versus-host disease (cGVHD) following unrelated donor hematopoietic stem cell transplantation (HSCT): higher response rate in recipients of unrelated donor (URD) umbilical cord blood (UCB). Biol Blood Marrow Transplant. 2007; 13(10):1145–52.
111. Verneris MR, et al. Relapse risk after umbilical cord blood transplantation: enhanced graft-versus-leukemia effect in recipients of 2 units. Blood. 2009;114(19):4293–9.
112. Rodrigues CA, et al. Analysis of risk factors for outcomes after unrelated cord blood transplantation in adults with lymphoid malignancies: a study by the Eurocord-Netcord and lymphoma working party of the European group for blood and marrow transplantation. J Clin Oncol. 2009;27(2):256–63.
113. Gluckman E, Rocha V. Donor selection for unrelated cord blood transplants. Curr Opin Immunol. 2006;18(5):565–70.
114. Rocha V, et al. Transplants of umbilical-cord blood or bone marrow from unrelated donors in adults with acute leukemia. N Engl J Med. 2004;351(22):2276–85.
115. Takahashi S, et al. Comparative single-institute analysis of cord blood transplantation from unrelated donors with bone marrow or peripheral blood stem-cell transplants from related donors in adult patients with hematologic malignancies after myeloablative conditioning regimen. Blood. 2007;109(3):1322–30.
116. Rocha V, et al. Reduced-intensity conditioning regimens before unrelated cord blood transplantation in adults with acute leukaemia and other haematological malignancies. Curr Opin Oncol. 2009;21 Suppl 1:S31–4.
117. Miyakoshi S, et al. Successful engraftment after reduced-intensity umbilical cord blood transplantation for adult patients with advanced hematological diseases. Clin Cancer Res. 2004;10(11):3586–92.
118. Yuji K, et al. Reduced-intensity unrelated cord blood transplantation for patients with advanced malignant lymphoma. Biol Blood Marrow Transplant. 2005;11(4):314–18.
119. Chao NJ, et al. Adult recipients of umbilical cord blood transplants after nonmyeloablative preparative regimens. Biol Blood Marrow Transplant. 2004;10(8):569–75.
120. Majhail NS, et al. Reduced-intensity allogeneic transplant in patients older than 55 years: unrelated umbilical cord blood is safe and effective for patients without a matched related donor. Biol Blood Marrow Transplant. 2008;14(3):282–9.

121. Ballen KK, et al. Double unrelated reduced-intensity umbilical cord blood transplantation in adults. Biol Blood Marrow Transplant. 2007;13(1):82–9.
122. Cutler C, Ballen K. Reduced-intensity conditioning and umbilical cord blood transplantation in adults. Bone Marrow Transplant. 2009;44(10):667–71.
123. Stanevsky A, Goldstein G, Nagler A. Umbilical cord blood transplantation: pros, cons and beyond. Blood Rev. 2009;23(5):199–204.
124. Bernaudin F, et al. Long-term results of related myeloablative stem-cell transplantation to cure sickle cell disease. Blood. 2007;110(7):2749–56.
125. Slatter MA, Gennery AR. Umbilical cord stem cell transplantation for primary immunodeficiencies. Expert Opin Biol Ther. 2006;6(6):555–65.
126. Staba SL, et al. Cord-blood transplants from unrelated donors in patients with Hurler's syndrome. N Engl J Med. 2004;350(19):1960–9.
127. Stein J, et al. Successful treatment of Wolman disease by unrelated umbilical cord blood transplantation. Eur J Pediatr. 2007;166(7):663–6.
128. Powles RL, et al. Mismatched family donors for bone-marrow transplantation as treatment for acute leukaemia. Lancet. 1983;1(8325):612–15.
129. Henslee PJ, et al. T cell depletion of HLA and haploidentical marrow reduces graft-versus-host disease but it may impair a graft-versus-leukemia effect. Transplant Proc. 1987;19(1 Pt 3):2701–6.
130. Ruggeri L, et al. Donor natural killer cell allorecognition of missing self in haploidentical hematopoietic transplantation for acute myeloid leukemia: challenging its predictive value. Blood. 2007;110(1):433–40.
131. Stern M, et al. Survival after T cell-depleted haploidentical stem cell transplantation is improved using the mother as donor. Blood. 2008;112(7):2990–5.
132. Rizzieri DA, et al. Partially matched, nonmyeloablative allogeneic transplantation: clinical outcomes and immune reconstitution. J Clin Oncol. 2007;25(6):690–7.
133. Ogawa H, et al. Unmanipulated HLA 2–3 antigen-mismatched (haploidentical) stem cell transplantation using nonmyeloablative conditioning. Biol Blood Marrow Transplant. 2006;12(10):1073–84.
134. Kasamon YL, et al. Nonmyeloablative HLA-haploidentical bone marrow transplantation with high-dose posttransplantation cyclophosphamide: effect of HLA disparity on outcome. Biol Blood Marrow Transplant. 2010;16(4):482–9.
135. Yoo KH, et al. Current status of pediatric umbilical cord blood transplantation in Korea: a multicenter retrospective analysis of 236 cases. Am J Hematol. 2011;86(1):12–7.
136. Kishi Y, et al. Early immune reaction after reduced-intensity cord-blood transplantation for adult patients. Transplantation. 2005;80(1):34–40.
137. Miyakoshi S, et al. Tacrolimus as prophylaxis for acute graft-versus-host disease in reduced intensity cord blood transplantation for adult patients with advanced hematologic diseases. Transplantation. 2007;84(3):316–22.
138. Uchida N, et al. Umbilical cord blood transplantation after reduced-intensity conditioning for elderly patients with hematologic diseases. Biol Blood Marrow Transplant. 2008;14(5):583–90.
139. Foeken LM, Green A, Hurley CK, Marry E, Wiegand T, Oudshoorn M; Donor Registries Working Group of the World Marrow Donor Association (WMDA). Monitoring the international use of unrelated donors for transplantation: the WMDA annual reports. Bone Marrow Transplant. 2010;45(5):811–8. Epub 2010 Feb 15.

Chapter 9
The Detection and Significance
of Minimal Residual Disease

Jerald P. Radich and Brent L. Wood

Abstract Minimal residual disease (MRD) is detected in many leukemia patients who have achieved complete remission. The detection of MRD by polymerase chain reaction (PCR) or flow cytometric assays is associated with a high risk of relapse following chemotherapy or hematopoietic stem cell transplantation (SCT). The systematic monitoring for MRD can identify cases at high risk of relapse that should be offered more aggressive or investigational therapy.

Keywords Minimal residual disease • Leukemia • Remission • Polymerase chain reaction • Flow cytometry • Chemotherapy • Hematopoietic stem cell transplantation • Relapse

Introduction

Relapse is the major obstacle to cure in leukemia, despite advances in combination chemotherapy, "targeted" therapy, and stem cell transplantation. Modern immunophenotyping and molecular biology allow us to detect residual leukemia in patients

J.P. Radich, M.D. (✉)
Department of Clinical Research and Oncology, University of Washington School of Medicine, Seattle, WA, USA

Clinical Research Division, Fred Hutchinson Cancer Research Center, 1100 Fairview Ave N, D5-100, 98109 Seattle, WA 98109, USA
e-mail: jradich@fhcrc.org

B.L. Wood, M.D., Ph.D.
Department of Laboratory Medicine, University of Washington Medical Center, 1959 NE Pacific St, Box 357110, Seattle, WA 98195, USA
e-mail: woodbl@u.washington.edu

E.H. Estey and F.R. Appelbaum (eds.), *Leukemia and Related Disorders: Integrated Treatment Approaches*, Contemporary Hematology,
DOI 10.1007/978-1-60761-565-1_9, © Springer Science+Business Media, LLC 2012

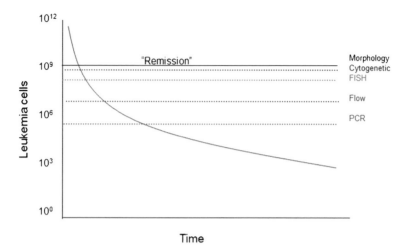

Fig. 9.1 The kinetics of response and MRD detection. At diagnosis, a patient may harbor up to 10^{12} leukemia cells. After induction therapy, conventional morphology defines remission as <5% blasts; at this point, up to 10^9 leukemia cells may be present. Other tests to define disease burden (corresponding to Table 9.1) can detect MRD. However, even when a patient has no detectable MRD, significant amounts of disease may still persist

who appear to be in remission by conventional morphology. The detection of minimal residual disease (MRD) has been shown to be predictive of relapse in leukemia in a variety of treatment settings.

An example of the kinetics of remission and relapse is shown in Fig. 9.1. At diagnosis, patients may have up to 10^{10}–10^{12} leukemia cells; thus in complete remission, potentially millions of leukemia cells still remain. The purpose of MRD detection is to estimate tumor burden as well as subsequent risk of relapse.

Methods of MRD Detection

Routine pathologic bone marrow examination relies on the morphologic differences between malignant and normal cells. Since the difference between normal and leukemia cells may be subtle, remission is defined by the practical (but somewhat arbitrary) cutoff of <5% blasts. As shown in Fig. 9.1, this level of detection means that enormous numbers of leukemia cells still may persist at morphological remission, so it is not surprising that some patients believed to be in remission subsequently relapse. Several more sensitive methods to detect residual disease are listed in Table 9.1.

Table 9.1 Methods to detect minimal residual disease

Detection method	Target	Sensitivity (%)
Pathologic examination	Cellular morphology	5
Cytogenetics	Chromosome structure	1–5
FISH	Specific genetic marker(s)	0.08–5
Flow cytometry	Surface antigen expression	0.01–0.1
PCR	DNA or RNA sequence	0.0001–0.1

Chromosomal Assays

Metaphase cytogenetics can detect approximately one leukemia cell in 100 normal cells ("10^{-1}" sensitivity) [1, 2]. However, most groups perform karyotyping based on only 20 metaphase preparations. Cytogenetics is the standard method to define cytogenetic remission and to find unanticipated genomic changes during therapy. Metaphase cytogenetics is limited by sampling only those few cells that divide in culture.

Fluorescence in situ hybridization (FISH) uses chromosome-specific or locus-specific probes to find tumor-specific genetic aberrations in metaphase or interphase cells. FISH can screen 200–10,000 cells for numerical chromosomal aberrations and can identify minor abnormal clones undetected by karyotypic study. The sensitivity of FISH is typically $2 \times 10^{-3} - 5 \times 10^{-3}$.

Flow Cytometry Assays

The pattern of cell surface antigen expression distinguishes malignant and normal hematopoietic cells [3]. "Multiparametric" flow cytometric assays use informative combinations of antibodies to identify patterns of aberrant antigen expression different in leukemia compared to normal cells of similar lineage (Fig. 9.2). The immunophenotypic abnormalities identified at diagnosis offer a "fingerprint" (the leukemia-associated immunophenotype) that can identify a residual leukemia population after therapy. However, changes in immunophenotype are common following therapy, particularly for acute leukemia [4–7], thus strict reliance on the pretreatment immunophenotype can lead to false-negative results. Current flow cytometric assays show a variable sensitivity that is typically 10^{-3}–10^{-4} in experienced hands. The old standard of using three to four simultaneous antigens (colors) is being displaced by techniques using at least eight to ten antigens/colors [8]. This progress means that flow cytometry rivals the sensitivity of PCR (see below) for MRD detection in many diseases.

Fig. 9.2 Minimal residual
disease in B lineage acute
lymphoblastic leukemia.
The gated B cell population
(CD19+) contains a mixture
of normal mature B cells
(CD20+, CD10–, *blue*),
immature B cells (CD10+,
variable CD20, *green*), and
residual leukemia (bright
CD10+, variable CD20+, *red*
and *arrow*). The leukemic
population is recognized by
the aberrant levels of
expression of CD10 and
CD20, distinguishing it from
all normal B cells

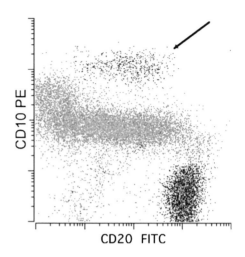

Polymerase Chain Reaction (PCR)

Nucleic acid amplification by the polymerase chain reaction (PCR) is often the most sensitive approach to detect MRD [9]. In PCR, a specific genetic lesion target is the "fingerprint" of the leukemia. Gene translocations, such as the t(9;22) in chronic myeloid leukemia (CML), the t(15:17), t(8;21), and inv(16)/t(16;16) found in acute myeloid leukemia (AML), are straightforward and sensitive leukemia-specific markers for MRD detection [10–16]. Nearly 40–50% of acute lymphocytic leukemia (ALL) and AML has some types of translocation that can be detected by PCR assays [17]. In ALL, the most used PCR markers involve the leukemia-specific "fingerprints" caused by the immunoglobulin heavy chain and T cell receptor rearrangement [18, 19]. These are potentially quite sensitive but are relatively labor intensive since unique primers to the leukemia-specific clonal rearrangement must be created for each individual patient.

Samples Suitable for MRD Detection

For CML, the detection of BCR-ABL is similar in either peripheral blood or bone marrow [20]. Similarly in pediatric T-ALL, there is good concordance between peripheral blood and marrow MRD [21–23]. In adult AML, there appears to be reasonably good concordance between peripheral blood and marrow MRD, although the absolute level is somewhat reduced in blood [24]. In Chronic Lymphocytic Leukemia (CLL) MRD persists in the marrow after it becomes undetectable in peripheral blood [25].

MRD Detection in Myeloid Leukemia

MRD Detection in AML Following Chemotherapy

Acute promyelocytic leukemia (APL) typically has the PML-RARα gene juxtaposition contained in the t(15;17). APL patients with MRD after induction or consolidation therapy have a significantly high risk of relapse [26, 27]. Serial PCR monitoring until completion of maintenance therapy allows for the identification of those patients at highest risk of relapse [28]. In a study of 70 APL patients, the MRD level after first consolidation was the most powerful predictor of relapse. Patients with an MRD level of $\geq 10^{-3}$ had a >tenfold higher relapse rate at 5 years compared to a level of $< 10^{-3}$ ($p = 0.001$). In APL, the analysis of peripheral blood is nearly as informative as bone marrow [29].

Disruptions of the core binding factor genes AML1 and CBFB are involved in the t(8;21) and inv. (16) "good" risk translocations. These occur in ~15–20% of adult and pediatric AML. The *qualitative* detection (presence or absence) of the AML1-MGT8 or CBFB-MYH11 mRNA has limited value in monitoring MRD and predicting relapse, since these transcripts often persist even in long-term complete remission [30–38]. However, quantification of MRD has been used to determine the critical level of MRD that segregates good and poor outcome [13, 35]. A posttherapy MRD level of <1% was associated with a relatively low risk of relapse [39–43]. MRD investigation at the end of treatment might have the best prognostic value in CBF-leukemia, including combining the transcription ratios at diagnosis and after 3–4 months during treatment [44].

The Wilm's tumor gene (WT1) is overexpressed at diagnosis of the majority of AML [45, 46]. Several studies showed that WT1 levels at diagnosis were associated with prognosis, with higher expression being associated with an inferior outcome [47]. WT1 is expressed at a low level in normal hematopoietic cells, which limits the utility of WT1 as a marker of MRD. However, the increase in WT1 levels during therapy has been associated with subsequent relapse in some studies [45], but not others [48].

The most common genetic mutations found in AML involve FLT3 and NPM, each occurring in $\geq 25\%$ of cases, especially concentrated in cases with normal cytogenetics. The most common mutations are activating insertion mutations. In FLT3, an internal tandem duplication (ITD) of 5–100 base pairs is inserted into the juxtamembrane domain, allowing for ligand-independent dimerization of the FLT3 receptor. Primers can be made for leukemia-specific amplification [49–52]. However, clonal evolution is common in AML, so that diagnostic and relapse cells are often discordant for FLT3 mutation status in ~20% of the time [53]. Mutation-specific PCR reactions have been constructed for the most common point mutations in NPM1; many potential mutations exist [54]. However, given the difficulty in constructing leukemia-specific primers for these cases, a far more practical solution is using flow cytometry as a means of MRD detection.

Immunophenotypic detection of MRD by flow cytometry can be used for identifying risk groups after induction and consolidation chemotherapy and for providing important information to postinduction treatment strategies. In adult AML, immunophenotypes sufficiently informative for MRD detection at a level of 10^{-3}–10^{-4} are found in 80–95% of cases [55] dependent on the reagent panel employed. In a study of 72 adults, repeat posttherapeutic evaluations enabled the identification of specific cutoff values of MRD associated with significant survival impact after induction and consolidation therapy [56]. A cutoff level of 1% after the first induction, of 0.14% after the second induction, and of 0.11% after consolidation resulted in a 6.1-fold, 3.4-fold, and 7.2-fold higher relative risk of relapse, respectively. Similar conclusions, albeit with slightly different cutoffs, can be drawn from other studies in adult AML [57, 58] with some suggesting a stronger association between relapse and end of consolidation MRD in comparison with end of induction MRD.

In childhood AML, Coustan-Smith et al. [59] found that 85% of cases had informative immunophenotypes with a detection sensitivity of 10^{-3}–10^{-4}. They found that 34% and 27% of patients had MRD after first and second induction, respectively, with a 2-year overall survival of approximately 30% compared with a survival of >70% in patients without detectable MRD. Sievers et al. [60] found immunophenotypic abnormalities in 41 (16%) of 252 children with AML who achieved morphologic CR with initial induction therapy, and MRD was highly associated with a poor outcome.

MRD in AML Following Stem Cell Transplantation

The significance of MRD following transplant depends on the specific genetic subtype of AML and generally follows the trends found after chemotherapy. In t(15;17) AML, the detection of the PML/RARα transcript following HCT strongly associated with relapse [58, 59], while in t(8;21), the AML1/ETO often remains after allogeneic transplant, without relapse [61–63].

WT1 has been used as a marker of MRD following HCT with variable results [64]; WT1 levels prior to transplant as a measure of disease burden have been studied to predict subsequent response following autologous transplant and suggest that high levels of WT1 transcripts in BM harvests are correlated with outcome. Patients with a low level of WT1 had a superior RFS compared to those with a high WT1 level [65]. Of note is that WT1 may be useful in the context of being a potential target for immunotherapy; in this context, WT1 levels might serve both as an indication of patients who might benefit from immunomodulation as well as a measure of response following immunotherapy [66].

The presence of pretransplant MRD in AML is associated with poor outcome. In an autologous transplant setting, the pretransplant MRD status, measured by multidimensional flow cytometry, reliably predicted outcome [67]. Patients ($n=19$) with $<3.5 \times 10^{-4}$ residual leukemia cells were assigned to as MRD low risk, those ($n=12$) with $\geq 3.5 \times 10^{-4}$ cells to as MRD high risk. One hundred percent of patients with high-risk disease relapsed versus 26% of the low risk group ($p=0.0004$). The median posttransplant RFS was 7 and 48 months for the MRD high-risk and MRD low-risk groups, respectively ($p=0.007$). Increasing MRD levels were shown in three of the five relapsing patients. A study of 99 adults undergoing allogeneic transplantation for AML in morphologic remission [61] showed 24% with detectable MRD pretransplant. Those with detectable MRD had a 30% 2-year overall survival with a 2-year estimate of relapse of 65% in comparison with those without detectable MRD having 77% 2-year overall survival and 18% 2-year estimate of relapse, yielding hazard ratios for positive MRD of 4 for overall mortality ($p<0.001$) and 8.5 for relapse ($p<0.001$).

Little data exist regarding AML MRD detection posttransplant and outcome, although one study of 41 patients suggests that MRD positivity $>10^{-3}$ at day 100 after allogeneic transplantation is associated with an increased risk of relapse [62]. It has also been suggested that AML MRD detection may be used in risk stratification to improve outcome with risk-directed therapy in a scheme including marrow transplantation [63].

Lastly, the measurement of the MRD burden of transplantation products may also be used to guide patient-tailored purging procedures [68]. An MRD level in the stem cell products of less than 0.05%, as measured by flow cytometry, was found to be associated with a remarkable RFS of 100% at 12 months.

MRD in CML Following Imatinib Therapy

In CML, quantitative PCR for the *BCR-ABL* transcript can be used to judge treatment response and give a strong prediction of future resistance or progression to accelerated or blast phase.

The iconic IRIS study compared the tyrosine kinase inhibitor imatinib (IM) against interferon and Ara-C in newly diagnosed chronic phase CML. At the 1-year mark, 68% of IM patients achieved a complete cytogenetic remission (CCyR), compared to only 7% in the patients receiving interferon/Ara-C [69, 70]. Quantitative *BCR-ABL* PCR of peripheral blood was performed in the patients who achieved a CCyR [71]. This study introduced the concept of the "major molecular response" (MMR), a 3-log reduction in *BCR-ABL* copy number from mean baseline of a subset of cases. MMR was found in 39% of imatinib-treated patients after 12 months of therapy, compared to only 2% in the IFN/Ara-C arm. Moreover, MMR at 12 months was associated with an improved progression-free survival: Patients with an MMR had a 0% risk of progression, compared to ~10% for cases in complete cytogenetic remission (CCyR) without an MMR, and ~25% in cases not achieving a CCyR. There has since been a plethora of studies on the use of BCR-ABL testing during TKI therapy. In sum: (1) MMR represents a "safe haven" with rare loss of CCyR or progression to advanced phase disease [64, 72]. (2) The rate of decline of BCR-ABL is important in predicting subsequent response and outcome [64, 73–75]. Patients who achieve MMR quickly are at a much higher probability to achieve a complete molecular remission (CMR). This is potentially highly important since studies have suggested that a subset of patients who have a prolonged CMR may have IM discontinued without subsequent relapse [76]. (3) The increase of BCR-ABL level is associated with the acquisition of ABL mutations, resistance, and relapse [72, 77].

MRD Detection in CML Posttransplant

Many studies have demonstrated the association of MRD and relapse in CML post-transplant [78–84]. Most of these studies were done in the pre-TKI era and, thus, were on a patient population largely skewed toward chronic phase. How these results relate to a new CML transplant population who have generally failed TKI and/or have progressed to advanced phase disease is unclear.

The highest risk of relapse associated with *BCR-ABL* detection appears to be associated "early" ($\leq$12 months post-SCT) after transplant [78, 83, 85]; positive patients 6–12 months posttransplant had an ~40% risk of relapse compared to <5% in patients without MRD. Qualitative tests earlier than 3 months post-SCT were not associated with relapse. Subsequent studies using *BCR-ABL* quantification by QPCR further defined the risk of MRD [86–92]. Low residual *BCR-ABL* posttransplant was associated with <1% relapse rate, compared to a 75% relapse rate in those with increasing or persistently high *BCR-ABL* levels [93]. CML patients "early" (3–5 months) posttransplant with undetectable *BCR-ABL* had a 9% risk of relapse, compared to patients with a "low" (<100 *BCR-ABL* transcripts/ug RNA) or "high" level of transcripts (>100 copies *BCR-ABL*/ug), who had a cumulative relapse rate of 30% and 74%, respectively [90]. CML patients studied "late" (>18 months) post-SCT [92] have a relatively high rate of MRD positivity (~25%), and 14% of these cases relapsed. However, only 1% of persistently negative patients relapsed. Curiously, MRD can be detected in patients who were years post-HCT; thus, MRD can occur in >25% of patients $\geq$3 years posttransplant, with subsequent relapse rates of ~10–20% [81, 85, 92, 94]. Rare patients in complete remission for >10 years post-HSCT have been found to be persistently MRD positive[95, 96].

MRD Detection in Lymphoid Leukemia

MRD Detection in ALL on Chemotherapy

In ALL, MRD detection can be performed by either flow cytometry or PCR. Flow cytometry assays rely on the aberrant expression of a constellation of surface antigens in the leukemia clone that differ from normal hematopoiesis, while PCR-based assays are based on clonal immunoglobulin heavy chain (IgH V-D-J) or T cell receptor (TCR) gene rearrangements. Both methods have excellent sensitivity, and both are susceptible to clonal shifts that occur with disease resistance in 10–20% of cases [97–100]. Potentially, the combined use of both methods will allow MRD detection in nearly all patients [101, 102]. Given the greater frequency of B compared to T cell ALL, most of the studies are biased toward B lineage ALL.

The clinical impact of MRD depends on the time where it is assessed. Early clearance of leukemia cells is a favorable prognostic indicator in childhood ALL [18, 103, 104]. Low or absent MRD in the bone marrow (BM) after the completion of induction therapy predicts a favorable outcome, as MRD-negative patients have an overall relapse rate of only 2–10% (Table 9.2) [18, 105–108]. On the other hand, high MRD levels at the end of induction treatment are associated with high relapse rates of 70–100% [18, 105–107, 109] with a graded risk of relapse related to the level of MRD detected down to 0.01% in B lineage ALL [110]. These patients at risk for relapse may benefit from considering alternative treatment approaches such as transplantation [18, 111, 112]. MRD status after induction therapy appears to be the most significant prognostic factor in pediatric ALL, independent of other clinically relevant risk factors, such as age, blast count, immunophenotype, presence of chromosome aberrations at diagnosis, and response to prednisone [18, 107, 113]. Following consolidation therapy, the presence of MRD >0.01%, while infrequent, is associated with a markedly poor outcome [110].

In pediatric ALL patients who relapse after achieving remission, MRD status after reinduction treatment is similarly important [112, 114], as the EFS of patients with less ($<10^{-30}$) MRD had a significantly better EFS than those with greater MRD (86% vs. 0%, respectively). In addition, in children who achieve a CR after first relapse, 54% had MRD level of $\geq 0.01\%$, and their subsequent relapse rate was 70%, compared with 28% for the MRD-negative patients [114]. In a three block reinduction protocol for children with relapsed ALL, both the level of MRD at the end of block 1 and the pattern of MRD measured at the end of each block were associated with outcome [115], with rising MRD being associated with the worst outcome. A poorer outcome and more frequent level of MRD >0.01% were also detected in patients with early relapse (<3 years from therapy) in comparison with late relapse, although MRD remained prognostic within both groups [115]. The value of continuing MRD monitoring during maintenance therapy and off therapy is less clear, since frequent monitoring has been difficult to employ [104, 107, 116].

MRD studies in adult ALL have lagged behind the pediatric studies, with most using PCR methods. There is increasing evidence that in adult ALL, as in children, an early decrease of MRD levels after induction therapy is an important predictor of prognosis and response to chemotherapy [117–119]. Thus, the assessment of the MRD kinetics at different follow-up time points defined risk groups based on a specific threshold MRD level in standard-risk adult ALL patients [120]. Patients with a rapid MRD decline to lower than 10^{-4} or under the detection limit at day 11 (during first induction) and day 24 (at the end of induction) were at low risk with a 3-year DFS and OS of 100%. In contrast, patients with persistent MRD of 10^{-4} until week 16 were at high risk with a 3-year DFS of 5.8% and a 3-year OS of 45.1%.

Flow cytometric studies of ALL MRD in adults are few but suggest findings similar to those seen in pediatric studies. In a study of 102 adolescent and adult patients with ALL [121], absence of MRD at day 35 following induction

Table 9.2 MRD in pediatric ALL

Study	EORTC [18]	iBFM [107]	St. Jude [105]	BFM-Austria [106]	NOPHO [29]	COG [110]
No. of patients	178	240	195	108	104	2,143
MRD method	Ig/TCR-PCR	Ig/TCR-PCR and TAL1 deletion	Flow cytometry	Flow cytometry	Ig/TCR-PCR	Flow cytometry
MRD study time point	After induction therapy	5 weeks after diagnosis	End of induction	Day 33 after start of induction therapy	Day 29 after start of induction therapy	Day 29 after start of induction therapy
		No. patients relapsing/No. with given MRD result				
MRD status						
Negative	7/88 (8%)	2/71 (3%)	9/123 (10%)	4/59 (7%)	1/53 (2%)	1,588 (6.8%)
$\leq 10^{-4}$	5/30 (17%)	8/33 (25%)	–/33 (23%, 43%)	1/5 (20%)		
$<10^{-2}, >10^{-4}$		12/38 (32%)		5/31 (16%)	9/32 (28%)	316 (28%)
$\geq 10^{-2}$	11/15 (73%)	20/27 (67%)	–/9 (72%)	3/3 (100%)	5/15 (33%)	67

chemotherapy (<0.05% cutoff) was associated with a significantly longer relapse-free survival (42 months vs. 16 months; $p=0.001$). A small subset of patients (11.8%) was also identified who obtained absence of MRD by day 14 after therapy and had an excellent prognosis (90% survival at 5 years). All cases with >0.1% MRD relapsed by 2 years. Similar to pediatric ALL, the presence of MRD at day 35 was the most relevant independent prognostic factor. One additional study confirms that MRD at end of induction is a strong independent risk factor in adults with ALL [122].

In the adult Ph+ ALL, MRD kinetics can be followed by measuring *BCR-ABL* levels with quantitative real-time PCR [123, 124]. Using this approach, 42 patients with complete hematological response following induction therapy were divided into two prognostic groups: good molecular responders (with >2 log reduction of BCR-ABL transcript levels after induction and >3 log reduction after consolidation therapy) and poor responders with higher MRD levels at both time points [124]. The probability of a 2-year survival was 48% for the good molecular responders compared to 0% ($p=0.0026$) for the poor molecular responders.

Krampera et al. demonstrated that frequent immunophenotypic MRD measurement in the first year of treatment is a useful outcome predictor for adult T-ALL patients [125]. MRD-positive patients prior to consolidation therapy had a probability of relapse at 2 years of 82%, compared to 39% ($p=0.00078$) in MRD-negative patients. In a larger study on 102 adolescent and adult ALL patients, MRD at day 35 was the most powerful independent prognostic parameter by multivariate analysis [126]. Patients in morphologic complete remission and a low MRD level (<0.05%) had a median RFS of 42 months versus 16 months ($p=0.001$) for patients with higher MRD levels. An excellent prognosis with a projected 5-year RFS of 90% was observed when MRD levels at day 14 were very low (<0.03%).

MRD in ALL Posttransplant

MRD detection prior to transplant and following transplantation is predictive of relapse and outcome [127–133]. Both PCR and flow cytometry have been used to detect MRD in these studies, with somewhat different criteria to determine "low" from "high" levels of MRD. The data suggest a very high risk of relapse (~75%) in cases with high levels of MRD prior to HSCT, intermediate risk of relapse in cases with low-level MRD (~50%), and a low risk of relapse in cases without MRD (~15%).

MRD detection following transplant is associated with an increased risk of relapse in both Ph− ALL and Ph+ ALL. In Ph− ALL, the relative risk of relapse in MRD+ cases posttransplant was five- to tenfold, with relapse occurring within months of MRD detection [82, 132]. In Ph+ ALL, the risk appears somewhat different, dependent whether the disease is p190 BCR-ABL or p210 BCR-ABL. All studies of Ph+ ALL demonstrate a strong association of MRD-positive cases detection and relapse after transplant [20, 80, 134, 135]. The data suggest that the risk of relapse associated with p190 *BCR-ABL* MRD is higher compared to p210 *BCR-ABL*.

Stirewalt et al. found the relative risk of relapse in all Ph+ ALL cases who were MRD+ compared to persistently MRD– posttransplant to be 4.4. However, the relative risk was 8.7 for p190 and 2.2 for p210 BCR-ABL disease [135].

MRD in Chronic Lymphocytic Leukemia (CLL)

Other B lineage hematologic malignancies (CLL, multiple myeloma, and non-Hodgkin lymphoma (NHL)) can be studied by similar strategies as ALL, using IgH V-D-J rearrangements to detect MRD. However, CLL is readily detectable by flow cytometry and may be the method of choice for MRD detection for CLL. In head-to-head comparisons of PCR and flow cytometry, PCR has been found to be slightly more sensitive at levels below 0.01%, with approximately 10% of flow cytometry negative cases being found to be PCR-positive for clonal IgH V-D-J rearrangements [136, 137]. However, this increased sensitivity must be weighed against the considerably greater ease, speed, and cost of flow cytometry compared to PCR technique.

The clinical significance of MRD in CLL depends on the treatment employed. In CLL cases treated with anti-CD52 antibody based therapy, autologous transplant, or allogeneic transplant, the presence of MRD is strongly associated with outcome and subsequent relapse [137]. Eradication of MRD from blood and bone marrow by anti-CD52 therapy is associated with longer treatment-free survival, although reappearance of MRD occurs in 50% and eradication appears to only be possible in patients without bulky disease [138]. In contrast, an absence of MRD at 12 months following allogeneic transplantation can be obtained in a majority of patients and appears to be associated with a very low rate of relapse [139].

After allogeneic transplant, a subset of patients remain with intermittent low-level positivity [140, 141]. This is reminiscent of the situation with CML, where some cases can remain MRD+ at low levels for greater than a decade following transplant. It remains to be seen if the allogeneic effect has a time limit, a concern since relapses do occur in CML greater than 10 years following transplant [142].

Conclusion

The detection of MRD is an important predictor of relapse following chemotherapy and transplantation. Following the example of CML, it may in the future be used as a primary outcome surrogate for longer-term relapse risk and outcome, thus dramatically shortening clinical trial time. In addition, MRD can be used to modify treatment strategies, allowing physicians to modify treatment plans to accommodate different drugs or methods (e.g., transplant vs. continuing chemotherapy) in cases with persistent disease. While the treatment of MRD is generally still investigational, it is important to move into the routine design of clinical studies, as it may be that we do not need many new drugs and treatment modalities but a better understanding of when to use them.

References

1. Arthur CK, Apperley JF, Guo AP, Rassool F, Gao LM, Goldman JM. Cytogenetic events after bone marrow transplantation for chronic myeloid leukemia in chronic phase. Blood. 1988;71(5):1179–86.
2. Hook EB. Exclusion of chromosomal mosaicism: tables of 90%, 95% and 99% confidence limits and comments on use. Am J Hum Genet. 1977;29(1):94–7.
3. Campana D, Coustan-Smith E. Advances in the immunological monitoring of childhood acute lymphoblastic leukaemia. Best Pract Res. 2002;15(1):1–19.
4. Dworzak J, Lamecker H, von Berg J, Klinder T, Lorenz C, Kainmuller D, et al. 3D reconstruction of the human rib cage from 2D projection images using a statistical shape model. Int J Comput Assist Radiol Surg. 2010;5(2):111–24.
5. Gaipa G, Basso G, Aliprandi S, Migliavacca M, Vallinoto C, Maglia O, et al. Prednisone induces immunophenotypic modulation of CD10 and CD34 in nonapoptotic B-cell precursor acute lymphoblastic leukemia cells. Cytometry B Clin Cytom. 2008;74(3):150–5.
6. Langebrake C, Brinkmann I, Teigler-Schlegel A, Creutzig U, Griesinger F, Puhlmann U, et al. Immunophenotypic differences between diagnosis and relapse in childhood AML: implications for MRD monitoring. Cytometry B Clin Cytom. 2005;63(1):1–9.
7. Voskova D, Schoch C, Schnittger S, Hiddemann W, Haferlach T, Kern W. Stability of leukemia-associated aberrant immunophenotypes in patients with acute myeloid leukemia between diagnosis and relapse: comparison with cytomorphologic, cytogenetic, and molecular genetic findings. Cytometry B Clin Cytom. 2004;62(1):25–38.
8. Wood B. 9-color and 10-color flow cytometry in the clinical laboratory. Arch Pathol Lab Med. 2006;130(5):680–90.
9. Saiki RK, Gelfand DH, Stoffel S, Scharf SJ, Higuchi R, Horn GT, et al. Primer-directed enzymatic amplification of DNA with a thermostable DNA polymerase. Science. 1988; 239(4839):487–91.
10. Claxton DF, Liu P, Hsu HB, Marlton P, Hester J, Collins F, et al. Detection of fusion transcripts generated by the inversion 16 chromosome in acute myelogenous leukemia. Blood. 1994;83(7):1750–6.
11. Hebert J, Cayuela JM, Daniel MT, Berger R, Sigaux F. Detection of minimal residual disease in acute myelomonocytic leukemia with abnormal marrow eosinophils by nested polymerase chain reaction with allele specific amplification. Blood. 1994;84(7):2291–6.
12. Kawasaki ES, Clark SS, Coyne MY, Smith SD, Champlin R, Witte ON, et al. Diagnosis of chronic myeloid and acute lymphocytic leukemias by detection of leukemia-specific mRNA sequences amplified in vitro. Proc Natl Acad Sci USA. 1988;85(15):5698–702.
13. Kusec R, Laczika K, Knobl P, Friedl J, Greinix H, Kahls P, et al. AML1/ETO fusion mRNA can be detected in remission blood samples of all patients with t(8;21) acute myeloid leukemia after chemotherapy or autologous bone marrow transplantation. Leukemia. 1994;8(5):735–9.
14. Lee MS, Chang KS, Cabanillas F, Freireich EJ, Trujillo JM, Stass SA. Detection of minimal residual cells carrying the t(14;18) by DNA sequence amplification. Science. 1987;237(4811): 175–8.
15. Maruyama F, Stass SA, Estey EH, Cork A, Hirano M, Ino T, et al. Detection of AML1/ETO fusion transcript as a tool for diagnosing t(8;21) positive acute myelogenous leukemia. Leukemia. 1994;8(1):40–5.
16. Miller Jr WH, Levine K, DeBlasio A, Frankel SR, Dmitrovsky E, Warrell Jr RP. Detection of minimal residual disease in acute promyelocytic leukemia by a reverse transcription polymerase chain reaction assay for the PML/RAR-alpha fusion mRNA. Blood. 1993;82(6): 1689–94.
17. Pallisgaard N, Hokland P, Riishoj DC, Pedersen B, Jorgensen P. Multiplex reverse transcription-polymerase chain reaction for simultaneous screening of 29 translocations and chromosomal aberrations in acute leukemia. Blood. 1998;92(2):574–88.

18. Cave H, van der Werff ten Bosch J, Suciu S, Guidal C, Waterkeyn C, Otten J, et al. Clinical significance of minimal residual disease in childhood acute lymphoblastic leukemia. European Organization for Research and Treatment of Cancer – Childhood Leukemia Cooperative Group. N Engl J Med. 1998;339(9):591–8.

19. Roberts WM, Estrov Z, Ouspenskaia MV, Johnston DA, McClain KL, Zipf TF. Measurement of residual leukemia during remission in childhood acute lymphoblastic leukemia. N Engl J Med. 1997;336(5):317–23.

20. Radich J, Gehly G, Lee A, Avery R, Bryant E, Edmands S, et al. Detection of bcr-abl transcripts in Philadelphia chromosome-positive acute lymphoblastic leukemia after marrow transplantation. Blood. 1997;89(7):2602–9.

21. Brisco MJ, Sykes PJ, Hughes E, Story CJ, Rice MS, Schwarer AP, et al. Molecular relapse can be detected in blood in a sensitive and timely fashion in B-lineage acute lymphoblastic leukemia. Leukemia. 2001;15(11):1801–2.

22. Coustan-Smith E, Sancho J, Hancock ML, Razzouk BI, Ribeiro RC, Rivera GK, et al. Use of peripheral blood instead of bone marrow to monitor residual disease in children with acute lymphoblastic leukemia. Blood. 2002;100(7):2399–402.

23. van der Velden VH, Jacobs DC, Wijkhuijs AJ, Comans-Bitter WM, Willemse MJ, Hahlen K, et al. Minimal residual disease levels in bone marrow and peripheral blood are comparable in children with T cell acute lymphoblastic leukemia (ALL), but not in precursor-B-ALL. Leukemia. 2002;16(8):1432–6.

24. Maurillo L, Buccisano F, Spagnoli A, Del Poeta G, Panetta P, Neri B, et al. Monitoring of minimal residual disease in adult acute myeloid leukemia using peripheral blood as an alternative source to bone marrow. Haematologica. 2007;92(5):605–11.

25. Rawstron AC, Kennedy B, Moreton P, Dickinson AJ, Cullen MJ, Richards SJ, et al. Early prediction of outcome and response to alemtuzumab therapy in chronic lymphocytic leukemia. Blood. 2004;103(6):2027–31.

26. Diverio D, Rossi V, Avvisati G, De Santis S, Pistilli A, Pane F, et al. Early detection of relapse by prospective reverse transcriptase-polymerase chain reaction analysis of the PML/RARalpha fusion gene in patients with acute promyelocytic leukemia enrolled in the GIMEMA-AIEOP multicenter "AIDA" trial. GIMEMA-AIEOP multicenter "AIDA" trial. Blood. 1998;92(3):784–9.

27. Mandelli F, Diverio D, Avvisati G, Luciano A, Barbui T, Bernasconi C, et al. Molecular remission in PML/RAR alpha-positive acute promyelocytic leukemia by combined all-trans retinoic acid and idarubicin (AIDA) therapy. Gruppo Italiano-Malattie Ematologiche Maligne dell'Adulto and Associazione Italiana di Ematologia ed Oncologia Pediatrica Cooperative Groups. Blood. 1997;90(3):1014–21.

28. Lee S, Kim YJ, Eom KS, Min CK, Kim HJ, Cho SG, et al. The significance of minimal residual disease kinetics in adults with newly diagnosed PML-RARalpha-positive acute promyelocytic leukemia: results of a prospective trial. Haematologica. 2006;91(5):671–4.

29. Gallagher RE, Yeap BY, Bi W, Livak KJ, Beaubier N, Rao S, et al. Quantitative real-time RT-PCR analysis of PML-RAR alpha mRNA in acute promyelocytic leukemia: assessment of prognostic significance in adult patients from intergroup protocol 0129. Blood. 2003; 101(7):2521–8.

30. Nucifora G, Larson RA, Rowley JD. Persistence of the 8;21 translocation in patients with acute myeloid leukemia type M2 in long-term remission. Blood. 1993;82(3):712–5.

31. Berger R. Differences between blastic chronic myeloid leukemia and Ph-positive acute leukemia. Leuk Lymphoma. 1993;11 Suppl 1:235–7.

32. Downing JR, Head DR, Curcio-Brint AM, Hulshof MG, Motroni TA, Raimondi SC, et al. An AML1/ETO fusion transcript is consistently detected by RNA-based polymerase chain reaction in acute myelogenous leukemia containing the (8;21)(q22;q22) translocation. Blood. 1993;81(11):2860–5.

33. Zhang T, Hillion J, Tong JH, Cao Q, Chen SJ, Berger R, et al. AML-1 gene rearrangement and AML-1-ETO gene expression as molecular markers of acute myeloblastic leukemia with t(8;21). Leukemia. 1994;8(5):729–34.

34. Sugimoto T, Das H, Imoto S, Murayama T, Gomyo H, Chakraborty S, et al. Quantitation of minimal residual disease in t(8;21)-positive acute myelogenous leukemia patients using real-time quantitative RT-PCR. Am J Hematol. 2000;64(2):101–6.
35. Jurlander J, Caligiuri MA, Ruutu T, Baer MR, Strout MP, Oberkircher AR, et al. Persistence of the AML1/ETO fusion transcript in patients treated with allogeneic bone marrow transplantation for t(8;21) leukemia. Blood. 1996;88(6):2183–91.
36. Marcucci G, Livak KJ, Bi W, Strout MP, Bloomfield CD, Caligiuri MA. Detection of minimal residual disease in patients with AML1/ETO-associated acute myeloid leukemia using a novel quantitative reverse transcription polymerase chain reaction assay. Leukemia. 1998;12(9):1482–9.
37. Gaiger A, Schmid D, Heinze G, Linnerth B, Greinix H, Kalhs P, et al. Detection of the WT1 transcript by RT-PCR in complete remission has no prognostic relevance in de novo acute myeloid leukemia. Leukemia. 1998;12(12):1886–94.
38. Costello R, Sainty D, Blaise D, Gastaut JA, Gabert J, Poirel H, et al. Prognosis value of residual disease monitoring by polymerase chain reaction in patients with CBF beta/MYH11-positive acute myeloblastic leukemia. Blood. 1997;89(6):2222–3.
39. Buonamici S, Ottaviani E, Testoni N, Montefusco V, Visani G, Bonifazi F, et al. Real-time quantitation of minimal residual disease in inv(16)-positive acute myeloid leukemia may indicate risk for clinical relapse and may identify patients in a curable state. Blood. 2002; 99(2):443–9.
40. Krauter J, Gorlich K, Ottmann O, Lubbert M, Dohner H, Heit W, et al. Prognostic value of minimal residual disease quantification by real-time reverse transcriptase polymerase chain reaction in patients with core binding factor leukemias. J Clin Oncol. 2003;21(23):4413–22.
41. Marcucci G, Caligiuri MA, Dohner H, Archer KJ, Schlenk RF, Dohner K, et al. Quantification of CBFbeta/MYH11 fusion transcript by real time RT-PCR in patients with INV(16) acute myeloid leukemia. Leukemia. 2001;15(7):1072–80.
42. Stentoft J, Hokland P, Ostergaard M, Hasle H, Nyvold CG. Minimal residual core binding factor AMLs by real time quantitative PCR–initial response to chemotherapy predicts event free survival and close monitoring of peripheral blood unravels the kinetics of relapse. Leuk Res. 2006;30(4):389–95.
43. Tobal K, Newton J, Macheta M, Chang J, Morgenstern G, Evans PA, et al. Molecular quantitation of minimal residual disease in acute myeloid leukemia with t(8;21) can identify patients in durable remission and predict clinical relapse. Blood. 2000;95(3):815–9.
44. Schnittger S, Weisser M, Schoch C, Hiddemann W, Haferlach T, Kern W. New score predicting for prognosis in PML-RARA+, AML1-ETO+, or CBFBMYH11+ acute myeloid leukemia based on quantification of fusion transcripts. Blood. 2003;102(8):2746–55.
45. Lapillonne H, Renneville A, Auvrignon A, Flamant C, Blaise A, Perot C, et al. High WT1 expression after induction therapy predicts high risk of relapse and death in pediatric acute myeloid leukemia. J Clin Oncol. 2006;24(10):1507–15.
46. Ostergaard M, Olesen LH, Hasle H, Kjeldsen E, Hokland P. WT1 gene expression: an excellent tool for monitoring minimal residual disease in 70% of acute myeloid leukaemia patients – results from a single-centre study. Br J Haematol. 2004;125(5):590–600.
47. Trka J, Kalinova M, Hrusak O, Zuna J, Krejci O, Madzo J, et al. Real-time quantitative PCR detection of WT1 gene expression in children with AML: prognostic significance, correlation with disease status and residual disease detection by flow cytometry. Leukemia. 2002;16(7): 1381–9.
48. Weisser M, Kern W, Rauhut S, Schoch C, Hiddemann W, Haferlach T, et al. Prognostic impact of RT-PCR-based quantification of WT1 gene expression during MRD monitoring of acute myeloid leukemia. Leukemia. 2005;19(8):1416–23.
49. Scholl C, Schlenk RF, Eiwen K, Dohner H, Frohling S, Dohner K. The prognostic value of MLL-AF9 detection in patients with t(9;11)(p22;q23)-positive acute myeloid leukemia. Haematologica. 2005;90(12):1626–34.
50. Scholl S, Loncarevic IF, Krause C, Kunert C, Clement JH, Hoffken K. Minimal residual disease based on patient specific Flt3-ITD and -ITT mutations in acute myeloid leukemia. Leuk Res. 2005;29(7):849–53.

51. Beretta C, Gaipa G, Rossi V, Bernasconi S, Spinelli O, Dell'Oro MG, et al. Development of a quantitative-PCR method for specific FLT3/ITD monitoring in acute myeloid leukemia. Leukemia. 2004;18(8):1441–4.

52. Stirewalt DL, Willman CL, Radich JP. Quantitative, real-time polymerase chain reactions for FLT3 internal tandem duplications are highly sensitive and specific. Leuk Res. 2001;25(12): 1085–8.

53. Chakraverty R, Peggs K, Chopra R, Milligan DW, Kottaridis PD, Verfuerth S, et al. Limiting transplantation-related mortality following unrelated donor stem cell transplantation by using a nonmyeloablative conditioning regimen. Blood. 2002;99(3):1071–8.

54. Gorello P, Cazzaniga G, Alberti F, Dell'Oro MG, Gottardi E, Specchia G, et al. Quantitative assessment of minimal residual disease in acute myeloid leukemia carrying nucleophosmin (NPM1) gene mutations. Leukemia. 2006;20(6):1103–8.

55. Kern W, Danhauser-Riedl S, Ratei R, Schnittger S, Schoch C, Kolb HJ, et al. Detection of minimal residual disease in unselected patients with acute myeloid leukemia using multiparameter flow cytometry for definition of leukemia-associated immunophenotypes and determination of their frequencies in normal bone marrow. Haematologica. 2003;88(6):646–53.

56. Feller N, van der Pol MA, van Stijn A, Weijers GW, Westra AH, Evertse BW, et al. MRD parameters using immunophenotypic detection methods are highly reliable in predicting survival in acute myeloid leukaemia. Leukemia. 2004;18(8):1380–90.

57. Kern W, Voskova D, Schoch C, Hiddemann W, Schnittger S, Haferlach T. Determination of relapse risk based on assessment of minimal residual disease during complete remission by multiparameter flow cytometry in unselected patients with acute myeloid leukemia. Blood. 2004;104(10):3078–85.

58. San Miguel JF, Vidriales MB, Lopez-Berges C, Diaz-Mediavilla J, Gutierrez N, Canizo C, et al. Early immunophenotypical evaluation of minimal residual disease in acute myeloid leukemia identifies different patient risk groups and may contribute to postinduction treatment stratification. Blood. 2001;98(6):1746–51.

59. Coustan-Smith E, Ribeiro RC, Rubnitz JE, Razzouk BI, Pui CH, Pounds S, et al. Clinical significance of residual disease during treatment in childhood acute myeloid leukaemia. Br J Haematol. 2003;123(2):243–52.

60. Sievers EL, Lange BJ, Alonzo TA, Gerbing RB, Bernstein ID, Smith FO, et al. Immunophenotypic evidence of leukemia after induction therapy predicts relapse: results from a prospective Children's Cancer Group study of 252 patients with acute myeloid leukemia. Blood. 2003;101(7):3398–406.

61. Walter RB, Gooley TA, Wood BL, Milano F, Fang M, Sorror ML, et al. Impact of pretransplantation minimal residual disease, as detected by multiparametric flow cytometry, on outcome of myeloablative hematopoietic cell transplantation for acute myeloid leukemia. J Clin Oncol. 2011;29:1190–7.

62. Diez-Campelo M, Perez-Simon JA, Perez J, Alcoceba M, Richtmon J, Vidriales B, et al. Minimal residual disease monitoring after allogeneic transplantation may help to individualize post-transplant therapeutic strategies in acute myeloid malignancies. Am J Hematol. 2009;84(3):149–52.

63. Rubnitz JE, Inaba H, Dahl G, Ribeiro RC, Bowman WP, Taub J, et al. Minimal residual disease-directed therapy for childhood acute myeloid leukaemia: results of the AML02 multicentre trial. Lancet Oncol. 2010;11(6):543–52.

64. Cortes J, Talpaz M, O'Brien S, Jones D, Luthra R, Shan J, et al. Molecular responses in patients with chronic myelogenous leukemia in chronic phase treated with imatinib mesylate. Clin Cancer Res. 2005;11(9):3425–32.

65. Osborne D, Frost L, Tobal K, Liu JAY. Elevated levels of WT1 transcripts in bone marrow harvests are associated with a high relapse risk in patients autografted for acute myeloid leukaemia. Bone Marrow Transplant. 2005;36(1):67–70.

66. Ogawa H, Tamaki H, Ikegame K, Soma T, Kawakami M, Tsuboi A, et al. The usefulness of monitoring WT1 gene transcripts for the prediction and management of relapse following allogeneic stem cell transplantation in acute type leukemia. Blood. 2003;101(5):1698–704.

67. Venditti A, Maurillo L, Buccisano F, Del Poeta G, Mazzone C, Tamburini A, et al. Pretransplant minimal residual disease level predicts clinical outcome in patients with acute myeloid leukemia receiving high-dose chemotherapy and autologous stem cell transplantation. Leukemia. 2003;17(11):2178–82.

68. Feller N, Jansen-van der Weide MC, van der Pol MA, Westra GA, Ossenkoppele GJ, Schuurhuis GJ. Purging of peripheral blood stem cell transplants in AML: a predictive model based on minimal residual disease burden. Exp Hematol. 2005;33(1):120–30.

69. O'Brien SG, Deininger MW. Imatinib in patients with newly diagnosed chronic-phase chronic myeloid leukemia. Semin Hematol. 2003;40(2 Suppl 2):26–30.

70. Kantarjian H, Talpaz M, Cortes J, Susan OB, Faderl S, Thomas D, et al. Quantitative polymerase chain reaction monitoring of BCR-ABL during therapy with imatinib mesylate (STI517; Gleevec) in chronic-phase chronic myelogenous leukemia. Clin Cancer Res. 2003;9:160–6.

71. Hughes TP, Kaeda J, Branford S, Rudzki Z, Hochhaus A, Hensley ML, et al. Frequency of major molecular responses to imatinib or interferon alfa plus cytarabine in newly diagnosed chronic myeloid leukemia. N Engl J Med. 2003;349(15):1423–32.

72. Marin D, Kaeda J, Szydlo R, Saunders S, Fleming A, Howard J, et al. Monitoring patients in complete cytogenetic remission after treatment of CML in chronic phase with imatinib: patterns of residual leukaemia and prognostic factors for cytogenetic relapse. Leukemia. 2005;19(4):507–12.

73. Branford S, Rudzki Z, Harper A, Grigg A, Taylor K, Durrant S, et al. Imatinib produces significantly superior molecular responses compared to interferon alfa plus cytarabine in patients with newly diagnosed chronic myeloid leukemia in chronic phase. Leukemia. 2003; 17(12):2401–9.

74. Merx K, Muller MC, Kreil S, Lahaye T, Paschka P, Schoch C, et al. Early reduction of BCR-ABL mRNA transcript levels predicts cytogenetic response in chronic phase CML patients treated with imatinib after failure of interferon alpha. Leukemia. 2002;16(9):1579–83.

75. Wang L, Pearson K, Ferguson JE, Clark RE. The early molecular response to imatinib predicts cytogenetic and clinical outcome in chronic myeloid leukaemia. Br J Haematol. 2003;120(6):990–9.

76. Mahon FX, Rea D, Guilhot J, Guilhot F, Huguet F, Nicolini F, et al. Discontinuation of imatinib in patients with chronic myeloid leukaemia who have maintained complete molecular remission for at least 2 years: the prospective, multicentre Stop Imatinib (STIM) trial. Lancet Oncol. 2010;11(11):1029–35.

77. Branford S, Rudzki Z, Walsh S, Parkinson I, Grigg A, Szer J, et al. Detection of BCR-ABL mutations in patients with CML treated with imatinib is virtually always accompanied by clinical resistance, and mutations in the ATP phosphate-binding loop (P-loop) are associated with a poor prognosis. Blood. 2003;102(1):276–83.

78. Hughes TP, Morgan GJ, Martiat P, Goldman JM. Detection of residual leukemia after bone marrow transplant for chronic myeloid leukemia: role of polymerase chain reaction in predicting relapse. Blood. 1991;77(4):874–8.

79. Lion T, Henn T, Gaiger A, Kalhs P, Gadner H. Early detection of relapse after bone marrow transplantation in patients with chronic myelogenous leukaemia. Lancet. 1993;341(8840): 275–6.

80. Miyamura K, Tahara T, Tanimoto M, Morishita Y, Kawashima K, Morishima Y, et al. Long persistent bcr-abl positive transcript detected by polymerase chain reaction after marrow transplant for chronic myelogenous leukemia without clinical relapse: a study of 64 patients. Blood. 1993;81(4):1089–93.

81. Pichert G, Roy DC, Gonin R, Alyea EP, Belanger R, Gyger M, et al. Distinct patterns of minimal residual disease associated with graft- versus-host disease after allogeneic bone marrow transplantation for chronic myelogenous leukemia. J Clin Oncol. 1995;13(7):1704–13.

82. Radich J, Ladne P, Gooley T. Polymerase chain reaction-based detection of minimal residual disease in acute lymphoblastic leukemia predicts relapse after allogeneic BMT. Biol Blood Marrow Transplant. 1995;1(1):24–31.

83. Roth MS, Antin JH, Ash R, Terry VH, Gotlieb M, Silver SM, et al. Prognostic significance of Philadelphia chromosome-positive cells detected by the polymerase chain reaction after allogeneic bone marrow transplant for chronic myelogenous leukemia. Blood. 1992;79(1): 276–82.
84. Sawyers CL, Timson L, Kawasaki ES, Clark SS, Witte ON, Champlin R. Molecular relapse in chronic myelogenous leukemia patients after bone marrow transplantation detected by polymerase chain reaction. Proc Natl Acad Sci USA. 1990;87(2):563–7.
85. Radich JP, Gehly G, Gooley T, Bryant E, Clift RA, Collins S, et al. Polymerase chain reaction detection of the BCR-ABL fusion transcript after allogeneic marrow transplantation for chronic myeloid leukemia: results and implications in 346 patients. Blood. 1995;85(9): 2632–8.
86. Branford S, Hughes TP, Rudzki Z. Monitoring chronic myeloid leukaemia therapy by real-time quantitative PCR in blood is a reliable alternative to bone marrow cytogenetics. Br J Haematol. 1999;107(3):587–99.
87. Lin YT, Lin DT, Jou ST, Lin KS, Lin KH. Allogeneic bone marrow transplantation for Philadelphia chromosome-positive chronic myelogenous leukemia in childhood. J Formos Med Assoc. 1997;96(5):320–4.
88. Mensink E, van de Locht A, Schattenberg A, Linders E, Schaap N, Geurts van Kessel A, et al. Quantitation of minimal residual disease in Philadelphia chromosome positive chronic myeloid leukaemia patients using real-time quantitative RT-PCR. Br J Haematol. 1998;102(3): 768–74.
89. Mughal TI, Yong A, Szydlo RM, Dazzi F, Olavarria E, van Rhee F, et al. Molecular studies in patients with chronic myeloid leukaemia in remission 5 years after allogeneic stem cell transplant define the risk of subsequent relapse. Br J Haematol. 2001;115(3):569–74.
90. Olavarria E, Kanfer E, Szydlo R, Kaeda J, Rezvani K, Cwynarski K, et al. Early detection of BCR-ABL transcripts by quantitative reverse transcriptase-polymerase chain reaction predicts outcome after allogeneic stem cell transplantation for chronic myeloid leukemia. Blood. 2001;97(6):1560–5.
91. Preudhomme C, Chams-Eddine L, Roumier C, Duflos-Grardel N, Denis C, Cosson A, et al. Detection of BCR-ABL transcripts in chronic myeloid leukemia (CML) using an in situ RT-PCR assay. Leukemia. 1999;13(5):818–23.
92. Radich JP, Gooley T, Bryant E, Chauncey T, Clift R, Beppu L, et al. The significance of bcr-abl molecular detection in chronic myeloid leukemia patients "late," 18 months or more after transplantation. Blood. 2001;98(6):1701–7.
93. Lin F, van Rhee F, Goldman JM, Cross NC. Kinetics of increasing BCR-ABL transcript numbers in chronic myeloid leukemia patients who relapse after bone marrow transplantation. Blood. 1996;87(10):4473–8.
94. Costello RT, Kirk J, Gabert J. Value of PCR analysis for long term survivors after allogeneic bone marrow transplant for chronic myelogenous leukemia: a comparative study. Leuk Lymphoma. 1996;20(3–4):239–43.
95. van Rhee F, Lin F, Cross NC, Reid CD, Lakhani AK, Szydlo RM, et al. Detection of residual leukaemia more than 10 years after allogeneic bone marrow transplantation for chronic myelogenous leukaemia. Bone Marrow Transplant. 1994;14(4):609–12.
96. Sobrinho-Simoes M, Wilczek V, Score J, Cross NC, Apperley JF, Melo JV. In search of the original leukemic clone in chronic myeloid leukemia patients in complete molecular remission after stem cell transplantation or imatinib. Blood. 2010;116(8):1329–35.
97. Szczepanski T, Willemse MJ, Brinkhof B, van Wering ER, van der Burg M, van Dongen JJ. Comparative analysis of Ig and TCR gene rearrangements at diagnosis and at relapse of childhood precursor-B-ALL provides improved strategies for selection of stable PCR targets for monitoring of minimal residual disease. Blood. 2002;99(7):2315–23.
98. Imashuku S, Terui K, Matsuyama T, Asami K, Tsuchiya S, Ishii E, et al. Lack of clinical utility of minimal residual disease detection in allogeneic stem cell recipients with childhood acute lymphoblastic leukemia: multi-institutional collaborative study in Japan. Bone Marrow Transplant. 2003;31(12):1127–35.

99. Szczepanski T, Pongers-Willemse MJ, Langerak AW, van Dongen JJ. Unusual immunoglobulin and T-cell receptor gene rearrangement patterns in acute lymphoblastic leukemias. Curr Top Microbiol Immunol. 1999;246:205–13. discussion 14–5.

100. Bjorklund E, Mazur J, Soderhall S, Porwit-MacDonald A. Flow cytometric follow-up of minimal residual disease in bone marrow gives prognostic information in children with acute lymphoblastic leukemia. Leukemia. 2003;17(1):138–48.

101. Kerst G, Kreyenberg H, Roth C, Well C, Dietz K, Coustan-Smith E, et al. Concurrent detection of minimal residual disease (MRD) in childhood acute lymphoblastic leukaemia by flow cytometry and real-time PCR. Br J Haematol. 2005;128(6):774–82.

102. Neale GA, Coustan-Smith E, Stow P, Pan Q, Chen X, Pui CH, et al. Comparative analysis of flow cytometry and polymerase chain reaction for the detection of minimal residual disease in childhood acute lymphoblastic leukemia. Leukemia. 2004;18(5):934–8.

103. Panzer-Grumayer ER, Schneider M, Panzer S, Fasching K, Gadner H. Rapid molecular response during early induction chemotherapy predicts a good outcome in childhood acute lymphoblastic leukemia. Blood. 2000;95(3):790–4.

104. Marshall GM, Haber M, Kwan E, Zhu L, Ferrara D, Xue C, et al. Importance of minimal residual disease testing during the second year of therapy for children with acute lymphoblastic leukemia. J Clin Oncol. 2003;21(4):704–9.

105. Coustan-Smith E, Sancho J, Hancock ML, Boyett JM, Behm FG, Raimondi SC, et al. Clinical importance of minimal residual disease in childhood acute lymphoblastic leukemia. Blood. 2000;96(8):2691–6.

106. Dworzak MN, Froschl G, Printz D, Mann G, Potschger U, Muhlegger N, et al. Prognostic significance and modalities of flow cytometric minimal residual disease detection in childhood acute lymphoblastic leukemia. Blood. 2002;99(6):1952–8.

107. van Dongen JJ, Seriu T, Panzer-Grumayer ER, Biondi A, Pongers-Willemse MJ, Corral L, et al. Prognostic value of minimal residual disease in acute lymphoblastic leukaemia in childhood. Lancet. 1998;352(9142):1731–8.

108. Nyvold C, Madsen HO, Ryder LP, Seyfarth J, Svejgaard A, Clausen N, et al. Precise quantification of minimal residual disease at day 29 allows identification of children with acute lymphoblastic leukemia and an excellent outcome. Blood. 2002;99(4):1253–8.

109. Vilmer E, Suciu S, Ferster A, Bertrand Y, Cave H, Thyss A, et al. Long-term results of three randomized trials (58831, 58832, 58881) in childhood acute lymphoblastic leukemia: a CLCG-EORTC report. Children Leukemia Cooperative Group. Leukemia. 2000;14(12):2257–66.

110. Borowitz MJ, Devidas M, Hunger SP, Bowman WP, Carroll AJ, Carroll WL, et al. Clinical significance of minimal residual disease in childhood acute lymphoblastic leukemia and its relationship to other prognostic factors: a Children's Oncology Group study. Blood. 2008;111(12):5477–85.

111. Uckun FM, Nachman JB, Sather HN, Sensel MG, Kraft P, Steinherz PG, et al. Clinical significance of Philadelphia chromosome positive pediatric acute lymphoblastic leukemia in the context of contemporary intensive therapies: a report from the Children's Cancer Group. Cancer. 1998;83(9):2030–9.

112. Eckert C, Biondi A, Seeger K, Cazzaniga G, Hartmann R, Beyermann B, et al. Prognostic value of minimal residual disease in relapsed childhood acute lymphoblastic leukaemia. Lancet. 2001;358(9289):1239–41.

113. Coustan-Smith E, Behm FG, Sanchez J, Boyett JM, Hancock ML, Raimondi SC, et al. Immunological detection of minimal residual disease in children with acute lymphoblastic leukaemia. Lancet. 1998;351(9102):550–4.

114. Coustan-Smith E, Gajjar A, Hijiya N, Razzouk BI, Ribeiro RC, Rivera GK, et al. Clinical significance of minimal residual disease in childhood acute lymphoblastic leukemia after first relapse. Leukemia. 2004;18(3):499–504.

115. Raetz EA, Borowitz MJ, Devidas M, Linda SB, Hunger SP, Winick NJ, et al. Reinduction platform for children with first marrow relapse of acute lymphoblastic leukemia: a Children's Oncology Group Study [corrected]. J Clin Oncol. 2008;26(24):3971–8.

116. Campana D, Neale GA, Coustan-Smith E, Pui CH. Detection of minimal residual disease in acute lymphoblastic leukemia: the St Jude experience. Leukemia. 2001;15(2):278–9.

117. Gameiro P, Mortuza FY, Hoffbrand AV, Foroni L. Minimal residual disease monitoring in adult T-cell acute lymphoblastic leukemia: a molecular based approach using T-cell receptor G and D gene rearrangements. Haematologica. 2002;87(11):1126–34.

118. Specchia G, Liso A, Pannunzio A, Albano F, Mestice A, Pastore D, et al. Molecular detection of minimal residual disease is associated with early relapse in adult acute lymphoblastic leukemia. Haematologica. 2004;89(10):1271–3.

119. Toubai T, Tanaka J, Ota S, Fukuhara T, Hashino S, Kondo T, et al. Minimal residual disease (MRD) monitoring using rearrangement of T-cell receptor and immunoglobulin H gene in the treatment of adult acute lymphoblastic leukemia patients. Am J Hematol. 2005;80(3):181–7.

120. Bruggemann M, Raff T, Flohr T, Gokbuget N, Nakao M, Droese J, et al. Clinical significance of minimal residual disease quantification in adult patients with standard-risk acute lymphoblastic leukemia. Blood. 2006;107(3):1116–23.

121. Vidriales MB, Orfao A, San-Miguel JF. Immunologic monitoring in adults with acute lymphoblastic leukemia. Curr Oncol Rep. 2003;5(5):413–8.

122. Holowiecki J, Krawczyk-Kulis M, Giebel S, Jagoda K, Stella-Holowiecka B, Piatkowska-Jakubas B, et al. Status of minimal residual disease after induction predicts outcome in both standard and high-risk Ph-negative adult acute lymphoblastic leukaemia. The Polish Adult Leukemia Group ALL 4–2002 MRD study. Br J Haematol. 2008;142(2):227–37.

123. Yokota H, Tsuno NH, Tanaka Y, Fukui T, Kitamura K, Hirai H, et al. Quantification of minimal residual disease in patients with e1a2 BCR-ABL-positive acute lymphoblastic leukemia using a real-time RT-PCR assay. Leukemia. 2002;16(6):1167–75.

124. Pane F, Cimino G, Izzo B, Camera A, Vitale A, Quintarelli C, et al. Significant reduction of the hybrid BCR/ABL transcripts after induction and consolidation therapy is a powerful predictor of treatment response in adult Philadelphia-positive acute lymphoblastic leukemia. Leukemia. 2005;19(4):628–35.

125. Krampera M, Vitale A, Vincenzi C, Perbellini O, Guarini A, Annino L, et al. Outcome prediction by immunophenotypic minimal residual disease detection in adult T-cell acute lymphoblastic leukaemia. Br J Haematol. 2003;120(1):74–9.

126. Vidriales MB, Perez JJ, Lopez-Berges MC, Gutierrez N, Ciudad J, Lucio P, et al. Minimal residual disease in adolescent (older than 14 years) and adult acute lymphoblastic leukemias: early immunophenotypic evaluation has high clinical value. Blood. 2003;101(12):4695–700.

127. Krejci O, van der Velden VH, Bader P, Kreyenberg H, Goulden N, Hancock J, et al. Level of minimal residual disease prior to haematopoietic stem cell transplantation predicts prognosis in paediatric patients with acute lymphoblastic leukaemia: a report of the Pre-BMT MRD Study Group. Bone Marrow Transplant. 2003;32(8):849–51.

128. Bader P, Hancock J, Kreyenberg H, Goulden NJ, Niethammer D, Oakhill A, et al. Minimal residual disease (MRD) status prior to allogeneic stem cell transplantation is a powerful predictor for post-transplant outcome in children with ALL. Leukemia. 2002;16(9):1668–72.

129. Knechtli CJ, Goulden NJ, Hancock JP, Grandage VL, Harris EL, Garland RJ, et al. Minimal residual disease status before allogeneic bone marrow transplantation is an important determinant of successful outcome for children and adolescents with acute lymphoblastic leukemia. Blood. 1998;92(11):4072–9.

130. Uzunel M, Mattsson J, Jaksch M, Remberger M, Ringden O. The significance of graft-versus-host disease and pretransplantation minimal residual disease status to outcome after allogeneic stem cell transplantation in patients with acute lymphoblastic leukemia. Blood. 2001;98(6):1982–4.

131. Sramkova L, Muzikova K, Fronkova E, Krejci O, Sedlacek P, Formankova R, et al. Detectable minimal residual disease before allogeneic hematopoietic stem cell transplantation predicts extremely poor prognosis in children with acute lymphoblastic leukemia. Pediatr Blood Cancer. 2007;48:93–100.

132. van der Velden VH, Joosten SA, Willemse MJ, van Wering ER, Lankester AW, van Dongen JJ, et al. Real-time quantitative PCR for detection of minimal residual disease before alloge-

neic stem cell transplantation predicts outcome in children with acute lymphoblastic leukemia. Leukemia. 2001;15(9):1485–7.

133. Sanchez J, Serrano J, Gomez P, Martinez F, Martin C, Madero L, et al. Clinical value of immunological monitoring of minimal residual disease in acute lymphoblastic leukaemia after allogeneic transplantation. Br J Haematol. 2002;116(3):686–94.

134. Miyamura K, Tanimoto M, Morishima Y, Horibe K, Yamamoto K, Akatsuka M, et al. Detection of Philadelphia chromosome-positive acute lymphoblastic leukemia by polymerase chain reaction: possible eradication of minimal residual disease by marrow transplantation. Blood. 1992;79(5):1366–70.

135. Stirewalt DL, Guthrie KA, Beppu L, Bryant EM, Doney K, Gooley T, et al. Predictors of relapse and overall survival in Philadelphia chromosome-positive acute lymphoblastic leukemia after transplantation. Biol Blood Marrow Transplant. 2003;9(3):206–12.

136. Bottcher S, Ritgen M, Pott C, Bruggemann M, Raff T, Stilgenbauer S, et al. Comparative analysis of minimal residual disease detection using four-color flow cytometry, consensus IgH-PCR, and quantitative IgH PCR in CLL after allogeneic and autologous stem cell transplantation. Leukemia. 2004;18(10):1637–45.

137. Rawstron AC, Kennedy B, Evans PA, Davies FE, Richards SJ, Haynes AP, et al. Quantitation of minimal disease levels in chronic lymphocytic leukemia using a sensitive flow cytometric assay improves the prediction of outcome and can be used to optimize therapy. Blood. 2001;98(1):29–35.

138. Moreton P, Kennedy B, Lucas G, Leach M, Rassam SM, Haynes A, et al. Eradication of minimal residual disease in B-cell chronic lymphocytic leukemia after alemtuzumab therapy is associated with prolonged survival. J Clin Oncol. 2005;23(13):2971–9.

139. Bottcher S, Ritgen M, Dreger P. Allogeneic stem cell transplantation for chronic lymphocytic leukemia: lessons to be learned from minimal residual disease studies. Blood Rev. 2011; 25(2):91–6.

140. Esteve J, Villamor N, Colomer D, Montserrat E. Different clinical value of minimal residual disease after autologous and allogenic stem cell transplantation for chronic lymphocytic leukemia. Blood. 2002;99(5):1873–4.

141. McSweeney PA, Niederwieser D, Shizuru JA, Sandmaier BM, Molina AJ, Maloney DG, et al. Hematopoietic cell transplantation in older patients with hematologic malignancies: replacing high-dose cytotoxic therapy with graft-versus-tumor effects. Blood. 2001;97(11): 3390–400.

142. Goldman JM, Majhail NS, Klein JP, Wang Z, Sobocinski KA, Arora M, et al. Relapse and late mortality in 5-year survivors of myeloablative allogeneic hematopoietic cell transplantation for chronic myeloid leukemia in first chronic phase. J Clin Oncol. 2010;28(11): 1888–95.

Chapter 10
Late Effects After Treatment for Leukemia

K. Scott Baker and Emily Jo Rajotte

Abstract As of January 2007, it is estimated that there were nearly 12 million people with a previous diagnosis of cancer living in the United States. Due to the fact that leukemia comprises only a small portion of all cancers, individuals successfully treated for leukemia account for approximately 2% of these survivors. Due to advances in leukemia treatment, over 50% of individuals diagnosed with leukemia today will be alive 5 years after diagnosis. Issues related to long-term effects of treatment are important to understand. Patients with acute leukemia are treated aggressively with chemotherapy and frequently hematopoietic cell transplantation (HCT) and are at higher risk for long-term consequences.

Keywords Leukemia • Treatment • Hematopoietic cell transplantation • Survival • Long-term effect • Acute leukemia • Chemotherapy • Disease-free survival • 5-year survival

Introduction

With advances in early detection and the development of more effective cancer therapies, the number of cancer survivors continues to increase. As of January 1, 2007, it is estimated that there were nearly 12 million people with a previous

K.S. Baker, M.D., M.S. (✉)
Department of Pediatrics, University of Washington School of Medicine, Seattle, WA, USA

Clinical Research Division, Fred Hutchinson Cancer Research Center,
1100 Fairview Ave N, Seattle, WA 98109, USA
e-mail: ksbaker@fhcrc.org

E.J. Rajotte, M.S., M.P.H.
Survivorship Program Manager, Clinical Research Division, Fred Hutchinson
Cancer Research Center, 1100 Fairview Ave N, LF-268, Seattle, WA 98109, USA
e-mail: erajotte@fhcrc.org

E.H. Estey and F.R. Appelbaum (eds.), *Leukemia and Related Disorders:*
Integrated Treatment Approaches, Contemporary Hematology,
DOI 10.1007/978-1-60761-565-1_10, © Springer Science+Business Media, LLC 2012

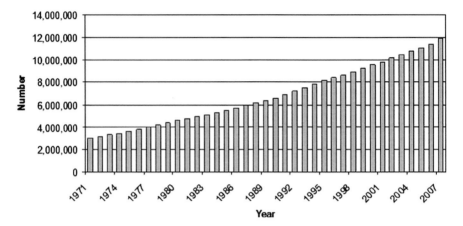

Fig. 10.1 Estimated number of cancer survivors in the United States from 1971 to 2007 [1]

diagnosis of cancer living in the United States (Fig. 10.1) [1]. Due to the fact that leukemia comprises only a small portion of all cancers, individuals successfully treated for leukemia account for approximately 2% of these survivors. However, due to advances in leukemia treatment that have been described elsewhere in this book, over 50% of individuals diagnosed with leukemia today will be alive 5 years after diagnosis, thus issues related to long-term effects of treatment in these patients are important to understand. Additionally, patients with acute leukemia are treated quite aggressively with chemotherapy and frequently hematopoietic cell transplantation (HCT) and thus are at higher risk for many long-term consequences.

The National Cancer Institute considers a person a cancer survivor from the time of diagnosis through the balance of his or her life. For many patients with chronic forms of leukemia, the survivorship continuum can include ongoing treatment throughout the remainder of their lifetime. In the case of chronic myeloid leukemia treated with tyrosine kinase inhibitors, the period of follow-up is still relatively short, and potential long-term effects of these medications are yet unknown. For patients treated as children or young adults, the long-term outcomes after follow-up of 30, 40, and 50 years are also not clearly defined, thus ongoing follow-up and surveillance of these individuals is very important.

Etiology of Long-Term and Late Effects

Long-term effects are generally considered to be conditions that develop during the active phase of a patient's treatment and then persist indefinitely, whereas late effects are conditions that develop after the completion of treatment but yet as a direct consequence of a specific treatment or combination of treatments. Patient-specific

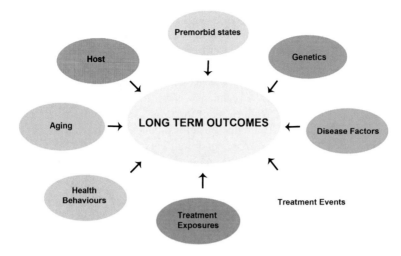

Fig. 10.2 Factors influencing late effects

factors, as well as treatment-specific factors and events, will have an impact on the risk for developing certain long-term outcomes, and each will be further discussed (Fig. 10.2).

Patient Factors

There are many patient-specific factors that impact the long-term outcome of leukemia survivors, although few have been very well studied. Age at diagnosis represents one of the most significant of these factors, and leukemia is one of the few malignancies that has little age predilection, with individuals being diagnosed from anytime from birth through geriatric adulthood. Obviously, both long-term and late effects of therapy can vary significantly in young children as compared to adults, or in middle aged adults compared to elderly adults. One of the best examples of this is the impact of cranial radiation for treatment or prophylaxis of central nervous system (CNS) leukemia on the developing brain of children compared to when this same therapy is delivered to a mature brain of an adult. After CNS radiation, children are at high risk for developing problems related to growth, development, endocrinopathies, and neurocognitive impairments [2]. Adults may experience some difficulties related to CNS radiation also (memory loss, fatigue), but the consequences may not be as severe or necessarily permanent. Other patient-related factors include other premorbid conditions (primarily in adult patients) such as obesity, hypertension, diabetes, preexisiting cardiovascular disease, or other organ system impairments that predispose these patients to complications related to chemotherapy on a short-term as well as long-term basis. These conditions may impact the ability to deliver effective treatment and may also lead to treatment-related morbidity that may persist after treatment is completed. Another factor that may in some cases also be related to premorbid conditions is that of underlying genetic phenotypes that can alter the risk for complications of therapy in one patient compared to another. Genetic polymorphisms have been shown to alter the metabolism of certain chemotherapy agents used in leukemia treatment which can lead to increased toxicity or alternatively to decreased effectiveness of the drug [3]. Polymorphisms may also impact the risk for cardiovascular complications, bone heath impairments, vitamin D metabolism, and likely many other conditions yet to be described. Lastly, certain health behaviors such as diet, lifestyle, exercise, nutrition, and others can also play a role in the protection from, or the risk for, the development of long-term and late effects in survivors and must be considered in a patient's overall long-term outcome risk profile.

Disease and Treatment Factors

Given that this chapter discusses the very broad range of acute and chronic leukemias, there are certainly disease characteristics of specific diagnoses that impact the presenting features of a particular patient, and that dictate the type and intensity of therapy which is delivered and the potential need for HCT. Treatment exposures themselves can be quantified, and potential risks determined, based upon known risks for late effects for the majority of agents that are commonly utilized. The risk of adverse effects from many treatment exposures are also cumulative in nature and/ or at times based on combined exposure to certain drugs or with radiation therapy. These will be discussed further below, although it is important to point out that there is very little published data on medical late effects in long-term survivors after successful treatment for leukemia with the exception of that which is published from pediatric cohorts and from studies in survivors after HCT. Additionally, long-term follow-up data on many newer agents is also currently lacking.

Common Issues on Long-Term Follow-up of Leukemia Survivors

Cardiovascular

In general, cardiovascular complications in leukemia survivors can be grouped into four main categories: (1) problems related to cardiomyopathy with or without congestive heart failure, (2) metabolic consequences that lead to increased CV risk (metabolic syndrome) including endothelial dysfunction or vascular effects that may lead to premature atherosclerotic changes, (3) valvular disease, and (4) pericardial disease and arrhythmias.

Table 10.1   Risk factors for anthracycline cardiac toxicity

Patient characteristics
Age: <18 or >65 at the time of treatment
Pregnancy
Comorbid conditions: hypertension, preexisting cardiac disease
Gender
Treatment characteristics
Cumulative dose of anthracyclines $\geq$300 mg/m^2, highest risk $\geq$450 mg/m^2
Combined with radiation therapy (mediastinal, total body)
Longer duration of follow-up

Anthracycline-induced cardiomyopathy is one of the most well-described chemotherapy-induced late effects with a vast array of literature describing its potential cardiac toxicity [4]. Anthracycline cardiotoxicity is dose dependent and results in a progressive decline in left ventricular systolic function [5, 6]. Other mediators of the risk of cardiomyopathy from anthracycline exposure exist and are shown in Table 10.1 [4–9]. Most standard leukemia protocols prescribe total cumulative doses of anthracyclines that fall below the threshold for significant cardiomyopathy risk; however, there is no dose below which the risk does not exist. There is not a great deal of data in the adult literature, and most of it from studies of breast cancer patients exposed to doxorubicin [4].

One of the few studies in lymphoma suggested that of patients who were exposed to a median dose of doxorubicin of 300 mg/m^2, 27% developed an asymptomatic fractional shortening of <25%. Beginning 5 years after treatment, the risk of cardiotoxicity among patients treated with doxorubicin has been shown to be increased compared to untreated individuals [5]. Patients who relapse and/or who subsequently undergo HCT generally have higher risks of cardiomyopathy as these patients are more likely to have higher cumulative anthracycline exposure and to subsequently receive high-dose cyclophosphamide and total body irradiation (TBI) which can also be associated with cardiac toxicity [10, 11]. Monitoring for the development of cardiomyopathy in asymptomatic individuals is controversial. Radionucleotide angiography, MUGA, or echocardiography can all be used for monitoring or detection of the development of left ventricular dysfunction, but there is no good evidence that early detection and treatment of asymptomatic individuals will alter the course towards progression to symptomatic disease.

Metabolic syndrome is a constellation of central obesity, insulin resistance, glucose intolerance, dyslipidemia, and hypertension and is associated with a substantially increased risk for type 2 diabetes mellitus and atherosclerotic cardiovascular disease (CVD) [12–14].

There is preliminary evidence to suggest that childhood cancer survivors are at an increased risk for premature development of metabolic syndrome [15–17]. In adult survivors of childhood acute lymphoblastic leukemia (ALL), various factors, including female sex [18], genetic predisposition [19], exposure to steroids [20], and cranial radiation therapy [18, 21], have been implicated in the development of obesity and other conditions characteristic of metabolic syndrome. The Childhood Cancer Survivor Study (CCSS) reports that childhood cancer survivors who have received >20 Gy of cranial radiation are 2.6-fold (females) and 1.9-fold (males) more likely to be obese, when compared with age- and race-matched siblings. The risk for obesity is greatest among females exposed to radiation exceeding 20 Gy at 0–4 years of age [18]. While the total dose of TBI exposure in HCT protocols is typically in the range of 10–14 Gy, the dose rate is higher, which may have a greater impact at the cellular level than a higher dose given over a longer time period [22].

In addition to significantly higher weight and body fat, childhood cancer survivors have been shown to have higher fasting plasma glucose and insulin levels and lower serum high-density lipoprotein (HDL) cholesterol [17]. A combination of obesity, hyperinsulinemia, and low HDL cholesterol was seen in 16% of the survivors but in none of the controls ($p=0.01$). Of the survivors with indicators of metabolic syndrome, 50% had received cranial radiation and also had markedly reduced spontaneous growth hormone (GH) secretion. Similar results were found in survivors of allogeneic HCT performed in childhood. Hyperinsulinemia, impaired glucose tolerance (by oral glucose tolerance test), hypertriglyceridemia, low HDL cholesterol, and abdominal obesity were more common among the HCT patients than among either the non-HCT group of leukemia patients or healthy controls [23]. Core signs of metabolic syndrome were found in 39% of HCT survivors vs. 8% of leukemia controls and 0% of healthy controls. Fifty-two percent of HCT patients were found to have hyperinsulinemia, and 43% had abnormal glucose metabolism, compared to none of the healthy controls ($p=0.0002$ and 0.001, respectively). Variables associated with hyperinsulinemia in the HCT patients were time from transplantation ($p=0.01$), presence of chronic graft vs. host disease (GVHD) ($p=0.01$), and hypogonadism ($p=0.04$). Another study found that the patients who received TBI had a significantly higher first-phase insulin response and insulinemia/glycemia ratio on glucose tolerance testing as compared to patients who received only lymphoid radiation, no radiation, or controls [24], suggesting that TBI may play a role in the development of insulin resistance.

In a large study of survivors after HCT, it was found that after adjustment for age, gender, and BMI, allogeneic HCT survivors were 3.7 times (95% CI: 1.8–7.3) more likely to report diabetes and 2.1 times (95% CI: 1.4–3.0) more likely to report hypertension compared to siblings. Allogeneic HCT survivors were also 2.3 times more likely to report hypertension (95% CI: 1.5–3.7) when compared with autologous recipients. Finally, TBI was associated with an increased risk of diabetes (OR=3.4, 95% CI: 1.6–7.5).

In an ongoing study, we have measured insulin resistance, fasting glucose, insulin, lipids, anthropometry, blood pressure, and carotid artery compliance and distensibility in 106 survivors of HCT performed in childhood for hematologic malignancies (current age 26.6 years) and 72 healthy sibling controls (current age 23.7 years). Preliminary analysis found two or more components of metabolic syndrome were present in 37% survivors and only 13.9% controls (OR, 2.7, 95% CI: 1.2–5.9, $p=0.02$). HCT survivors who had TBI with or without cranial radiation had significantly higher total cholesterol, LDL cholesterol, triglycerides, and insulin and lower

HDL cholesterol levels, and they were also more insulin resistant. However, for the subjects who did not receive any radiation prior to or during HCT, there were no differences in any of the cardiovascular risk factors compared to controls. Carotid artery distensibility was decreased in survivors who received TBI compared to controls with even greater negative impact in those who received TBI and pre-HCT cranial radiation. These findings are concerning and suggest that even at a relatively young age, and independent of obesity, HCT survivors of childhood hematologic malignancies have increased cardiovascular risk factors present as well as adverse vascular changes, which are associated with exposure to TBI, with or without cranial radiation. These abnormalities may ultimately contribute to a higher risk of early cardiovascular morbidity and mortality, and thus early screening and management of modifiable cardiovascular risk factors should be considered in these young HCT survivors.

Screening and Treatment Recommendations

Presence of metabolic syndrome places survivors at an elevated risk for a number of adverse health outcomes, such as overt diabetes and cardiovascular disease, which when combined with prior exposure to cardiotoxic agents such as chest radiation and anthracyclines and cyclophosphamide [25, 26], could have a potentially devastating consequence on the survivors. [27] Monitoring of CV risk parameters (lipid profile, fasting blood sugar, blood pressure, weight) are all important as these are all potentially modifiable risk factors. Also important is counseling regarding diet and lifestyle factors (smoking, exercise) as these too play a role in modifying CV risk.

Endocrine

In children, endocrine-related late effects are primarily seen in patients who receive cranial radiation for treatment or prophylaxis of CNS leukemia, and typically there are not significant consequences from standard protocols utilized for leukemia treatment. In a large cohort of children with ALL in the Childhood Cancer Survivor Study ($n=4{,}151$), ALL survivors were three times more likely to report a chronic endocrine condition compared to a sibling control group [28]. However, this only represented 4.4% of the ALL survivors, and for those who had not relapsed and who did not ever receive any radiation as part of their therapy, they were no more likely to report endocrine conditions than were their siblings. ALL survivors who received radiation were four times more likely to report chronic endocrine conditions than nonirradiated survivors. Whole brain irradiation in doses $\geq$18 Gy in children can lead to short stature from hypothalamic-pituitary axis damage with resultant growth hormone deficiency [29–31]. Adults may also develop GH deficiency after CNS-directed radiation, but there have been no studies to document this. Adult survivors of childhood leukemia that have received cranial radiation have been found to have GH deficiency with a higher risk of metabolic syndrome features [32].

Survivors after HCT who have received more intensive therapy (myeloablative conditioning regimens), particularly protocols that include total body irradiation, are at risk for long-term endocrine impairments. Data from the Bone Marrow Transplant Survivor Study (BMT-SS) has shown that survivors more than 2 years after myeloablative HCT (autologous and allogeneic combined) for chronic myeloid leukemia ($n=248$, median follow-up 7 years, range 2–27) were over three times more likely to report an endocrine impairment compared to a sibling control group [33]. This included a higher risk of hypothyroidism (odds ratio [OR] 2.7, 95% confidence interval [CI] 1.6–4.5, $p<0.001$) and diabetes (OR 4.9, 95% CI: 2.3–10.5). After allogeneic HCT, the risk of hypothyroidism was higher in recipients who developed chronic GVHD (cGVHD), but the higher risk of diabetes was present whether cGVHD had developed or not. The cumulative incidence of hypothyroidism at 10 years after HCT was 13% for survivors of autologous HCT, 8% after related donor HCT, and 19% after unrelated donor HCT.

In an analysis of survivors after HCT for AML and ALL from the BMT-SS, endocrine impairments were reported by nearly 30% of survivors compared to 11% in sibling controls ($p<0.001$) [34]. Hypothyroidism and diabetes were both significantly more likely to develop in survivors. In an analysis that examined risk factors for developing adverse outcomes including diagnosis, transplant type, exposure to TBI, cGVHD, and sex, no factors were identified that increased the risk of hypothyroidism. For diabetes, the only risk factor that was identified was allogeneic HCT compared to autologous (OR 3.9, 95% CI: 1.09–14.01, $p=0.04$).

Screening and Treatment Recommendations

While there are no good data to guide the long-term surveillance for adverse endocrine outcomes of adult survivors of leukemia who have not received a transplant, data from the transplant literature would certainly support the ongoing surveillance for hypothyroidism and also for the presence of hyperglycemia/diabetes in survivors after HCT. Children should also be considered for growth hormone testing if growth parameters begin to demonstrate abnormalities.

Bone

Bone health is becoming an increasing concern in leukemia survivors. The risks of osteopenia and avascular necrosis have been well described in relation to exposure to steroids but less so in relation to other cancer treatments. The duration of osteopenia has not been well documented. There is an increasing amount of data, however, indicating that recovery of osteopenia or osteoporosis may not always occur, and that reduction in bone mineral density can be detected many years after therapy has been completed [35]. There have been many studies in the pediatric literature that have addressed the issue of bone health in childhood cancer survivors, but few that have looked at this issue in adults. In chronic myeloid leukemia (CML) survivors, data from the BMT-SS found that the risk of osteoporosis was over seven times higher compared to siblings, and the risk for avascular necrosis was 12 times higher [33]. Both outcomes were significantly more frequent in survivors who had cGVHD, presumably from greater exposure to steroids although actual exposure was not quantified. As noted above, data from the BMT-SS has also examined bone health and found that AML and ALL survivors after HCT were also more likely than siblings to report osteoporosis and avascular necrosis. Risk factors for osteoporosis included allogeneic donor and female sex. For avascular necrosis, a higher risk was also seen in recipients of allogeneic HCT and a trend towards a higher risk in patients who had ALL (presumably from higher pretransplant cumulative steroid exposure).

Screening and Treatment Recommendations

For any patient who has had a significant steroid exposure or total body irradiation, consideration of bone density screening should be given. Additional risk factors to consider include: older age at time of treatment, concurrent growth hormone deficiency, hypogonadism, hyperthyroidism, vitamin D deficiency, smoking, and alcohol. In the HCT population, current recommendations are for bone density screening in all patients at 1 year post-HCT with reassessment if abnormal at that time [36]. Treatment of osteopenia or osteoporosis in leukemia survivors can be approached in a similar fashion to what is done in the general population with interventions such as calcium and vitamin D supplementation, weight-bearing exercise, smoking cessation, and limits of alcohol intake. In more severe cases, or for those who do not respond to conservative measures, treatment with bisphosphonates has been utilized successfully, although this approach would require ruling out any other underlying endocrinologic abnormality, as noted above, that is present.

Functional Outcomes

An increasingly important issue in survivors is the impact that the cancer diagnosis and treatment has on their overall functional status, including such issues as ability to carry out activities of daily living, ability to do household chores, ability to work or attend school, etc. Impairment of their functional status can have a tremendous impact on a survivor's quality of life also and ultimately may impact the development of other health-related complications. Most of the data that has been published on functional outcomes is from studies of adult survivors of childhood cancer or from studies in survivors after HCT (most with hematologic malignancies) with a few focusing on the breast cancer survivor population. In survivors after HCT for CML, patients were compared to a sibling control group and were found to be more likely to report the need for assistance with routine activities such as housework or shopping and to report that their current health prevented them from attending school or work. Siblings were also more likely than survivors to report their health as excellent, very good, or good (94% vs. 78%, $p < 0.001$) [33]. In this same study, when comparing recipients of unrelated donor (URD) transplants to either related donor (RD) or autologous transplants, survivors after URD HCT were more likely to report limitations in their ability to perform routine activities, and that their current health was preventing them from attending school or work. In this cohort who had received allogeneic HCT, those with cGVHD were 2.4 times more likely to report poor overall health. In a similar study that was restricted to survivors 2 or more years after HCT for AML or ALL, leukemia survivors were significantly more likely than siblings to report that they required assistance with routine activities or with activities of daily living. They also were more likely to not attend school or work secondary to their health, and nearly 17% reported their health to be fair or poor compared to 5% of siblings ($p < 0.001$) [34]. Similar to the study in CML patients, the only significant predictor of these outcomes was the presence of cGVHD in patients who had received allogeneic HCT.

In a longitudinal study of recovery and long-term function after HCT for leukemia or lymphoma, investigators prospectively followed 319 adults from pretransplant until 5 years post-HCT with serial assessments of physical limitations, return to work, depression, and distress related to treatment or disease [37]. They found that physical recovery occurred earlier than psychological or work recovery. Eighty-four percent of survivors without recurrent malignancy who had a history of work or school outside the home had returned to work or school full time by 5 years. Patients who had cGVHD, females, and those with less social support prior to HCT were all more depressed after HCT. Full recovery after HCT was found to be a 3- to 5-year process. The incidence of cGVHD in participants was 54%, of whom 46% reported active cGVHD. In multivariable analyses, subjects with active cGVHD were more likely to report adverse general health, mental health, functional impairments, activity limitation, and pain than were those with no history of cGVHD. However, health status did not differ between those with resolved cGVHD and those who never had cGVHD. Therefore, it is reasonable to conclude that active cGVHD has a significant impact on many aspects of the overall health status of HCT survivors, and that, most importantly, those successfully treated for cGVHD do not appear to have long-term impairments.

Screening and Treatment Recommendations

Increased awareness of the issues related to impairments in functional capabilities, delayed recovery, and limitations in returning to school and work will be the first step towards developing effective surveillance and treatments for these issues. Routine evaluation from a physical and occupational therapy standpoint with ongoing intervention is very useful at improving recovery of physical function after HCT and would be of benefit to patients undergoing intensive therapy without HCT. Currently, this avenue is frequently offered to only the most significantly impaired patients. Additionally, screening for psychological distress during therapy and in long-term follow-up is very important and should include referral for appropriate mental health services as this psychological distress may adversely impact the functional status of patients also. Simple self-report screening tools that can be filled out prior to off-therapy follow-up visits are an easy way to help determine what concerns patients are experiencing related to these issues.

Psychosocial

From a long-term follow-up, standpoint psychosocial issues are common in cancer survivors, but again there are no data available specific to individuals who have been treated for leukemia. Psychological distress, including depression and anxiety, can be experienced during therapy as well as after therapy in long-term follow-up, and this can be influenced by many factors, including a patient's psychological adjustment prior to the cancer diagnosis. The prevalence of depression in cancer survivors has been estimated to range between 10% and 50% [38, 39]. Other psychological issues such as posttraumatic distress syndrome can affect survivors after the completion of their cancer treatment [40, 41]. Fear of recurrence can lead to ongoing anxiety in survivors and impact their psychological health even years after diagnosis [42]. Other stressors to the overall well-being of survivors include financial difficulties, inability to work or attend school, sexual dysfunction, and the psychological impact of physical long-term or late effects. Due to the intensity of the therapy, survivors after HCT may be at higher risk for impaired psychological dysfunction. The recovery period is longer [37] and may be complicated by chronic GVHD with a resultant higher level of psychological and physical distress.

Screening and Treatment Recommendations

The long-term follow-up of survivors should include screening for psychological health including depression, anxiety, sexual health, status of relationships, and for financial or insurance concerns or problems with insurance. At a minimum, this can be accomplished with questionnaire-based tools. At the time of follow-up visits, some survivorship programs provide social work services to provide a brief psychosocial screening of survivors during clinic visits. These issues should be reviewed by providers, and appropriate referrals made for psychological or psychiatric evaluations, as well as for sexual dysfunction, or financial counseling.

Second Malignant Neoplasms (SMN)

Despite successful cure of their primary malignancy, cancer survivors face a lifelong higher risk of developing new malignancies. The etiology of these second cancers is not entirely known but has been linked to treatment exposures including certain chemotherapy agents and ionizing radiation, as well as from the effects of prolonged immunosuppression. It is also likely that in some patients, there may exist an underlying genetic susceptibility to the effects of these treatments or to the development of cancer itself. This certainly is the case in patients with underlying syndromes that predispose to DNA breakage such as Fanconi anemia where the effects of exposure to radiation lead to a significantly higher risk of developing new solid tumors in those patients undergoing HCT [43]. There have been no studies that have examined the risk of SMN in adult patients with leukemia undergoing standard chemotherapy. Data from adult survivors of childhood leukemia have shown that the cumulative incidence of SMN at 25 years was 5.2% overall and 6.2% in irradiated patients vs. 3.1% in patients who did not receive radiation [28]. Eighty-one percent of the SMN that were reported occurred in irradiated patients and 53% of those in the central nervous system highlighting this unique risk in childhood ALL patients. Risk factors that have been identified related to the exposure to specific chemotherapy agents include a risk of secondary AML in patients who have been exposed to topoisomerase I inhibitors [44, 45], alkylating agents, and radiation [46–48].

There are more studies that have examined the risk of SMN in patients after HCT; in most of these studies, patients with hematologic malignancies comprise the majority of patients who had received a transplant. Data from single institutional analyses have shown that the cumulative incidence for the development of any post-transplant malignancy was 6.9% at 20 years post-HCT, and the cumulative incidence for invasive solid cancers was 3.8% [49]. There were 34 patients who had developed a new distinct hematologic malignancy as their SMN, and 30 of those developed in patients who had received an autologous transplant for lymphoma ($n=26$), other solid tumors ($n=4$), and four developed new morphologic and cytogenetically distinct cases of AML or MDS after their original allogeneic HCT for AML or CML. The donor/host origins of the leukemia in these patients were not reported, but cases of donor-derived leukemia after HCT have also been reported [50]. In a large study published recently from the Center for International Blood and Marrow Transplant examining the development of new solid tumors in over 28,000 recipients of allogeneic HCT, it was found that survivors after HCT developed new solid cancers at twice the rate that was expected based on general population rates [51]. This risk increased to threefold for patients who were followed for over 15 years. The risk of non-squamous cell carcinoma was higher in patients who had received radiation at ages less than 30, and cGVHD and male sex were the main risk factors for squamous cell carcinomas.

Screening and Treatment Recommendations

No published guidelines for screening of cancer survivors for SMN exist. Patients should be informed of the potential risk for developing an SMN based upon their treatment exposures. This information should also be conveyed to their primary care physician. They should be strongly encouraged to comply with age-appropriate screening and early detection strategies (breast and testicular self-exams, mammography, Pap smears, colonoscopy) and avoidance of any additional exposures that impact the risk of cancer (sunburn, smoking). For individuals exposed to cranial radiation as children, periodic MRI screening for the development of secondary brain tumors may be indicated if the exposure dose has been significant or if any neurologic symptoms or concerns develop.

Late Mortality

There are now two major studies that have examined the issue of late mortality in patients who were treated with HCT. The first of these examined 1,479 individuals who had survived 2 or more years after allogeneic HCT [52]. These survivors were at a median age of 25.9 years at the time of HCT and had a median length of follow-up of 9.5 years. The probability of survival at 15 years from HCT was 80.2%, and the relative mortality was 9.9 (95% confidence interval, 8.7–11.2). Mortality did decrease with time from HCT but still remained significantly elevated at 15 years after HCT. Relapse of primary disease (29%) and cGVHD (22%) were the leading causes of premature death, but risk of death from second malignancies and cardiac or pulmonary causes were also elevated. Nonrelapse-related mortality was increased among patients older than 18 years at HCT and among those with cGVHD. The second study examined 2,574 patients who had survived for at least 5 years after HCT without recurrence of their primary disease and found that survival at 20 years after HCT was 80.4% [53]. Mortality rates were four- to nine fold higher for at least 30 years, and this yielded a 30% reduction in life expectancy. The most common causes of late deaths were SMN and recurrent disease, but deaths due to infection, cGVHD, respiratory diseases, and cardiovascular disease were also more common than in the general population. Survivors need to be counseled regarding these issues, but it is likely that some of these deaths could potentially be prevented with closer long-term follow-up and monitoring of HCT survivors that continues throughout their lifetime.

Clinical Follow-up of Survivors

Treatment Summaries and Survivorship Care Plans

With survivorship now recognized as a distinct phase of care in the cancer continuum, the focus turns to surveillance for and management of long-term and late effects that occur as a result of cancer and its treatment, as well as routine health promotion and prevention of disease.

In 2004, the President's Cancer Panel issued *Living Beyond Cancer: Finding a New Balance*, providing a review of the effects of cancer treatment over a life span and among separate age groups [54]. The advisory group's report was based on a yearlong series of meetings with nearly 200 cancer survivors, their caregivers, health-care providers, and insurers. The report recommended that cancer patients completing treatment be provided with a comprehensive care plan that would detail the nature of the cancer diagnosed, what therapies were given, complications that might result, and recommended follow-up care.

A few years later, the Institute of Medicine (IOM) published an influential report, *From Cancer Patient to Cancer Survivor: Lost in Transition*, which examined a broad range of medical and psychosocial issues faced by cancer survivors as a consequence of their diagnosis and its treatment and has probably been the publication most responsible for drawing attention to the survivorship phase of care [55]. The report's 17-member committee, along with more than 30 cancer professionals from all parts of the cancer community, recommended that patients completing primary treatment should be provided with a comprehensive care summary and follow-up care plan that is clearly and effectively explained. This "Survivorship Care Plan" would summarize critical information needed for the survivor's long-term care and would include:

- Cancer type, treatments received, and their potential consequences
- Specific information about the timing and content of recommended follow-up
- Recommendations regarding preventive practices and how to maintain health and well-being
- Information on legal protections regarding employment and access to health insurance
- The availability of psychosocial services in the community

These content areas, adapted from those recommended by the President's Cancer Panel report are elaborated upon in Table 10.2.

A number of organizations have worked on versions of such a plan, including the American Society of Clinical Oncology (ASCO), the Lance Armstrong Foundation, and Journey Forward, many of whom make these tools available online. The ASCO Cancer Treatment Plan and Summary (http://www.asco.org/treatmentsummary) template is intended to be completed by the treating oncologist as a brief record of cancer treatment and includes recommendations for follow-up tests that are based on the best available scientific evidence from ASCO's clinical practice guidelines. The LIVESTRONG Care Plan (http://www.livestrongcareplan.org/), provided through the Lance Armstrong Foundation and maintained by Penn Medicine's OncoLink, focuses on the medical consequences a survivor may face based on the National Comprehensive Cancer Network Guidelines and the Children's Oncology Group Long-Term Follow-up Guidelines. Journey Forward (http://www.journeyforward. org/) provides another version of an online tool designed by oncologists to help medical professionals create custom survivorship care plans, adapted in part from ASCO Chemotherapy Treatment Summary templates and Surveillance Guidelines. All of these treatment plans and summary templates were developed to help improve documentation and coordination of cancer treatment and survivorship care and are intended to facilitate provider-to-provider and provider-to-patient communication.

Table 10.2 Survivorship care plan

Upon discharge from cancer treatment, including treatment of recurrences, every patient should be given a record of all care received and important disease characteristics. This should include, at a minimum:

1. Diagnostic tests performed and results
2. Tumor characteristics (e.g., site[s], stage and grade, hormone receptor status, marker information)
3. Dates of treatment initiation and completion
4. Surgery, chemotherapy, radiotherapy, transplant, hormonal therapy, or gene or other therapies provided, including agents used, treatment regimen, total dosage, identifying number and title of clinical trials (if any), indicators of treatment response, and toxicities experienced during treatment
5. Psychosocial, nutritional, and other supportive services provided
6. Full contact information on treating institutions and key individual providers
7. Identification of a key point of contact and coordinator of continuing care

Upon discharge from cancer treatment, every patient and his/her primary health-care provider should receive a written follow-up care plan incorporating available evidence-based standards of care. This should include, at a minimum:

1. The likely course of recovery from treatment toxicities, as well as the need for ongoing health maintenance/adjuvant therapy
2. A description of recommended cancer screening and other periodic testing and examinations, and the schedule on which they should be performed (and who should provide them)
3. Information on possible late and long-term effects of treatment and symptoms of such effects
4. Information on possible signs of recurrence and second tumors
5. Information on the possible effects of cancer on marital/partner relationship, sexual functioning, work, and parenting and the potential future need for psychosocial support
6. Information on the potential insurance, employment, and financial consequences of cancer and, as necessary, referral to counseling, legal aid, and financial assistance
7. Specific recommendations for healthy behaviors (e.g., diet, exercise, healthy weight, sunscreen use, immunizations, smoking cessation, osteoporosis prevention). When appropriate, recommendations that first-degree relatives be informed about their increased risk and the need for cancer screening (e.g., breast cancer, colorectal cancer, prostate cancer)
8. As appropriate, information on genetic counseling and testing to identify high-risk individuals who could benefit from more comprehensive cancer surveillance, chemoprevention, or risk-reducing surgery
9. As appropriate, information on known effective chemoprevention strategies for secondary prevention (e.g., tamoxifen in women at high risk for breast cancer; aspirin for colorectal cancer prevention)
10. Referrals to specific follow-up care providers (e.g., rehabilitation, fertility, psychology), support groups, and/or the patient's primary care provider
11. A listing of cancer-related resources and information (e.g., Internet-based sources and telephone listings for major cancer support organizations)

Source: Adapted from the President's Cancer Panel [54]

Long-Term Follow-up Guidelines

The "Survivorship Care Plan" is designed to inform clinicians involved in the subsequent care of cancer survivors about treatment exposures, signs and symptoms of late effects, and recommended care for the future. To carry out this plan, an organized set of clinical practice guidelines based on the best available evidence is needed to help ensure appropriate follow-up care. Unfortunately, the status of cancer-related guidelines for follow-up of adult cancer survivors fails these ideals. The research necessary to understand and frame these concerns and to structure a plan of care for adult cancer survivors has not been adequate, and follow-up recommendations have been based primarily on consensus in the absence of evidence. Despite this lack of empirical guidelines, the IOM report maintained that survivorship care plans "have strong face validity and can reasonably be assumed to improve care unless and until evidence accumulates to the contrary" [55].

Pediatric oncology has taken the lead in developing treatment summaries and guidelines for follow-up care plans for patients and their families and in communicating this information to other health-care providers. The Children's Oncology Group *Long-Term Follow-Up Guidelines for Survivors of Childhood, Adolescent, and Young Adult Cancers* were developed and maintained and updated by the Children's Oncology Group's Long-Term Follow-Up Guidelines Core Committee and its associated Task Forces [56]. Although generally consensus-based rather than data-driven, these recommendations provide consistency for follow-up care of childhood cancers, a feature lacking in long-term follow-up care provided to adult cancer survivors.

The National Marrow Donor Program (http://www.marrow.org/), a nonprofit organization dedicated to providing resources for all patients receiving bone marrow or umbilical cord blood transplant, provides a brief guide to the stages of recovery after transplant. These guidelines may be of particular assistance among hematopoietic cell transplantation (HCT) recipients for leukemia.

Conclusions

Leukemia survivors are at risk for multiple different adverse outcomes that can have an impact on their physical, mental, and functional well-being and quality of life. However, for the majority of these potential late complications, most are amenable to either prevention or treatment. Follow-up care is too often focused on possible recurrence rather than on a survivor's overall health status, and the need for standardized guidelines for long-term follow-up of adult survivors that goes beyond surveillance for recurrence is greatly needed. Survivors in particular, need to maintain close adherence to preventive screening practices for other chronic diseases as well as for the development of second malignancies. When available, dedicated survivorship programs provide an excellent means of evaluating a survivor's overall health care needs and for establishing a specific care plan for them moving forward that can be utilized by the survivor and their health-care providers. There is still a great deal of research that needs to be done for cancer survivors, particularly focused on underlying mechanisms that determine who is at risk for certain complications and why, and how identical treatments can have a vastly differing impact on one individual compared to another. Additionally, as new therapies are developed, there will be a continuous learning curve regarding their long-term impact.

References

1. Howlader N, Noone AM, Krapcho M, Neyman N, Aminou R, Waldron W, Altekruse SF, Kosary CL, Ruhl J, Tatalovich Z, Cho H, Mariotto A, Eisner MP, Lewis DR, Chen HS, Feuer EJ, Cronin KA, Edwards BK, editors. SEER cancer statistics review, 1975–2008. Bethesda: National Cancer Institute. http://seer.cancer.gov/csr/1975_2008/, based on November 2010 SEER data submission, posted to the SEER web site, 2011.
2. Baker KS, Bresters D, Sande JE. The burden of cure: long-term side effects following hematopoietic stem cell transplantation (HSCT) in children. Pediatr Clin North Am. 2010;57:323–42.
3. Shimasaki N, Mori T, Torii C, et al. Influence of MTHFR and RFC1 polymorphisms on toxicities during maintenance chemotherapy for childhood acute lymphoblastic leukemia or lymphoma. J Pediatr Hematol Oncol. 2008;30:347–52.
4. Carver JR, Shapiro CL, Ng A, et al. American society of clinical oncology clinical evidence review on the ongoing care of adult cancer survivors: cardiac and pulmonary late effects. J Clin Oncol. 2007;25:3991–4008.
5. Doyle JJ, Neugut AI, Jacobson JS, Grann VR, Hershman DL. Chemotherapy and cardiotoxicity in older breast cancer patients: a population-based study. J Clin Oncol. 2005;23: 8597–605.
6. Shapiro CL, Hardenbergh PH, Gelman R, et al. Cardiac effects of adjuvant doxorubicin and radiation therapy in breast cancer patients. J Clin Oncol. 1998;16:3493–501.
7. Hequet O, Le QH, Moullet I, et al. Subclinical late cardiomyopathy after doxorubicin therapy for lymphoma in adults. J Clin Oncol. 2004;22:1864–71.
8. Lipshultz SE, Colan SD, Gelber RD, Perez-Atayde AR, Sallan SE, Sanders SP. Late cardiac effects of doxorubicin therapy for acute lymphoblastic leukemia in childhood. N Engl J Med. 1991;324:808–15.
9. Lipshultz SE, Lipsitz SR, Mone SM, et al. Female sex and drug dose as risk factors for late cardiotoxic effects of doxorubicin therapy for childhood cancer. N Engl J Med. 1995;332: 1738–43.
10. Braverman AC, Antin JH, Plappert MT, Cook EF, Lee RT. Cyclophosphamide cardiotoxicity in bone marrow transplantation: a prospective evaluation of new dosing regimens. J Clin Oncol. 1991;9:1215–23.
11. Sakata-Yanagimoto M, Kanda Y, Nakagawa M, et al. Predictors for severe cardiac complications after hematopoietic stem cell transplantation. Bone Marrow Transplant. 2004;33: 1043–7.
12. Reusch JE. Current concepts in insulin resistance, type 2 diabetes mellitus, and the metabolic syndrome. Am J Cardiol. 2002;90:19G–26.
13. Trevisan M, Liu J, Bahsas FB, Menotti A. Syndrome X and mortality: a population-based study. Risk Factor and Life Expectancy Research Group. Am J Epidemiol. 1998;148:958–66.
14. Lakka HM, Laaksonen DE, Lakka TA, et al. The metabolic syndrome and total and cardiovascular disease mortality in middle-aged men. JAMA. 2002;288:2709–16.
15. Nuver J, van den Belt-Dusebout AW, Gietema JA. Long-term survivors of acute lymphoblastic leukemia. N Engl J Med. 2003;349:1973. author reply 1973.

16. Talvensaari K, Knip M. Childhood cancer and later development of the metabolic syndrome. Ann Med. 1997;29:353–5.

17. Talvensaari KK, Lanning M, Tapanainen P, Knip M. Long-term survivors of childhood cancer have an increased risk of manifesting the metabolic syndrome. J Clin Endocrinol Metab. 1996;81:3051–5.

18. Oeffinger KC, Mertens AC, Sklar CA, et al. Obesity in adult survivors of childhood acute lymphoblastic leukemia: a report from the childhood cancer survivor study. J Clin Oncol. 2003;17:1359–65.

19. Högler W, Shaw N. Bone mineral density in young adult survivors of acute lymphoblastic leukemia. Cancer. 2009;115:4885. author reply 4885–4886.

20. Reilly JJ, Brougham M, Montgomery C, Richardson F, Kelly A, Gibson BE. Effect of glucocorticoid therapy on energy intake in children treated for acute lymphoblastic leukemia. J Clin Endocrinol Metab. 2001;86:3742–5.

21. Sklar CA, Mertens AC, Walter A, et al. Changes in body mass index and prevalence of overweight in survivors of childhood acute lymphoblastic leukemia: role of cranial irradiation. Med Pediatr Oncol. 2000;35:91–5.

22. Down JD, Boudewijn A, van Os R, Thames HD, Ploemacher RE. Variations in radiation sensitivity and repair among different hematopoietic stem cell subsets following fractionated irradiation. Blood. 1995;86:122–7.

23. Taskinen M, Saarinen-Pihkala UM, Hovi L, Lipsanen-Nyman M. Impaired glucose tolerance and dyslipidaemia as late effects after bone-marrow transplantation in childhood. Lancet. 2000;356:993–7.

24. Lorini R, Cortona L, Scaramuzza A, et al. Hyperinsulinemia in children and adolescents after bone marrow transplantation. Bone Marrow Transplant. 1995;15:873–7.

25. Sorensen K, Levitt G, Bull C, Chessells J, Sullivan I. Anthracycline dose in childhood acute lymphoblastic leukemia: issues of early survival versus late cardiotoxicity. J Clin Oncol. 1997;15:61–8.

26. Colvin M, Hilton J. Pharmacology of cyclophosphamide and metabolites. Cancer Treat Rep. 1981;65 Suppl 3:89–95.

27. Nuver J, Smit AJ, Postma A, Sleijfer DT, Gietema JA. The metabolic syndrome in long-term cancer survivors, an important target for secondary preventive measures. Cancer Treat Rev. 2002;28:195–214.

28. Mody R, Li S, Dover DC, et al. Twenty-five-year follow-up among survivors of childhood acute lymphoblastic leukemia: a report from the childhood cancer survivor study. Blood. 2008;111:5515–23.

29. Bongers ME, Francken AB, Rouwe C, Kamps WA, Postma A. Reduction of adult height in childhood acute lymphoblastic leukemia survivors after prophylactic cranial irradiation. Pediatr Blood Cancer. 2005;45:139–43.

30. Brownstein CM, Mertens AC, Mitby PA, et al. Factors that affect final height and change in height standard deviation scores in survivors of childhood cancer treated with growth hormone: a report from the childhood cancer survivor study. J Clin Endocrinol Metab. 2004;89:4422–7.

31. Huma Z, Boulad F, Black P, Heller G, Sklar C. Growth in children after bone marrow transplantation for acute leukemia. Blood. 1995;86:819–24.

32. Gurney JG, Ness KK, Sibley SD, et al. Metabolic syndrome and growth hormone deficiency in adult survivors of childhood acute lymphoblastic leukemia. Cancer. 2006;107:1303–12.

33. Baker KS, Gurney JG, Ness KK, et al. Late effects in survivors of chronic myeloid leukemia treated with hematopoietic cell transplantation: results from the bone marrow transplant survivor study. Blood. 2004;104:1898–906.

34. Baker KS, Ness K, Weisdorf D, et al. Late effects in survivors of acute leukemia treated with hematopoietic cell transplantation (HCT): a report from the bone marrow transplant survivor study (BMT-SS). Biol Blood Marrow Transplant. 2007;13:21–2.

35. Thomas IH, Donohue JE, Ness KK, Dengel DR, Baker KS, Gurney JG. Bone mineral density in young adult survivors of acute lymphoblastic leukemia. Cancer. 2008;113:3248–56.

36. Rizzo JD, Wingard JR, Tichelli A, et al. Recommended screening and preventive practices for long-term survivors after hematopoietic cell transplantation: joint recommendations of the

European Group for Blood and Marrow Transplantation, the Center for International Blood and Marrow Transplant Research, and the American Society of Blood and Marrow Transplantation. Biol Blood Marrow Transplant. 2006;12:138–51.

37. Syrjala KL, Langer SL, Abrams JR, et al. Recovery and long-term function after hematopoietic cell transplantation for leukemia or lymphoma. JAMA. 2004;291:2335–43.

38. Pirl WF. Evidence report on the occurrence, assessment, and treatment of depression in cancer patients. J Natl Cancer Inst Monogr. 2004;32:32–9.

39. Pasquini M, Biondi M. Depression in cancer patients: a critical review. Clin Pract Epidemiol Ment Health. 2007;3:2.

40. Kangas M, Henry JL, Bryant RA. Posttraumatic stress disorder following cancer. A conceptual and empirical review. Clin Psychol Rev. 2002;22:499–524.

41. Black EK, White CA. Fear of recurrence, sense of coherence and posttraumatic stress disorder in haematological cancer survivors. Psychooncology. 2005;14:510–5.

42. Lee-Jones C, Humphris G, Dixon R, Hatcher MB. Fear of cancer recurrence – a literature review and proposed cognitive formulation to explain exacerbation of recurrence fears. Psychooncology. 1997;6:95–105.

43. Deeg HJ, Socie G, Schoch G, et al. Malignancies after marrow transplantation for aplastic anemia and fanconi anemia: a joint Seattle and Paris analysis of results in 700 patients. Blood. 1996;87:386–92.

44. Andersen MK, Christiansen DH, Jensen BA, Ernst P, Hauge G, Pedersen-Bjergaard J. Therapy-related acute lymphoblastic leukaemia with MLL rearrangements following DNA topoisomerase II inhibitors, an increasing problem: report on two new cases and review of the literature since 1992. Br J Haematol. 2001;114:539–43.

45. Kantidze OL, Razin SV. Chemotherapy-related secondary leukemias: a role for DNA repair by error-prone non-homologous end joining in topoisomerase II – induced chromosomal rearrangements. Gene. 2007;391:76–9.

46. Hawkins MM, Wilson LM, Stovall MA, et al. Epipodophyllotoxins, alkylating agents, and radiation and risk of secondary leukaemia after childhood cancer. BMJ. 1992;304:951–8.

47. Kantarjian HM, Keating MJ, Walters RS, et al. Therapy-related leukemia and myelodysplastic syndrome: clinical, cytogenetic, and prognostic features. J Clin Oncol. 1986;4:1748–57.

48. Tucker MA, Meadows AT, Boice Jr JD, et al. Leukemia after therapy with alkylating agents for childhood cancer. J Natl Cancer Inst. 1987;78:459–64.

49. Baker KS, DeFor TE, Burns LJ, Ramsay NK, Neglia JP, Robison LL. New malignancies after blood or marrow stem-cell transplantation in children and adults: incidence and risk factors. J Clin Oncol. 2003;21:1352–8.

50. Fraser CJ, Hirsch BA, Dayton V, et al. First report of donor cell-derived acute leukemia as a complication of umbilical cord blood transplantation. Blood. 2005;106:4377–80.

51. Rizzo JD, Curtis RE, Socie G, et al. Solid cancers after allogeneic hematopoietic cell transplantation. Blood. 2009;113:1175–83.

52. Bhatia S, Francisco L, Carter A, et al. Late mortality after allogeneic hematopoietic cell transplantation and functional status of long-term survivors: report from the bone marrow transplant survivor study. Blood. 2007;110:3784–92.

53. Martin PJ, Counts Jr GW, Appelbaum FR, et al. Life expectancy in patients surviving more than 5 years after hematopoietic cell transplantation. J Clin Oncol. 2010;28:1011–6.

54. Reuben SH. Living beyond cancer: finding a new balance. President's Cancer panel 2003–2004 annual report, vol. 2010. Bethesda: National Cancer Institute. 2004.

55. National Cancer Policy Board Committee on Cancer Survivorship: Improving Care and Quality of Life. From cancer patient to cancer survivor: lost in transition. Washington, DC: National Academies Press; 2006.

56. Landier W, Bhatia S, Eshelman DA, et al. Development of risk-based guidelines for pediatric cancer survivors: the Children's Oncology Group Long-Term Follow-Up Guidelines from the Children's Oncology Group Late Effects Committee and Nursing Discipline. J Clin Oncol. 2004;22:4979–90.

Chapter 11
Transfusion Support of the Patient with Hematologic Malignancy

Terry B. Gernsheimer and Meghan Delaney

Abstract Recent advances have markedly improved survival outcomes in the treatment of leukemia and other hematologic malignancies, but despite new techniques in growth factor and stem cell technology, chronic or prolonged periods of pancytopenia remain a significant problem, and transfusion is a cornerstone of management. An evidence-based approach to best practice must take into account indications for transfusions as well as their risks.

Keywords Platelet transfusion • Red cell transfusion • Granulocyte transfusion • Transfusion-associated graft versus host disease • Anemia • Thrombocytopenia • Transfusion reactions • Allergic transfusion reaction • Febrile nonhemolytic transfusion reaction • Hemolytic transfusion reaction • Transfusion-associated acute lung injury (TRALI) • CMV infection • Leukocyte reduction • Hemostasis • Transfusion threshold • Bleeding • Hemorrhage • Platelet refractoriness

T.B. Gernsheimer, M.D. (✉)
Division of Hematology, Department of Medicine,
University of Washington School of Medicine, Seattle, WA, USA

Transfusion Services, Seattle Cancer Care Alliance, Seattle, WA, USA

Puget Sound Blood Center, 921 Terry Avenue, 98104 Seattle, WA, USA
e-mail: bldbuddy@u.washington.edu

M. Delaney, DO, PMH,
Department of Laboratory Medicine, Assistant Medical Director,
Puget Sound Blood Center, 921 Terry Avenue, 98104 Seattle, WA, USA
e-mail: meghand@psbc.org

E.H. Estey and F.R. Appelbaum (eds.), *Leukemia and Related Disorders:*
Integrated Treatment Approaches, Contemporary Hematology,
DOI 10.1007/978-1-60761-565-1_11, © Springer Science+Business Media, LLC 2012

Introduction

Recent advances have markedly improved survival outcomes in the treatment of leukemia and other hematologic malignancies, but despite new techniques in growth factor and stem cell technology, chronic or prolonged periods of pancytopenia remain a significant problem, and transfusion is a cornerstone of management. An evidence-based approach to best practice must take into account indications for transfusions as well as their risks.

Platelet Transfusion

Patients undergoing induction chemotherapy or HSCT for acute leukemia have a significant incidence of hemorrhage [1] which can be fatal [2]. More intensive chemotherapy and radiation therapy result not only in more prolonged periods of thrombocytopenia but also cause significant damage to mucosa and other tissues with rapid cell turnover further impacting the need for hemostatic support. Platelets are consumed in the presence of sepsis, malignancy, inflammation [3], and other clinical factors and are often the last hematopoietic line to recover or engraft, and megakaryocytes are also most likely to fail to engraft following hematopoietic stem cell transplantation (HSCT). Patients may also become refractory to platelet transfusions and require special support to maintain platelet counts at a safe level. The increasing demand for platelet components has had a substantial impact on this limited resource [4] and is expensive, costing on average $4,000 for autologous peripheral blood stem cell and $11,000 for bone marrow transplant patients.

Platelet Transfusion Thresholds

Platelets play a vital role in normal homeostasis by maintaining vascular integrity, supporting the vascular endothelium by plugging gaps, and preventing the thinning of the vessel wall and extravasation of red blood cells [5]. In 1962, Gaydos et al. [6] found the incidence of all bleeding increases in patients with acute leukemia as the platelet count falls below 100,000/μL, but gross hemorrhage does not increase significantly until the count falls below 20,000/μL. Autopsy studies on 57 patients with acute leukemia found bleeding to be the proximate cause of death in 20 (65%) of the 30 patients who were not transfused with platelets but in only 4 (15%) of 27 transfused patients, [7] implying that bleeding could be prevented with transfusion. When platelets became routinely available in the 1970s, prophylactic transfusion at platelet counts of 20,000–30,000/μL became the standard; however, aspirin administration was routine for pain and fever when these early studies were conducted, and increasing knowledge of drug effects on platelet function has called into question practice guidelines based on those data.

Harker and Slichter quantitated bleeding by measuring radioactivity in the stool of thrombocytopenic patients who had been injected with Cr-labeled red blood cells [8]. An obligate amount of blood loss from gastrointestinal mucosa appears to occur at all platelet counts and does not increase until the count falls to levels of 5–10,000/μL. Prophylactic platelet transfusion triggers vary widely among practitioners [9]. Lower trigger levels may lead to decreased platelet use [10], and multiple studies have not shown detrimental effects of lowering platelet transfusion thresholds to 10,000 [11–14] or even 5,000/μL (10)[10] in otherwise stable patients. Risk of bleeding may be related to the duration of thrombocytopenia, which may be a surrogate for the severity of the illness and intensity of therapy [2] This raises the questions of whether prophylactic platelet transfusion is required at all [15, 16] and whether a therapeutic transfusion strategy, that is, transfusing for signs of bleeding only, in patients undergoing less toxic therapy and more rapid recovery such as autologous stem cell transplantation may be a safe alternative. The TOPPS study [9], being conducted in the United Kingdom, will evaluate the proportion of patients who experience a major bleeding event up to 30 days postrandomization to receive either prophylactic platelet transfusions at a threshold of 10,000/μL or for WHO bleeding grade 2 or higher [17].

Platelet Transfusion Dose

There is a direct relationship between platelet count and platelet survival when the count falls to less than 100,000/μL with an increasing percentage of platelet loss from the circulation, suggesting a physiologic requirement for platelets. The number of platelets required for endothelial support and maintenance of hemostasis has been calculated to be 7,100 platelets/μL/day [8, 18], but this does not take into account platelets consumed in the presence of sepsis, malignancy, inflammation [19], and other clinical factors.

Numerous transfusion trials have compared low and/or high doses of platelets to standard doses [20–22]. The SToP study [23], a prospective international randomized controlled trial randomizing patients with platelet counts less than 10,000/μL to receive prophylactic platelet transfusions with either a "low dose" ($1.5–2.9 \times 10^{11}$ platelets/component) or a "standard dose" ($3.0–6.0 \times 10^{11}$) platelet transfusion, was stopped due to safety concerns after enrolling less than half the patients needed.

The Platelet Dose Trial (PLADO) [1], the largest platelet transfusion trial ever undertaken, enrolled approximately 1,300 patients in a multicenter prospective blinded trial, comparing bleeding events according to the WHO scale between patients transfused prophylactically for platelet counts less than or equal to 10,000/μL with low dose, medium dose, or high dose platelet transfusions (1.1×10^{11},

2.2×10^{11}, or 4.4×10^{11} platelets per square meter of body surface area, respectively). Although grade 2 or higher bleeding differed significantly between each clinical group (79% of allogeneic SCT patients, 73% of patients receiving chemotherapy for a hematologic malignancy, and 57% of autologous or syngeneic SCT patients), platelet dose had no effect on bleeding rates within any of these clinical groups. In addition, the time from first platelet transfusion to onset of grade 2 or higher bleeding was not significantly different among the arms. Bleeding risk was significantly higher at 25%, with morning platelet counts of ≤5,000/μL; was stable at 17% with platelet counts between 6,000/μL and 80,000/μL; and was further reduced at platelet counts of ≥81,000/μL, confirming the safety of a platelet transfusion threshold of 10,000/μL. Platelet transfusion increments were lower, and platelet transfusions were required more frequently in patients receiving smaller doses (median time between transfusion 1.1, 1.9, and 2.9 days for the low, medium, and high dose arms), making a low dose transfusion strategy inefficient for outpatient care. Patients in the lower dose arm used fewer platelets overall prior to recovery of their platelet counts $(9.25, 11.25, 19.63 \times 10^{11}$, respectively).

Prevention of Platelet Alloimmunization

Recognition of alloantigen requires the expression of both class I and class II HLA antigens on the surface of transfused cells [24, 25]. Platelets express only class I HLA antigens, while WBCs express both class I and class II HLA antigens, and RBCs effectively express neither. Studies in rats and mice have demonstrated that reducing the number of leukocytes in platelet transfusions could prevent alloimmunization [24, 26]. Multiple prospective randomized clinical trials have evaluated the efficacy of leukocyte reduction of RBCs and platelets compared with unmodified blood components to prevent alloimmunization to platelets [27–29]. The largest of these, the Trial to Reduce Platelet Alloimmunization (TRAP) [30], compared the rate of development of lymphocytotoxic antibodies and platelet refractoriness in patients undergoing induction chemotherapy for acute myeloid leukemia randomized to receive unmodified (control) random pooled platelet transfusions, UVB-irradiated platelet transfusions, pooled platelet transfusions filtered to remove leukocytes, and apheresis single-donor platelet transfusion filtered to remove leukocytes. Forty-five percent of patients who received unmodified platelet transfusions developed lymphocytotoxic antibodies, and 13% of these became refractory to platelet transfusions. In contrast, only 17–21% of patients who received any of the modified platelet components developed lymphocytotoxic antibodies ($P<0.001$), and only 3–5% became refractory ($P≤0.03$). Patients who had previously been pregnant developed antibodies at a higher rate but still could be shown to derive a benefit from modified blood components. Patients with hematologic malignancy who will require ongoing platelet support should be transfused with leukocyte-reduced cellular blood components to prevent alloimmunization and refractoriness to platelet transfusions.

Refractoriness to Platelet Transfusion

Chronically thrombocytopenic patients who have received multiple red blood cell (RBC) and platelet transfusions become refractory to pooled random-donor platelet concentrates at a rate of 30–70% [31]. Refractoriness to platelet transfusion is associated with poor outcome following HSCT [32], at least partially related to the morbidity and mortality associated with bleeding. HLA alloimmunization is preventable in a majority of patients with acute leukemia by leukocyte filtration of cellular blood components [30]. However, many patients still become refractory to platelet transfusions as HLA alloimmunization or a variety of clinical factors that have been associated with poor platelet increments including sepsis; splenomegaly; medications such as amphotericin B, tacrolimus, and cyclosporine; venoocclusive disease; conditioning regimens that include total body irradiation; and bone marrow transplant for chronic myeloid leukemia [33–35]. However, limiting the exposure to donors by utilizing single-donor apheresis platelets has not consistently shown a decrease in the rate of platelet refractoriness and lymphocytotoxic antibody formation [30, 36–38].

Refractoriness is generally defined as a lack of response in posttransfusion platelet increments after two or more consecutive transfusions. The corrected count increment (CCI) takes into account both platelet dose and the patient's size and is defined as follows [39]:

$$CCI = \frac{(\text{Platelet increment per } \mu L) \times (\text{Body surface area in square meters})}{\text{Number of platelets transfused } (\times 10^{11})}$$

Values below 7,500/μL at 1 h following transfusion have been associated with accelerated platelet destruction.

Refractoriness due to antibodies directed against class I HLA antigens can be diagnosed by antibody identification against a panel of cells or HLA-laden beads. Selecting antigen-compatible donors or HLA-matched donors often makes platelet support possible [40], but patients with HLA types rare in the donor population may be difficult to support. Cross matching the patient's serum with a panel of platelet antibodies may be helpful in selection of donors that are compatible with the patient [41]; however, because of the short shelf life (5 days) of platelets, these have limited availability. Platelet-specific antibodies have been identified in multiply transfused patients at varying frequency [30], but their contribution to platelet refractoriness has not been clearly defined. Leukoreduction does not appear to affect the rate of alloimmunization to platelet-specific antigens [42]. The use of intravenous immunoglobulin therapy for platelet refractoriness is controversial because of cost and variable benefit [42–44]. Patients with high titers of anti-A or anti-B isoagglutinins (e.g., >1:64) may have inadequate response to ABO-incompatible platelet transfusions [45], and a trial of ABO-compatible platelets to determine the role of ABO in refractoriness is indicated.

Nontransfusion Support of Hemostasis

In the patient with severe refractoriness to platelet transfusion for whom HLA-selected donors are unavailable or unsuccessful, adjunctive strategies to support hemostasis may be helpful [46]. Corticosteroids and estrogens have both been used to enhance hemostatic function. Maintaining the hemoglobin level at higher values may have positive effects on platelet function [47]. The use of antifibrinolytic agents such as epsilon aminocaproic acid and tranexamic acid has been reported to be of value in support of the thrombocytopenic patient to both treat and prevent bleeding [48, 49]. Bleeding in the urinary tract, especially the upper urinary tract, is a contraindication and disseminated intravascular coagulation (DIC) is a relative contraindication to the use of these agents. Randomized trials are needed to determine their effectiveness in the prevention of bleeding and decreasing the use of platelet transfusions in patients with hypoproliferative thrombocytopenia. DDAVP [50] and recombinant Factor VIIa [51] have also been used to control thrombocytopenic bleeding, but their usefulness is unclear, and recombinant Factor VIIa, in particular, is an expensive option.

Many of the clinical factors that contribute to a poor posttransfusion increment have a more marked effect when stored as opposed to when fresh (<24 h after collection) platelets are transfused [52]. These patients may have a better response to fresh platelets if available.

The use of platelet growth factors has not been shown to decrease the duration of thrombocytopenia significantly and has been associated with an accelerated malignant transformation in patients with myelodysplastic syndromes [53]. Their use should be considered experimental at this time, but they represent a potentially effective new modality for increasing platelet counts in patients with some marrow reserve. Platelet substitutes and new methods of storing platelets remain a focus of research to meet the challenges to provide platelet support in the future.

Red Blood Cell (RBC) Transfusion

Anemia is common in patients with hematological malignancies and may be seen in up to 70% of patients [54]. In addition to marrow invasion and ineffective hematopoiesis, suppression of EPO production [55], inflammatory block in iron mobilization, and marrow suppression due to chemotherapy may all contribute to anemia in malignancy [56].

Anemia not only affects quality of life but may negatively impact survival [57], particularly when associated with marrow involvement [58].

Red Blood Cell Transfusion Thresholds

There are no randomized studies in leukemia patients that address red cell transfusion thresholds. In a multicenter trial of 838 critically ill, hemodynamically stable patients randomized to an RBC transfusion threshold of 7.0 g of hemoglobin had a significantly lower mortality rate when compared to those randomized to a transfusion threshold of 9.0 g of hemoglobin (22.2% vs. 28.1% [$P=0.05$]) [59]. However, the appropriate hemoglobin threshold to allow a reasonable quality of life with manageable symptoms may need to be individualized in a patient with chronic anemia. In addition, bleeding times are prolonged at lower hemoglobin levels [42, 60], likely due to effects of red cells on platelet-endothelial interaction. For these reasons, higher hemoglobin triggers for transfusion of 9 or 10 g have been chosen at some centers.

Red Blood Cell Alloimmunization

Sensitization to foreign red cell antigens may lead to the production of red cell alloantibodies, increasing the risk of hemolytic transfusion reactions due to incompatible blood transfusion. The presence of red blood cell antibodies complicates the process of cross matching and locating compatible units for transfusion.

Red blood cell antigens are relatively weak immunogens with only 2–6% of the transfused population becoming sensitized [61]. The reason why some patients are at higher risk of red cell alloimmunization is not understood, but the acquired immune status may be important [61]. Mice injected with nucleotides that stimulate immune response had a higher rate of sensitization to foreign red cell antigens than those that were not immune stimulated.

Patients with lymphoproliferative disorders and acute myeloid leukemia have a relatively low rate of red blood cell alloimmunization of 1.8%. Patients with other hematological diseases, such as chronic myeloid leukemia, pancytopenia, and aplastic anemia, have a 5.7–13.6% rate of red cell alloimmunization, while patients with autoimmune hemolytic anemia, cirrhosis, and myelodysplasia have the high rate of 16–33.4% [62, 63]. These differential rates suggest immune competence and immune dysregulation, disease factors and genetic variability all play a role in determining the risk of red blood cell alloimmunization in the individual patient.

Granulocyte Transfusion

The degree of granulocytopenia is directly related to the risk of infection [64]. Although antibiotics have improved morbidity and mortality of prolonged periods of neutropenia, most drugs are less effective in the presence of granulocytopenia.

Bacterial and, more particularly, fungal infections remain major causes of death despite shortening of the period of neutropenia with hematopoietic growth factors [65]. Granulocytes collected by continuous flow centrifugation and filtration leukapheresis function normally in vitro in the quantitative nitroblue tetrazolium, oxygen consumption, and chemotaxis assays [66]. Bacterial killing is only slightly decreased in filtration leukapheresis granulocytes and circulate for several hours posttransfusion, and transfused granulocytes rapidly migrate to sites of infection [67].

Early studies showed promise for the use of granulocyte transfusion for treatment of documented infections in neutropenic patients [68–70]; however, their usefulness in the prevention of infection has been more controversial [71]. Usefulness of granulocyte transfusions has been limited by the inability to collect cells in sufficient amounts to provide an effective transfusion dose; poor response to granulocytes in heavily transfused, alloimmunized patients [72]; and the early development of alloimmunization in patients transfused with granulocytes [73].

Granulocyte donors are administered with corticosteroids prior to granulocyte collection to increase yield with some limited success. More recently, the administration of granulocyte colony-stimulating factor (G-CSF) has been administered to donors prior to collection with an aim of increasing collections and posttransfusion increments [74, 75], and an evaluation of their clinical usefulness in patients with diagnosed infection is ongoing [76].

Adverse Events

Transfusion Reactions

Transfusion reactions far exceed viral disease transmission in transfusion complication rates. Reactions are classified as allergic, febrile nonhemolytic, hemolytic, septic, or transfusion-associated acute lung injury (TRALI). A transfusion must be stopped immediately if a reaction is suspected, and supportive treatment, including medications, oxygen, positioning, and intravenous fluids, should be administered as indicated. Severe reactions may require ventilator support and transfer to critical care level of support. All transfusion reactions must have a postreaction investigation, including a clerical check, blood sample to rule out mistransfusion, and culture if sepsis is suspected.

Allergic transfusion reactions range from very mild localized urticaria to severe and life-threatening anaphylaxis. Allergic reactions are common, complicating 2–5% of transfusion and are caused by preformed IgE antibodies to antigens in the donor plasma which stimulate mast-cell degranulation and histamine release, although host factors have also been implicated [77, 78]. The presence of one allergic reaction usually does not predict future reactions, as donor-derived foreign plasma proteins that stimulated the reaction are not likely to be the same from one blood donor to the next [78], but some patients appear to be more prone to these reactions. Patients with IgA deficiency and preformed anti-IgA antibodies are at risk for anaphylaxis.

Febrile nonhemolytic transfusion reactions (FNHTR) are one of the most common types of transfusion reactions and are associated with high-plasma-containing blood products, such as platelets [78]. FNHTRs usually include fever and/or chills and rigors, hypertension, and increased heart rate. In a study by Heddle, patients with leukemia transfused plasma supernatant from platelet concentrates had significantly more reactions than those transfused the platelet pellet [79]. Because febrile reactions are common, many patients are premedicated prior to transfusion; however, premedication did not reduce the rate of FNHTR, complicating transfusion of leukocyte-reduced apheresis platelet versus placebo in a study of leukemia patients [80]. Premedication may mask a fever, which can be the first sign of a more serious reaction or sepsis. Leukocyte reduction decreases the incidence of febrile transfusion reactions and, if not already part of the transfusion plan to prevent HLA alloimmunization or CMV transmission, may be added for patients with recurrent febrile reactions [81–83].

Hemolytic transfusion reactions are rare (1 in 250–600,000) but can be fatal. Hemolysis may occur immediately at the time of transfusion (acute hemolytic transfusion reaction) or be delayed as much as 7–14 days following transfusion. Acute hemolytic transfusion reactions are usually severe with pain at the infusion site, flank pain, and feeling of impending doom. The laboratory evaluation supports intravascular hemolysis with a positive direct Coombs test and plasma hemoglobinemia. Disseminated intravascular coagulation may occur. These reactions are often attributed to ABO mistransfusions due to clerical mistakes [84, 85]. The rate of fatal septic reactions differs by the type of blood product. Red blood cells have an estimated fatality rate due to bacterial contamination of one in 8,000,000; platelet components which are kept at room temperature have a rate of one in 50–500,000 [86].

Transfusion-related acute lung injury (TRALI) has been the leading cause of transfusion-related fatality reported to the FDA since 2001 [87]. There are two proposed pathophysiological models for TRALI: (1) donor-derived antileukocyte antibodies activate recipient pulmonary leukocytes or (2) a two-hit theory in which patients with a predisposing condition are transfused with blood products containing biologically active lipids [88, 89]. The diagnosis of TRALI requires the clinical symptoms of acute lung injury (ALI) with hypemia with $PaO_2/FiO_2 < 300$ mmHg, decreased pulmonary compliance despite normal cardiac function within 6 h of transfusion, bilateral pulmonary infiltrates, and exclusion of other causes of lung injury [90]. Treatment of TRALI is supportive only, as other interventions do not alter the course of the lung injury which begins to recover spontaneously 48–72 h after transfusion. The mortality rate from TRALI is 5–25% [91]. In a cohort study of 2,297 critically ill patients, there were 24 instances of TRALI, and of these, six were in patients with hematological malignancy which is significantly higher than in matched controls [92]. Hematological malignancy was the second most common diagnosis associated with TRALI. A case report suggests that drugs used in the management of leukemia may prime recipient neutrophils and predispose to the development of TRALI [93].

Transfusion-Associated Graft Versus Host Disease

Transfusion-associated graft versus host disease (TA-GVHD) is a potential complication of transfusion of any blood component containing viable T lymphocytes. It is rare in immunocompetent individuals but fatal in >90% of cases within 2–3 weeks [94]. These cells may engraft and proliferate in the patient, targeting bone marrow, skin, thymus, gastrointestinal tract, liver, and spleen. The risk is higher when donor and patient share an HLA haplotype, for example, in family members or in populations with a restricted number of haplotypes, but severely immunosuppressed patients such as those undergoing chemotherapy for acute leukemia or HSCT patients are especially susceptible [95]. Ionizing radiation inhibits lymphocyte mitotic activity and blast transformation [96] and can prevent TA-GVHD. Doses of gamma irradiation below 50 Gy do not appear to have any major adverse effect on platelet function, although there is some evidence that irradiation causes a modest leakage of potassium and shortened posttransfusion recovery and survival. RBC, platelet, and granulocyte components should be irradiated with at least 25 Gy [97] prior to transfusion to patients with hematologic malignancy. Buffy coats and donor lymphocyte transfusions from the marrow donor given to enhance engraftment should not be irradiated. Irradiation of fresh frozen plasma, cryoprecipitate, deglycerolized frozen RBCs, and washed RBCs is unnecessary since these products have no viable lymphocytes. Photochemical treatment of platelets with psoralens and ultraviolet A light which inactivates transfusion-transmitted pathogens [98] may also prevent TA-GVHD by inactivating leukocytes [99], but further study is needed. Although leukocyte filtration removes more than 99% of WBCs, the residual leukocyte load may still result in transfusion-associated GVHD [100].

Prevention of Transfusion-Transmitted Cytomegalovirus (CMV) Infection

CMV is a DNA virus acquired as a primary infection with body secretions, blood products, or organ allografts. Infection in a normal host usually is asymptomatic but remains latent for life and can cause recurrent infection upon reactivation. CMV infection and seropositivity are extremely common, 40% in highly industrialized areas, higher in warmer climates and densely populated areas, and may be close to100% in developing countries [101].

Transfusion-associated CMV infection in the immunocompetent patient with a normal immune system is usually asymptomatic, occurring 4–12 weeks after blood component exposure in 0.9–17% of patients [102], but CMV infection is a common cause of morbidity and mortality in patients undergoing autologous and allogeneic HSCT [103–106]. The use of prophylactic antiviral agents in patients who are CMV seropositive or soon after the first sign of infection has led to significant reductions in the incidence of CMV disease and CMV-related mortality [107, 108]; however, these agents may have significant marrow toxicity, and patients who are CMV seronegative should be prevented from seroconverting prior to transplantation if possible. Individuals identified as possible candidates for HSCT should be tested early to determine their CMV status. The risk of transfusion-transmitted CMV infection can be reduced by transfusing only CMV-seronegative blood; however, because the virus is harbored within white blood cells, reduction of the number of leukocytes can reduce the viral load passed to the patient during transfusion. Leukocyte reduction, by any method capable of achieving a residual leukocyte count of $<5 \times 10^6$, allows for the reduction of transfusion-transmitted CMV to a level at least equivalent to the level occurring with the use of CMV-seronegative components transfused to seronegative recipients [109–111] and can be safely substituted for CMV-seronegative blood components when these are not available or when leukocyte-reduced blood components are also indicated.

Conclusions

Transfusion remains a key part of management of the patient with hematologic malignancy. Advances in our understanding of the risk factors for bleeding have helped develop best practices to prevent and treat its occurrence. Moreover, knowledge about indications for red blood cell transfusion and the utility of granulocyte transfusions, along with improvements in transfusion safety, are necessary to keep pace with the challenges of more intensive therapies and long-term support of this patient population.

References

1. Slichter SJ, Kaufman RM, Assman SF, et al. Dose of prophylactic platelet transfusions and prevention of hemorrhage. N Engl J Med. 2010;362:600–13.
2. Heddle NM, Cook RJ, Sigouin C, et al. A descriptive analysis of international transfusion practice and bleeding outcomes in patients with acute leukemia. Transfusion. 2006; 46:903–11.
3. George T, Ho-Tin-Noe B, Carbo C, et al. Inflammation induces hemorrhage in thrombocytopenia. Blood. 2008;111:4958–64.
4. Bernstein S, Nademanee A, et al. A multicenter study of platelet recovery and utilization in patients after myeloablative therapy and hematopoietic stem cell transplantation. Blood. 1998;9:3509–17.
5. Kitchens CS, Weiss L. Ultrastructural changes of endothelium associated with thrombocytopenia. Blood. 1975;46:567–78.
6. Gaydos LA, Freireich EJ, Mantel N. The quantitative relation between platelet count and hemorrhage in patients with acute leukemia. N Engl J Med. 1962;266:905–9.
7. Han T, Stutzman L, Cohen E. Effect of platelet transfusion on hemorrhage in patients with acute leukemia. Cancer. 1966;1919:37–42.
8. Harker LA, Slichter SJ. The bleeding time as a screening test for evaluation of platelet function. N Engl J Med. 1972;287:155–9.

9. Blajchman MA, Slichter SJ, Heddle NM, Murphy MF. New strategies for the optimal use of platelet transfusions. Hematology Am Soc Hematol Educ Program 2008;198–204.

10. Slichter SJ, LeBlanc R, Jones MK, et al. Quantitative analysis of bleeding risk in cancer patients prophylactically transfused at platelet counts of 5,000, 10,000, or 20,000 platelets/μl. Blood. 1999;94:376a.

11. Heckman KD, et al. Randomized study of prophylactic platelet transfusion threshold during induction therapy for adult acute leukemia: 10,000/uL Vs 20,000/uL. J Clin Oncol. 1997;15:1143–9.

12. Wandt H, et al. Safety and cost effectiveness of a 10 X 109/L trigger for prophylactic platelet transfusions compared to the traditional 20 X 109/L: a prospective comparative trial in 105 patients with acute myeloid leukemia. Blood. 1998;91:3601–6.

13. Gmur J, et al. Safety of stringent prophylactic platelet transfusion policy for patients with acute leukemia. Lancet. 1991;338:1223–6.

14. Rebulla P, Finazzi G, Marangoni R, et al. A multicenter randomized trial of the threshold for prophylactic platelet transfusions in adults with acute myeloid leukemia. N Engl J Med. 1997;337:1870–5.

15. Wandt H, Schaefer-Eckart K, Frank M, et al. A therapeutic platelet transfusion strategy is safe and feasible in patients after autologous peripheral blood stem cell transplantation. Bone Marrow Transplant. 2006;37:387–92.

16. Pisciotto PT, Benson K, Hume H, et al. Prophylactic versus therapeutic platelet transfusion practices in hematology and/or oncology patients. Transfusion. 1995;35:498–502.

17. Miller AB, Hoogstraten B, Staquat M, Winkler A. Reporting results of cancer treatment. Cancer. 1981;47:207–14.

18. Hanson SR, Slichter SJ. Platelet kinetics in patients with bone marrow hypoplasia: evidence for a fixed platelet requirement. Blood. 1985;66:1105–9.

19. George T, Ho-Tin-Noe B, Carbo C, et al. Inflammation induces hemorrhage in thrombocytopenia. Blood. 2008;111:4958–64.

20. Klumpp TR, Herman JH, Gaughan JP, et al. Clinical consequences of alterations I platelet transfusion dose: a prospective, randomized, double-blinded trial. Transfusion. 1999;39:674–81.

21. Norol F, Bierling P, Roudot-Thoraval F, et al. Platelet transfusion: a dose–response study. Blood. 1998;92:1448–53.

22. Sensebé L, Giraudeau B, Bardiau L, et al. The efficiency of transfusion high doses of platelets in hematologic patients with thrombocytopenia: results of a prospective, randomized, open, blinded end point (PROBE) study. Blood. 2005;105:862–4.

23. Heddle NM, Cook RJ, Tinmouth A, et al. A randomized controlled trial comparing standard-and low-dose strategies for transfusion of platelets (SToP) to patients with thrombocytopenia. Blood. 2009;113:1564–73.

24. Welsh KI, Burgos H, Batchelor JR. The immune response to allogeneic rat platelets: Ag-B antigens in matrix lacking Ia. Eur J Immunol. 1977;7:267–72.

25. Batchelor JR, Welsh KI, Burgos H. Transplantation antigens per se are poor immunogens within a species. Nature. 1978;273:54–6.

26. Claas FHJ, Smeenk RJT, Schmidt R, et al. Alloimmunization against the MHC antigens after platelet transfusion is due to contaminating leukocytes in the platelet suspension. Exp Hematol. 1981;9:84–9.

27. Sniecinski I, O'Donnell MR, Nowicki B, Hill LR. Prevention of refractoriness and HLA-alloimmunization using filtered blood products. Blood. 1988;5:1402–7.

28. Schiffer CA, Dutcher JP, Aisner J, Hogge D, Wiernik PH, Reilly JP. A randomized trial of leukocyte depleted platelet transfusion to modify alloimmunization in patients with leukemia. Blood. 1983;62:815–20.

29. Murphy MF, Metcalfe P, Thomas H, et al. Use of leucocyte-poor blood components and HLA-matched-platelet donors to prevent HLA alloimmunization. Br J Haematol. 1986;62:529–34.

30. Trial to Reduce Alloimmunization to Platelets (TRAP) Trial Study Group. A randomized trial evaluating leukocyte-reduction and UV-B irradiation of platelets to prevent alloimmunization and refractoriness to platelet transfusions. N Engl J Med. 1997;337:1861–9.
31. Slichter SJ. Principles of platelet transfusion therapy. In: Hoffman R, Benz Jr EJ, Shattil SJ, Furie B, Cohen HJ, Silberstein LE, editors. Hematology: basic principles and practice. 2nd ed. New York: Churchill Livingstone; 1995. p. 1987–2006.
32. Toor A, Choo S, et al. Bleeding risk and platelet transfusion refractoriness in patients with acute myelogenous leukemia who undergo autologous stem cell transplantation. Bone Marrow Transplant. 2000;26:315–20.
33. Ishida A, Handa M, et al. Clinical factors influencing posttransfusion platelet increment in patients undergoing hematopoietic progenitor cell transplantation – a prospective analysis. Transfusion. 1998;38:839–47.
34. Bishop J, McGrath K, et al. Clinical factors influencing efficacy of pooled platelet transfusions. Blood. 1988;71:383–7.
35. Alcorta I, Pereira A, et al. Clinical and laboratory factors associated with platelet transfusion refractoriness: a case–control study. Br J Haem. 1996;93:220–4.
36. Gmur J, von Felten A, et al. Delayed alloimmunization using random single donor platelet transfusions: a prospective study in thrombocytopenic patients with acute leukemia. Blood. 1983;62:473–9.
37. Sintnicolaas K, Vriesendorp H, et al. Delayed alloimmunization by random single donor platelet transfusions. Lancet. 1981;317:750–4.
38. Kakaiya RM, Hezzey AJ, Bove JR, et al. Alloimmunization following apheresis platelets vs. pooled platelet concentrate transfusion-a prospective randomized study. Transfusion. 1981; 21:600a.
39. Delaflor-Weiss E, Mintz PD. The evaluation and management of platelet refractoriness and alloimmunization. Transfus Med Rev. 2000;14:180–96.
40. Pai S-C, Lo S-C, Lin Tsai S-J, et al. Epitope-based matching for HLA-alloimmunized platelet refractoriness in patients with hematologic diseases. Transfusion. 2010;50:2318–27.
41. Friedberg RC, Donnelly SF, Mintz PD. Independent roles for platelet crossmatching and HLA in the selection of platelets for alloimmunized patients. Transfusion. 1994;34:215–20.
42. Bierling P, Cordonnier C, Rodet M, et al. High dose intravenous gammaglobulin and platelet transfusions in leukaemic HLA-immunized patients. Scand J Haematol. 1984;33:215–20.
43. Kickler T, Braine HG, Piantadosi S, et al. A randomized placebo-controlled trial of intravenous gammaglobulin in alloimmunized thrombocytopenic patients. Blood. 1990;75:313–6.
44. Lee EJ, Norris D, Schiffer CA. Intravenous immune globulin for patients alloimmunized to random donor platelet transfusion. Transfusion. 1987;27:245–7.
45. Carr R, Hutton J, et al. Transfusion of ABO-mismatched platelets leads to early platelet refractoriness. Br J Haem. 1990;75:408–13.
46. Cattaneo M, Mannucci PM. Current status of non-transfusional haemostatic agents. Haematologica. 1999;84(Suppl EHA-4):120–3.
47. Valeri CR, Cassidy G, Pivacek LE, et al. Anemia-induced increase in the bleeding time: implications for treatment of nonsurgical blood loss. Transfusion. 2001;41:977–83.
48. Bartholomew JR, Salgia R, Bell WR. Control of bleeding in patients with immune and non-immune thrombocytopenia with aminocaproic acid. Arch Intern Med. 1989;149:1959–61.
49. Garewal HS, Durie BGM. Antifibrinolytic therapy with aminocaproic acid for the control of bleeding in thrombocytopenic patients. Scand J Haematol. 1985;35:497–500.
50. Mannucci PM. Desmopressin: a nontransfusional hemostatic agent. Annu Rev Med. 1990;41:55–64.
51. Poon MC. The evidence for the use of recombinant human activated factor VII in the treatment of bleeding patients with quantitative and qualitative platelet disorders. Transfus Med Rev. 2007;21:223–36.
52. Norol F, Kuentz M, et al. Influence of clinical status on the efficiency of stored platelet transfusion. Br J Haem. 1994;86:125–9.

53. Kantarjian HM, Giles FJ, Greenberg PL, et al. Phase 2 study of romiplostim in patients with low- or intermediate-risk myelodysplastic syndrome receiving azacitidine therapy. Blood. 2010;116:3163–70.
54. Birgegard G, Gascon P, Ludwig H. Evaluation of anaemia in patients with multiple myeloma and lymphoma: findings of the European CANCER ANAEMIA SURVEY. Eur J Haematol. 2006;77(5):378–86.
55. Spivak JL, Gascon P, Ludwig H. Anemia management in oncology and hematology. Oncologist. 2009;14 Suppl 1:43–56.
56. Coiffier B, Guastalla JP, Pujade-Lauraine E, Bastit P, Anemia Study Group. Predicting cancer-associated anaemia in patients receiving non-platinum chemotherapy: Results of a retrospective survey. Eur J Cancer. 2001;37(13):1617–23.
57. Hellstrom-Lindberg E, Gulbrandsen N, Lindberg G, Ahlgren T, Dahl IM, Dybedal I, Grimfors G, Hesse-Sundin E, Hjorth M, Kanter-Lewensohn L, Linder O, Luthman M, Lofvenberg E, Oberg G, Porwit-MacDonald A, Radlund A, Samuelsson J, Tangen JM, Winquist I, Wisloff F, Scandinavian MDS Group. A validated decision model for treating the anaemia of myelodysplastic syndromes with erythropoietin + granulocyte colony stimulating factor: significant effects on quality of life. Br J Haematol. 2003;120(6):1037–46.
58. Moullet I, Salles G, Ketterer N, Dumontet C, Bouafia F, Neidhart-Berard EM, Thieblemont C, Felman P, Coiffier B. Frequency and significance of anemia in non Hodgkin's lymphoma patients. Ann Oncol. 1998;9(10):1109–15.
59. Hebert PC, Wells G, Blajchman MA, Marshall J, Martin C, Pagliarello G, Tweeddale M, Schweitzer I, Yetisir E. A multicenter, randomized, controlled clinical trial of transfusion requirements in critical care. Transfusion requirements in critical care investigators, Canadian critical care trials group. N Engl J Med. 1999;340(6):409–17.
60. Blajchman MA, Bordin JO, Bardossy L, Heddle NM. The contribution of the haematocrit to thrombocytopenic bleeding in experimental animals. Br J Haematol. 1994;86(2):347–50.
61. Hendrickson JE, Desmarets M, Deshpande SS, Chadwick TE, Hillyer CD, Roback JD, Zimring JC. Recipient inflammation affects the frequency and magnitude of immunization to transfused red blood cells. Transfusion. 2006;46(9):1526–36.
62. Seyfried H, Walewska I. Analysis of immune response to red blood cell antigens in multi-transfused patients with different diseases. Mater Med Pol. 1990;22(1):21–5.
63. Arriaga F, Bonanad S, Larrea L, de la Rubia J, Lopez F, Sanz MA, Sanz G, Marty ML. Immunohematologic study in 112 patients with myelodysplastic syndromes: 10-year analysis. Sangre (Barc). 1995;40(3):177–80.
64. Pizzo PA. Management of fever in patients with cancer and treatment-induced neutropenia. N Engl J Med. 1993;328:1323–32.
65. Engels EA, Ellis CA, Supran SE, et al. Early infection in bone marrow transplantation: quantitative study of clinical factors that affect risk. Clin Infect Dis. 1999;28:256–66.
66. McCullough J, Weiblen B, et al. In vitro function and post-transfusion survival of granulocytes collected by continuous-flow centrifugation and by filtration leukapheresis. Blood. 1976;2:315–26.
67. Dutcher J, Schiffer C, Johnston G. Rapid migration of indium-labeled granulocytes to sites of infection. N Engl J Med. 1981;304:586–9.
68. Lowenthal RM, Grossman L, Goldman JM, et al. Granulocyte transfusions in treatment of infections in patients with acute leukemia and aplastic anemia. Lancet. 1975;1(7903): 353–8.
69. Alavi J, Root R, et al. A randomized clinical trial of granulocyte transfusions for infection in acute leukemia. N Engl J Med. 1977;13:706–11.
70. Vogler W, Winton E. A controlled study of the efficacy of granulocyte transfusions in patients with neutropenia. Am J Med. 1977;4:548–55.
71. Clift RA, Sanders JE, Thomas ED, et al. Granulocyte transfusions for the prevention of infection in patients receiving bone marrow transplants. N Engl J Med. 1978;298:1052–7.
72. Adkins D, Goodnough L, et al. Effect of leukocyte compatibility on neutrophil increment after transfusion of granulocyte colony-stimulating factor-mobilized prophylactic

granulocyte transfusions and on clinical outcomes after stem cell transplantation. Blood. 2000;11:3605–12.

73. Schiffer C, Aisner J, et al. Alloimmunization following prophylactic granulocyte transfusion. Blood. 1979;54:766–74.

74. Caspar CB, Seger RA, Burger J, Gmur J. Effective stimulation of donors for granulocyte transfusion with recombinant methionyl granulocyte colony-stimulating factor. Blood. 1993;81:2866–71.

75. Price TH, Bowden RA, Boeckh M, et al. Phase I/II trial of neutrophil transfusions from donors stimulated with G-CSF and dexamethasone for treatment of patients with infections in hematopoietic stem cell transplantation. Blood. 2000;95:3302–9.

76. Dzik WH. The NHLBI clinical trials network in transfusion medicine and hemostasis: an overview. J Clin Apheresis. 2006;21:57–9.

77. Savage WJ, Tobian AA, Fuller AK, Wood RA, King KE, Ness PM. Allergic transfusion reactions to platelets are associated more with recipient and donor factors than with product attributes. Transfusion. 2011;51(8):1716–22. Epub 2011 Jan 7.

78. Tobian AA, Savage WJ, Tisch DJ, Thoman S, King KE, Ness PM. Prevention of allergic transfusion reactions to platelets and red blood cells through plasma reduction. Transfusion. 2011;51(8):1716–22. Epub 2011 Jan 7.

79. Heddle NM, Klama L, Singer J, Richards C, Fedak P, Walker I, Kelton JG. The role of the plasma from platelet concentrates in transfusion reactions. N Engl J Med. 1994;331(10):625–8.

80. Wang SE, Lara Jr PN, Lee-Ow A, Reed J, Wang LR, Palmer P, Tuscano JM, Richman CM, Beckett L, Wun T. Acetaminophen and diphenhydramine as premedication for platelet transfusions: A prospective randomized double-blind placebo-controlled trial. Am J Hematol. 2002;70(3):191–4.

81. Geiger TL, Howard SC. Acetaminophen and diphenhydramine premedication for allergic and febrile nonhemolytic transfusion reactions: good prophylaxis or bad practice? Transfus Med Rev. 2007;21(1):1–12.

82. Patterson BJ, Freedman J, Blanchette V, Sher G, Pinkerton P, Hannach B, Meharchand J, Lau W, Boyce N, Pinchefsky E, Tasev T, Pinchefsky J, Poon S, Shulman L, MacK P, Thomas K, Blanchette N, Greenspan D, Panzarella T. Effect of premedication guidelines and leukoreduction on the rate of febrile nonhaemolytic platelet transfusion reactions. Transfus Med. 2000;10(3):199–206.

83. Couban S, Carruthers J, Andreou P, Klama LN, Barr R, Kelton JG, Heddle NM. Platelet transfusions in children: results of a randomized, prospective, crossover trial of plasma removal and a prospective audit of WBC reduction. Transfusion. 2002;42(6):753–8.

84. Ahrens N, Pruss A, Kiesewetter H, Salama A. Failure of bedside ABO testing is still the most common cause of incorrect blood transfusion in the barcode era. Transfus Apher Sci. 2005;33(1):25–9.

85. Janatpour KA, Kalmin ND, Jensen HM, Holland PV. Clinical outcomes of ABO incompatible RBC transfusions. Am J Clin Pathol. 2008;129(2):276–81.

86. Wagner SJ. Transfusion-transmitted bacterial infection: risks, sources and interventions. Vox Sang. 2004;86(3):157–63.

87. Holness L, Knippen MA, Simmons L, Lachenbruch PA. Fatalities caused by TRALI. Transfus Med Rev. 2004;18(3):184–8.

88. Popovsky MA, Moore SB. Diagnostic and pathogenetic considerations in transfusion related acute lung injury. Transfusion. 1985;25(6):573–7.

89. Silliman CC, Paterson AJ, Dickey WO, Stroneck DF, Popovsky MA, Caldwell SA, Ambruso DR. The association of biologically active lipids with the development of transfusion-related acute lung injury: a retrospective study. Transfusion. 1997;37(7):719–26.

90. Kleinman S, Caulfield T, Chan P, Davenport R, McFarland J, McPhedran S, Meade M, Morrison D, Pinsent T, Robillard P, Slinger P. Toward an understanding of transfusion related acute lung injury: statement of a consensus panel. Transfusion. 2004;44(12):1774–89.

91. Silliman CC, Ambruso DR, Boshkov LK. Transfusion-related acute lung injury. Blood. 2005;105(6):2266–73.
92. Rana R, Fernandez-Perez ER, Khan SA, Rana S, Winters JL, Lesnick TG, Moore SB, Gajic O. Transfusion-related acute lung injury and pulmonary edema in critically ill patients: a retrospective study. Transfusion. 2006;46(9):1478–83.
93. Jeddi R, Mansouri R, Kacem K, Gouider E, Abid HB, Belhadjali Z, Meddeb B. Transfusion-related acute lung injury (TRALI) during remission induction course of acute myeloid leukemia: a possible role for all-transretinoic-acid (ATRA)? Pathol Biol (Paris). 2009;57(6): 500–2.
94. Anderson KC, Weinstein HJ. Transfusion-associated graft-versus-host disease. N Engl J Med. 1990;323:315–21.
95. Greenbaum BH. Transfusion-associated graft-versus-host disease: historical perspectives, incidence, and current Use of irradiated blood products. J Clin Oncol. 1991;9:1889–902.
96. Sprent J, Anderson RE, Miller JFAP. Radiosensitivity of T and B lymphocytes. II. Effect of irradiation on response of T cells to alloantigens. Eur J Immunol. 1974;4:204–10.
97. BCSH Blood Transfusion Task Force. Guidelines on gamma irradiation of blood components for the prevention of transfusion-associated graft-versus-host disease. Transfus Med. 1996;6:261–71.
98. Lin L, Dikeman R, Molini B, et al. Photochemical treatment of platelet concentrates with amotosalen and UVA inactivates a broad spectrum of pathogenic bacteria. Transfusion. 2004;44:1496–504.
99. Grass JA, Wafa T, Reames A, et al. Prevention of transfusion associated graft-versus-host disease by photochemical treatment. Blood. 1999;93:3140–7.
100. Akahoshi M, Takanashi M, Masuda M, et al. A case of transfusion-associated graft-versus-host disease not prevented by white cell-reduction filters. Transfusion. 1992;32:169–72.
101. Clair P, Embil J, Fahey J. A seroepidemiologic study of cytomegalovirus infection in a Canadian recruit population. Mil Med. 1990;155:489–92.
102. Tegtmeier GE. Post transfusion cytomegalovirus infections. Arch Pathol Lab Med. 1989;113:236–45.
103. Meyers J, Flournoy N, et al. Risk factors for cytomegalovirus infection after human marrow transplantation. J Infect Dis. 1986;153:478–88.
104. Konoplev S, Champlin RE, et al. Cytomegalovirus pneumonia in adult autologous blood marrow transplant recipients. Bone Marrow Transplant. 2001;27:877–81.
105. Enright H, Haake R, et al. Cytomegalovirus pneumonia after bone marrow transplantation. Transplantation. 1993;55:1339–45.
106. Reusser P. The challenge of cytomegalovirus infection after bone marrow transplantation: epidemiology, prophylaxis and therapy. Bone Marrow Transplant. 1996;18:107–9.
107. Goodrich J, Bowden R, et al. Ganciclovir prophylaxis to prevent cytomegalovirus disease after allogeneic marrow transplant. Ann Intern Med. 1993;118:173–8.
108. Winston D, Ho W, et al. Ganciclovir prophylaxis of cytomegalovirus infection and disease in allogeneic bone marrow transplant recipients. Ann Intern Med. 1993;118:179–84.
109. Bowden R, Slichter S, et al. A comparison of filtered leukocyte-reduced and cytomegalovirus (CMV) seronegative blood products for the prevention of transfusion-associated CMV infection after marrow transplant. Blood. 1995;86:3598–603.
110. DeWitte T, Schattenberg A, et al. Prevention of primary cytomegalovirus infection after allogeneic bone marrow transplantation by using leukocyte-poor random blood products from cytomegalovirus-unscreened blood bank donors. Transplantation. 1990;50:964–8.
111. de Graan-Hentzen Y, Gratama J, et al. Prevention of primary cytomegalovirus infection in patients with hematologic malignancies by intensive white cell depletion of blood products. Transfusion. 1989;29:757–60.

Chapter 12
Infections in Leukemia and Hematopoietic Stem Cell Transplantation

Steven A. Pergam, Debra K. Mattson, and Michael Boeckh

Abstract Infections are one of the most common complications in patients diagnosed with leukemia and serve as a major obstacle to treatment. Through the early 1970s, infections were the most common cause of death in patients diagnosed with acute leukemia, but improvement in treatment and supportive care over the past few decades, coupled with expanded prophylaxis and prevention regimens, have led to reduction in both the frequency and severity of infections. Regardless, due in part to an aging cancer population and the diversity of cancer treatments and procedures, infectious diseases remain a major cause of morbidity and mortality in patients with leukemia.

S.A. Pergam, M.D., MPH (✉)
Vaccine and Infectious Diseases and Clinical Research Divisions, Fred Hutchinson Cancer Research Center, 1100 Fairview Ave N, D3-100, Seattle, WA 98109, USA

Allergy and Infectious Diseases Division, University of Washington School of Medicine, Seattle, WA, USA
e-mail: spergam@fhcrc.org

D.K. Mattson, PA-C
Vaccine and Infectious Diseases and Clinical Research Divisions, Fred Hutchinson Cancer Research Center, 1100 Fairview Ave N, D3-100, Seattle, WA 98109, USA
e-mail: dmattson@fhcrc.org

M. Boeckh, M.D.
Vaccine and Infectious Diseases and Clinical Research Divisions, Fred Hutchinson Cancer Research Center, 1100 Fairview Ave N, D3-100, Seattle, WA 98109, USA

Allergy and Infectious Diseases Division, University of Washington School of Medicine, Seattle, WA, USA
e-mail: mboeckh@fhcrc.org

E.H. Estey and F.R. Appelbaum (eds.), *Leukemia and Related Disorders:*
Integrated Treatment Approaches, Contemporary Hematology,
DOI 10.1007/978-1-60761-565-1_12, © Springer Science+Business Media, LLC 2012

Keywords Infection • Leukemia • Hematopoietic stem cell transplantation • Prophylaxis • Viral infection • Bacterial infection • Fungal infection • Neutropenia • Drug-resistant pathogens • Mortality • Transplant-associated infection

Introduction

Infections are one of the most common complications in patients diagnosed with leukemia and serve as a major obstacle to treatment [1]. Through the early 1970s, infections were the most common cause of death in patients diagnosed with acute leukemia [2, 3], but improvement in treatment and supportive care over the past few decades, coupled with expanded prophylaxis and prevention regimens, have led to reduction in both the frequency and severity of infections [4– 6]. Regardless, due in part to an aging cancer population and the diversity of cancer treatments and procedures, infectious diseases remain a major cause of morbidity and mortality in patients with leukemia.

Leukemia is associated with marked alterations in humoral and cellular immunity which enhance the ability of microorganisms to evade detection and destruction. As the bone marrow is replaced with malignant cells, myeloid and lymphoid cell production fall, and those available have weakened responses to pathogens. Peripheral leukocytes in patients with acute leukemia have impaired phagocytosis [7, 8] which can lead to increased risk of bacterial and fungal infections, while chronic leukemias demonstrate reduced immunoglobulin production [9, 10]. Due to these immune deficits, it is not uncommon for infections to be a primary reason for patients to seek care, and uncontrolled or uncommon infections are known to portend an undiagnosed hematologic malignancy [11].

In addition to direct effects, treatment leads to further decrements in the ability of patients to fight infection. Chemotherapy-associated marrow toxicity is unavoidable, and neutropenia and/or lymphopenia is nearly universal during therapy for acute leukemia. Protracted periods of agranulocytosis and delayed recovery of adaptive immunity are more common following aggressive therapy for relapsed disease and/or conditioning prior to hematopoietic cell transplantation (HCT) [12–14]. Furthermore, alterations in normal gut flora [15], destruction of mucosal barriers [16, 17], transfusion-associated iron overload [18], and loss of skin integrity further increase the risk of infection. All told, the multiple negative effects of therapy further compromise the immune response, placing these patients at added risk for severe and life-threatening infections.

The development of prophylactic strategies for viral [6, 19, 20] and bacterial infections [4], as well as broad-spectrum antifungals [21, 22], has improved prevention and treatment options for these high-risk patients. Novel laboratory techniques, such as molecular diagnostics for viral infections [23], have also allowed for earlier detection of major infections [24]. Hematologic support through the use of colony-stimulating factors has helped to shorten neutropenia and further limit infectious complications [25]. However, even as diagnostic and therapeutic options have evolved, novel treatment options for leukemia, biologic immune-modulating therapies, expanded transplant protocols for high-risk patients, and alternate stem cell donor sources have led to additional immune dysfunction and infectious risk. Not surprisingly, prevention regimens have also led to the emergence of drug-resistant pathogens [26–30], many of which are associated with increased infection-related mortality.

In this chapter, we review the most prevalent infections seen in leukemia, but we will focus primarily on transplant-associated infections. We review timing of infections and then common infections by organ systems. We also discuss the management of neutropenic fever and assess important prevention strategies. This chapter should serve as a reference for clinicians on common infectious complications; however, the sheer number of potential infections is too large to allow for a comprehensive review. In addition, when addressing this topic, there is a large variation on the strength of clinical evidence in the literature. Randomized clinical trials evaluating treatment and prevention of infections, for example, are the strongest for cytomegalovirus (CMV) and fungal infections, but the majority of data are based either on retrospective clinical studies or on expert opinion. In this overview, we do not address the strength of evidence and instead refer you to more comprehensive guidelines and reviews whenever possible throughout the chapter [31, 32]. Finally, when providing care for these complex patients, we recommend close collaboration with colleagues in Infectious Diseases, Pulmonary/Critical Care, Surgery, and with local Clinical Microbiology and Virology laboratories.

Timing of Infections (Reviewed in Reference [31])

Pretransplant/Preinduction

Patients with underlying leukemia are at high risk for infections, and many present to primary care providers with infections as the first sign of their underlying hematologic malignancy. Prolonged neutropenia prior to transplant has also been shown to be a predictor of posttransplant infectious risk and mortality [33]. Providers must assess patients at presentation for infection symptoms such as recurrent fevers, chronic cough, skin nodules, or upper respiratory symptoms prior to starting treatment, and all patients with infectious symptoms should undergo pretransplant evaluation. Some infections may even require delay in transplant conditioning (e.g., respiratory syncytial virus [RSV]) [34–36]. All patients should also have standard pretransplant serologic testing as recommended in updated guidelines [31].

Preengraftment (Days 0–15)

During the early period postchemotherapy and conditioning, patients have abnormalities in barrier and innate responses which dramatically increase the risk of infection. Significant mucositis, long-term catheters, and prolonged periods of hospitalization all increase risk. Early bacterial infections are typically associated with mucositis, such as *Streptococcus* species and enteric gram-negative rods (GNRs), or related to central catheters. Viral infections are infrequent in the early preengraftment phase, except for HSV and HHV-6, which commonly occur in this time frame. Respiratory pathogens are less frequent during this period due to the more limited outpatient exposure. Patients are at high risk for Candida and invasive moulds during this period [31].

Postengraftment (Days 16–100)

In this period after neutrophil recovery, adaptive and humoral immune responses remain impaired [31]. Patients continue to be at risk for bacteremia with gram-positive and GNR organisms, but viral and fungal infections become more prominent. Cytomegalovirus (CMV) usually occurs in weeks 3–4, and EBV in the second and third months posttransplant [37]. Respiratory viral infections increase in frequency with the move to more outpatient therapy. Aspergillus, Candida, and other fungal infections continue through the postengraftment phase due to the development of graft-versus-host disease (GVHD) and associated treatments.

Late Period (Days 100–1 Year)

After day 100, patients more commonly develop infections with encapsulated (e.g., *Streptococcus pneumoniae*) and community-acquired bacterial infections. Respiratory viruses remain major pathogens. Late T-cell recovery and lymphopenia also allow for continued development of CMV and other viral-related complications. Varicella-zoster virus (VZV) reactivation primarily occurs as a late complication [37]. Late fungal infections occur in patients with ongoing GVHD issues. *Pneumocystis jiroveci* (PCP) occurs in posttransplant patients not receiving appropriate PCP prophylaxis.

Infections by Organ System

Empiric therapy for neutropenic fever during leukemia treatment and transplantation is reviewed in detail in other sources [31, 32, 39]. In order to address the multiple possible infections that can occur during treatment for leukemia, we have divided infections into specific organ systems (Fig. 12.1). In this section, we focus on clinical signs/symptoms, differential diagnosis, and diagnostic strategies, followed by a brief review of treatment options.

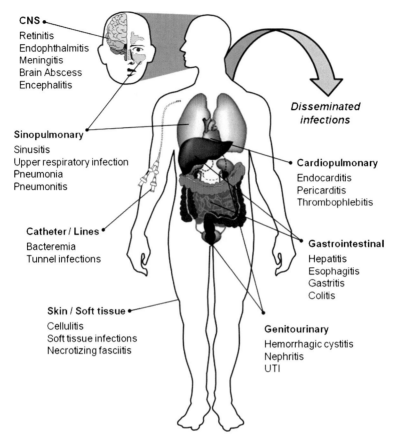

CNS
Retinitis
Endophthalmitis
Meningitis
Brain Abscess
Encephalitis

Disseminated infections

Sinopulmonary
Sinusitis
Upper respiratory infection
Pneumonia
Pneumonitis

Cardiopulmonary
Endocarditis
Pericarditis
Thrombophlebitis

Catheter / Lines
Bacteremia
Tunnel infections

Gastrointestinal
Hepatitis
Esophagitis
Gastritis
Colitis

Skin / Soft tissue
Cellulitis
Soft tissue infections
Necrotizing fasciitis

Genitourinary
Hemorrhagic cystitis
Nephritis
UTI

Fig. 12.1 Locations and types of common infections in leukemia and transplant recipients (*Figure drawn by Kyoko Kurosawa*)

Line-Associated and Bloodstream Infections

Signs and Symptoms

Patients who develop bloodstream infections present with a wide spectrum of symptoms which vary from asymptomatic (usually detected by surveillance cultures) [40] to fulminant septic shock. Patients with bloodstream infections are usually febrile, but fever may be masked in some patients on immunosuppression, particularly those on high-dose steroids. Hypothermia is an infrequent presentation. Careful examination of the central venous catheter (CVC) may provide visual clues that suggest infection, such as erythema or purulence around the line or exit site; some patients may complain of chest wall pain or numbness at sites of catheter placement. A thorough skin exam is also important, as some patients develop skin

S.A. Pergam et al.

nodules, ecthyma gangrenosum, or other lesions during episodes of bacteremia [41, 42] or fungemia [43, 44]. The development of hypoxia, renal insufficiency, and liver function abnormalities are ominous signs of developing septic shock and multiorgan failure.

Differential Diagnosis

Bacterial

Central lines can be a source for infection for leukemia patients, but more frequently, patients can develop infections due to the breakdown of mucosal barriers. Once bacteria gain access to the bloodstream, either through mucosal breakdown or through central catheters, they adhere to synthetic material by developing complex biofilms. These foreign bodies can thus become foci for infections and allow bacteria to escape immune control [45] without altering their pathogenicity [46]. Neutropenia and innate immune dysfunction following postinduction therapy and transplantation may also help facilitate biofilm formation [47–49]. The development of mucositis and GVHD facilitates bacterial translocation and increases the risk for bloodstream infections [50].

Guidelines for line-associated infections and specific recommendations for transplant recipients are reviewed in greater detail in other sources [31, 51]. Line-site and bloodstream infections occur during therapy for leukemia; they occur most commonly during the first week after line placement and during neutropenia and in patients with GVHD [52]. The majority of cases are due to chemotherapy-associated bacterial translocation from mucosal sites. Most early infections in these patients are caused by gram-positive organisms; however, GNRs are not infrequent in patients with severe mucositis or lower gastrointestinal GVHD. GNR resistance to prophylactic antibiotics is increasing [43, 54]. Nontuberculous mycobacteria (NTM) are a rare cause of tunnel- and line-associated infections; line removal is required for cure [55].

Specific gram-positive bacterial species are commonly associated with leukemia therapy and transplantation. Coagulase-negative *Staphylococcus* species (CoNS) are the most common cause of bacteremia in most studies [54, 56–59]. *Staphylococcus aureus* (including methicillin-resistant *S. aureus* [MRSA]) is associated with the development and treatment of GVHD and with significantly more morbidity than CoNS [60]. *Streptococcus viridans* bacteremia often occurs following conditioning and can be associated with the development of septic shock, multiorgan failure, and death [61–63]. Leukemic patients are at high risk for *S. pneumonia* and may be more likely to develop invasive complications [64–66]. *Enterococcal* species, particularly vancomycin-resistant *Enterococcus* (VRE), are a major problem in patients with leukemia and transplantation and are an increasing cause of bacteremia [67, 68]. Risk is increased with prolonged hospitalization, high-dose steroids, gut GVHD, prior cephalosporin therapy, and prior VRE colonization [68, 69].

Less frequent gram-positive species such as *Corynebacterium jeikeium* can also cause disease in this population [70].

A variety of GNR organisms cause bloodstream infections, but *Pseudomonas aeruginosa* remains one of the most important GNRs. *P. aeruginosa*'s intrinsic virulence leads to additional mortality, and it is often associated with high-level resistance [71, 72]. *Stenotrophomonas maltophilia* is resistant to carbepenems and other standard neutropenic treatment options and is often preferentially selected in this population [73–75]. With the continued emergence of multidrug-resistant GNR pathogens, providers need to be cautious in choosing empiric regimens [52, 72] as these organisms are associated with prolonged bacteremia and increased morbidity and mortality [76]. Due to bacterial translocation during episodes of severe mucositis and gut GVHD, enteric GNRs and gram-positive clostridial species are more frequent. In particular, *C. perfringens* bacteremia can lead to severe life-threatening intravascular hemolysis [77], and *C. septicum* bacteremia is associated with gastrointestinal complications [78].

Fungal

Candida species can also lead to bloodstream infections, particularly in patients who either are receiving broad-spectrum antibiotics or have clinically significant mucositis [79]. *Candida* species that are detected in patients receiving antifungal prophylaxis are more likely to be resistant species, particularly *C. krusei* and *C. glabrata* [79, 80]. Data suggest that rates of candidemia may be decreasing [81]. Other yeasts, such as Rhodotorula [78], are a less frequent cause of bloodstream infections.

Although moulds can spread hematogenously, they are rare causes of bloodstream infections [82, 83]. *Fusarium*, however, are the one mould species that routinely can present with fungemia [84]. Typical "banana-shaped" conidia seen on gram stain from blood cultures are pathognomonic for fusariosis. At sites of skin breakdown, fungal infections can invade damaged tissue, so exit infections can sometimes be caused by fungal pathogens [85, 86].

Diagnostics

Blood cultures are the mainstay of any work-up for patients suspected of having an infection. It is recommended that patients with central catheters have cultures drawn from their lines; peripheral cultures should also be drawn if possible [51]. A meta-analysis found that line cultures were a better diagnostic test for bacteremia with better sensitivity and negative predictive value when compared to a peripheral culture [87]. Current guidelines suggest that if a peripheral culture is not possible, it is recommended that ≥2 blood samples should be drawn from each catheter lumen [51, 88]. Differential time to positivity and quantitative blood cultures are other techniques to help identify catheter-associated infections that are beyond the scope of this chapter but are reviewed elsewhere [89–91].

Line tips should be sent for culture at the time of removal if at all possible [51]. Skin biopsies can also be helpful in patients with suspicious skin lesions in some infections [70].

Treatment

Treatment options vary by pathogen and site (see Table 12.1). Tunnel infections require line removal [51], but exit-site infections can sometimes be managed with antibiotic therapy, particularly if they are not associated with bacteremia. Exit-site infections that do not improve with systemic antibiotic therapy should lead to line removal [51]. Antibiotic therapy for any bloodstream infections should be based on culture and sensitivity testing, and patients should have repeat cultures to assure that the organism has cleared. Most bacterial infections require at least 2 weeks of IV therapy, but some pathogens (e.g., *Listeria monocytogenes*) may need more prolonged courses. Patients with NTM should be treated for at least 3 months with a combination of at least 2–3 agents [55]. Patients with candidemia should be treated with fluconazole, lipid amphotericin B formulations, or an echinocandin, and any central catheter should be removed [92]. All patients with candidemia should undergo an ophthalmologic evaluation. Recommendations regarding the management of Candida infections are reviewed in reference by Pappas et al. [92]. Decisions regarding tunneled line or port removal should be done in collaboration with Infectious Diseases, Interventional Radiology, or Surgery and are reviewed by Mermel [51].

Central Nervous System

Signs and Symptoms

Patients undergoing HCT and those who are receiving leukemia therapy are more likely to have neurologic complications [93]. Up to 30% of patients undergoing HCT can develop delirium during follow-up, with the nearly half occurring in the first 4 weeks posttransplant [94]. Infections may present with symptoms that are subtle (e.g., mild confusion) and rarely may be asymptomatic [95]. More common manifestations are headache, memory loss, focal weakness, or imbalance. Patients with eye infections can present with visual loss, eye pain, proptosis, changes in ocular movements (e.g., cranial nerve dysfunction), pupillary changes, or periorbital edema, all of which should lead to urgent ophthalmologic evaluation.

While certain symptoms such as anterograde amnesia [96] and personality changes [97] are classically associated with specific infections (HHV-6 and HSV, respectively), symptoms are not diagnostic of the underlying disorder. Patients with

Table 12.1 Treatment options for selected pathogens*

Pathogen	Treatment		Prevention	Notes
	First line	Second line		
Bacterial				
S. epidermidis[†]	IV vancomycin	IV daptomycin or linezolid	–	–
S. aureus				
Methicillin sensitive	IV nafcillin	IV cefazolin	• Nares swab for MRSA screening	• Infection control
MRSA	IV vancomycin	IV daptomycin or linezolid		
Enterococcus species				
Non-VRE[†]	IV ampicillin +/– gent or IV vancomycin		–	–
VRE	IV daptomycin or linezolid	IV quinupristin/ dalfopristin‡	• Pretransplant rectal screening	• Infection control
Viridans strep.	IV vancomycin	IV penicillin	• Penicillin or vancomycin preemptively during periods of high risk	• Caution for resistance to fluoroquinolones in centers that use as prophylaxis for neutropenia
C. jeikeium	IV vancomycin	–	–	–
L. monocytogenes	IV ampicillin	–	• Avoid high-risk foods	–
S. maltophilia	IV TMP/S	Varies	–	–
P. aeruginosa and other GNR	Varies	Varies	• Fluoroquinolone prophylaxis for neutropenic fever	• Empiric treatment should be based on institutional antimicrobial rate of resistance
Nocardia species	IV TMP/S	IV imipenem	• TMP/S prophylaxis	• Patients with CNS disease should likely receive dual therapy initially • Treatment should be based on sensitivity testing
C. difficile	Metronidazole (IV or oral [preferred])	Vancomycin (oral)	–	• Oral vancomycin may have better outcomes in severe infections • Infection control

(continued)

Table 12.1 (continued)

Pathogen	Treatment		Prevention	Notes
	First line	Second line		
Fungal				
Aspergillus species	Voriconazole (IV or oral) or IV amphotericin B§	Posaconazole (oral)	• Posaconazole prophylaxis	• Benefits of combination therapy are not clear
Mucorales species	IV Amphotericin B§ or posaconazole (oral)	–	–	• Benefits of combination therapy are not clear • Treatment should be based on sensitivity testing when possible • Unclear if posaconazole or IV amphotericin is the best first choice
Candida species				
Azole sensitive	IV fluconazole	IV echinocandins‖	• Fluconazole prophylaxis	• Azole-resistant strains are more likely in patients receiving fluconazole or other azole prophylaxis
Azole resistant	IV echinocandins‖	IV amphotericin B§		
P. jiroveci	IV TMP/S	IV clarithromycin/primaquine (oral) or IV pentamidine	• Oral TMP/S, dapsone, or atovaquone prophylaxis	–
Viral				
Cytomegalovirus	IV ganciclovir	IV foscarnet or cidofovir	• Surveillance and preemptive therapy • High-dose acyclovir prophylaxis	• Patients with ganciclovir-resistant strains should receive foscarnet
EBV	IV rituximab	–	• Preemptive screening in high-risk patients	–
HSV/VZV	IV acyclovir	IV foscarnet	• Oral acyclovir/valacyclovir prophylaxis	–
HHV-6	IV foscarnet or IV ganciclovir	–	–	–

Infection	Treatment	Alternative	Prophylaxis/Prevention	Comments
Adenovirus	IV cidofovir	Ribavirin (oral or IV)	• Preemptive screening in high-risk patients	• IV ribavirin only available through FDA EIND • T-cell immunotherapy can be considered if available
Influenza A and B	Oseltamivir (oral)	Zanamivir (inhaled)	• Vaccination	• Developing resistance has been reported to oseltamivir • Combination therapy can be considered in high-risk patients • Infection control
RSV	Ribavirin (inhaled) +/- IV palivizumab for treatment of lower tract disease	—	• Seasonal palivizumab prophylaxis in high-risk children • Inhaled ribavirin is thought to prevent development of lower tract disease (prophylaxis) in high-risk patients	• Use of palivizumab in adults is unclear but may provide benefits in severely ill patients IVIG may also be considered in high-risk cases. • Infection control
Other infections				
T. gondii	Pyrimethamine (oral) + IV sulfadiazine + folinic acid	TMP/S(oral or IV) or clindamycin (oral of IV) w/pyrimethamine (oral) + folinic acid	• TMP/S prophylaxis • Dapsone prophylaxis +/- pyrimethamine • Consider surveillance in high-risk patients	• Other PCP prevention agents and low-dose TMP/S are not as effective at preventing
Strongyloidiasis	Ivermectin (oral)	Albendazole (oral)	• Pretransplant serology and evaluation • Consider pretransplant empiric treatment if patient considered from high-risk area	—

Abbreviations: IV, intravenous; MRSA, Methicillin-resistant *Staphylococcus aureus*; VRE, Vancomycin-resistant Enterococcus; TMP/S, Trimethoprim/Sulfamethoxazole; GNR, Gram negative rods; CNS, Central Nervous System; EBV, Ebstein-Barr virus; HSV, Herpes simplex virus; VZV, Varicella zoster virus; HHV-6, Human herpesvirus-6; FDA, Federal Drug Administration; EIND, Emergency Investigational Drug Authorization; RSV, Respiratory syncytial virus; IVIG, intravenous immunoglobulin. *These are based on standard recommendations. All decision regarding therapy should be developed based on current clinical practice, resistance testing and institutional policies. † non-VRE Enterococcus are not always sensitive to Ampicillin, so decisions regarding first line therapy should be based on sensitivity testing. ‡ Only effective against *E. faecium* (*E. faecalis* intrinsically resistant). §Typically use lipid formulations of Amphotericin B to reduce side effects. ‖Includes caspofungin, micafungin, and anidulafungin.

more severe infections can present with more ominous symptoms such as seizures, encephalitis, or focal weakness. Perhaps most importantly, fever may not always be present to suggest an infectious etiology [98, 99]. Since these patients have numerous noninfectious etiologies that can lead to CNS dysfunction, it is even more important to aggressively pursue a diagnosis.

Differential Diagnosis

Bacterial

Bacterial infections are a relatively uncommon cause of CNS infections in an age where prophylactic antibiotics are standard practice. Gram-negative and gram-positive organisms can get into the CNS and lead to meningitis during treatment, and although rare, resistant bacteria may be more common due to prior antibiotic exposure. Community-acquired meningitis caused by bacteria such as *S. pneumoniae* is infrequent, but due to alterations in humoral immunity, emerging microbial resistance and a move to more outpatient care can occur late posttransplant and during periods of treatment for GHVD [100, 101]. *Rothia mucilaginosa*, a gram-positive organism that is a commensal organism in oral flora, is associated with a rare, but severe, meningitis that occurs almost exclusively during periods of severe mucositis [102]. Central line–associated bacteremia rarely leads to ophthalmic infection causing sight-threatening endophthalmitis or brain involvement [103, 104], and even less frequently, bacteria can gain access through intracranial interventions such as Ommaya port placement [105].

Some bacteria have a known predilection for the CNS and may not be addressed by standard prophylaxis strategies. *Listeria monocytogenes* is a non-spore-forming gram-positive rod that is most commonly acquired as a food-borne illness with a particular penchant for involving the CNS [106]. Nearly 50% of immunocompromised patients who develop listeriosis develop CNS disease [107], which can present as acute cerebritis or brain abscesses (Fig. 12.2). *Nocardia* species are filamentous bacteria that usually lead to pulmonary infections, of which over 30% develop CNS lesions; most commonly single or multiple abscesses. Many with CNS involvement are asymptomatic at the time of diagnosis, so routine brain imaging is recommended in all patients diagnosed with *Nocardia* [108].

Fungal

Cryptococcus neoformans is a cause of meningitis in immunocompromised hosts and leads to occasional infections in leukemic patients [109]. Fluconazole prophylaxis has limited this infection, but late disease can occur in transplant recipients. Similarly, *Candida* species ophthalmic infections (endophthalmitis or retinitis) can occur in leukemia patients undergoing chemotherapy or transplant, but CNS infections are almost universally associated with systemic fungemia. Resistant species, such as *C. krusei* and *C. glabrata*, should be considered in patients who develop CNS involvement while on prophylactic therapy [110].

Fig. 12.2 Patient presented with fever, seizures, dysarthria, and right-sided weakness. An MRI of the brain demonstrated an abscess (*yellow arrow*) with surrounding edema. Blood cultures were positive for gram-positive rods which were later indentified to be *Listeria monocytogenes.* Symptoms improved after institution of ampicillin and gentamicin therapy. The patient improved after a prolonged course of antibiotics

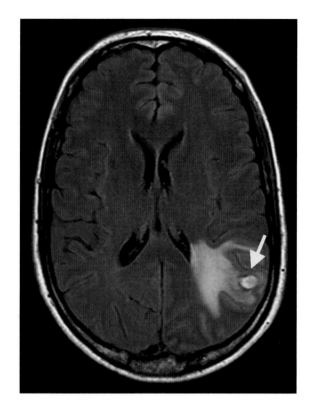

Mould infections, particularly *Aspergillus* species, can also lead to serious and life-threatening CNS infections. Involvement of the CNS usually develops from a primary pulmonary source, through hematogenous spread or through direct invasion from involved sinuses. Mould infections primarily lead to space-occupying lesions, but can also present as cerebral infarctions or meningitis [111, 112]. Retrospective reviews of brain abscesses in transplant patients suggest that *Aspergillus* is the most common cause [99, 113, 114] and that fungal etiologies make up close to 90% of episodes [113, 114]. While Aspergillus may be the most common fungus, CNS infection can also be caused by other opportunistic moulds such as the *Mucorales* (zygomyces) species [115, 116] and *Scedosporium* [117]. Rhinocerebral involvement and cavernous sinus involvement are unique presentations nearly always associated with the Mucorales [118]. Endemic moulds, such as *Histoplasma capsulatum* [119] and *Coccidiodomycosis immitis* [120], are infrequent and develop only in patients with travel or residence in areas of endemicity [121–123].

Viral

Latent viruses can cause CNS-related disease, particularly in patients undergoing HCT [124]. During the early posttransplant period, HHV-6 is the most common viral cause of CNS infection [94, 124]. HHV-6 reactivation usually occurs between 2 and

4 weeks posttransplant, and symptoms can range from mild delirium and cognitive dysfunction to seizures and encephalitis [125]. Varicella-zoster virus (VZV) is another neurotropic virus primarily associated with encephalitis, though vasculopathy can also be associated with CNS involvement [126]. Interestingly, although VZV reactivation usually presents with prominent skin involvement (herpes zoster), patients with CNS disease may present without rash [127, 128]. Herpes simplex (HSV) encephalitis can also occur in leukemia and transplant recipients, though patients are more likely to present with personality changes and focal abnormalities [129]. Additionally, both HSV and VZV can present with involvement in the otic branch presenting with unilateral facial paralysis, ear pain, and vesicles in the auditory canal and auricle (Ramsay Hunt syndrome) [130, 131]. CNS involvement of both VZV and HSV usually occurs only after the discontinuation of prophylactic acyclovir; such prophylaxis has not been shown to prevent HHV-6. Other latent herpesvirus infections, such as Epstein-Barr virus (EBV) [132] and cytomegalovirus (CMV) [133, 134], can also cause CNS disease and, in EBV's case, can be associated with both encephalitis and posttransplant lymphoproliferative disorder (PTLD) [37, 135].

The polyomaviruses, particularly JC virus, are less frequent CNS pathogens in this population. JC virus is the causative agent of progressive multifocal leukoencephalopathy (PML), which occurs late in the posttransplant period and presents with focal neurologic findings and altered mental status as a result of white matter demyelination [136–138]. Other viral pathogens such as West Nile virus [139, 140] and enteroviruses [141] cause sporadic cases of CNS disease.

Other Infections

Toxoplasmosis is most commonly found in patients who are seropositive prior to starting therapy [142], but has been rarely reported in patients who were seronegative [143, 144]. When toxoplasmosis does develop in the posttransplant period, nearly all cases are associated with CNS involvement [144]. Symptoms are varied, diagnosis is difficult, and outcomes are very poor [144, 145]. *Strongyloides stercoralis* hyperinfection, which occurs from a reactivation of a clinically silent infection, can lead to a polymicrobial meningitis and direct parasite invasion into the CNS [146, 147]. Patients with prior exposure to areas of high endemicity of Strongyloides are at risk, but this is a rare complication.

Diagnostics

The mainstay of any work-up for CNS-related symptoms is first and foremost a thorough neurologic exam. Early findings can be subtle and missed on cursory review, but a focal neurologic exam can identify subtle cranial nerve abnormalities, unsuspected confusion, and/or focal weakness. It is important to pay special attention to the oropharynx, sinuses, auditory canals, and nasal passageways, as lesions in these locations (e.g., a black eschar or vesicles) can suggest either a route of infection and/or a specific pathogen. Patients with nuchal rigidity, mental status changes, fever, and other classic signs for bacterial meningitis should be considered for urgent lumbar puncture and empiric antibiotics to avoid major delays in treatment.

Radiologic imaging is critical to assessing high-risk immunocompromised patients, as clinical symptoms vary in these patients. Both computed tomography (CT) and magnetic resonance imaging (MRI) provide important diagnostic data; an MRI provides better resolution, but CT scans are often more readily available. Radiologic imaging can evaluate for space-occupying lesions or evidence of increased intracranial pressure which would preclude cerebrospinal fluid (CSF) analyses. Specific radiologic manifestations of certain infections, such as herpes simplex (temporal lobe involvement), HHV-6 (mesial temporal lobes, limbic encephalitis) [148], and JC virus (single or multifocal white matter lesions without mass effect) [149], can be suggestive of the underlying diagnosis. These patients may also present with atypical findings on imaging. Toxoplasmosis for example, may not present with classic ring-enhancing lesions [150, 151]. Additionally, imaging can suggest other noninfectious etiologies which can lead to CNS symptoms. An excellent review of radiologic findings associated with hematopoietic transplantation is reviewed by Nishiguchi [151].

CSF analyses are critically important for a diagnosis. Standard cell counts, glucose, total protein as well as gram stain, cultures, polymerase chain reaction (PCR) testing, and molecular analyses can potentially lead to a diagnosis. Specific tests that can be considered during CSF analysis are listed in Table 12.3. Serologic tests can be beneficial in patients who are considered to be at risk for endemic mycoses or parasitic disease, and blood cultures can provide additional data for potential bacterial and fungal processes. Patients with symptoms at other locations (e.g., cough) should undergo additional imaging to help complete a diagnostic work-up. Other data to rule out other noninfectious etiologies should also be considered, such as drug levels to assess for CNS drug toxicity and CSF cytologic review and flow cytometry to assess for CNS involvement of leukemia if appropriate. Toxoplasmosis PCR from serum should be assessed in patients who are known to be seropositive for toxoplasmosis [152]. Finally, brain biopsy may be necessary in some rare cases to make the diagnosis.

Treatment

Due to the poor outcome of infections that occur in the CNS, it is important to consider early antimicrobial therapy while awaiting the results of diagnostic testing, as delay can lead to major morbidity with severe infections. Bacterial infections need aggressive IV therapy with duration dependent on the diagnosis (see Table 12.1). Dual therapy for CNS *Nocardia* species infections should be considered initially (e.g., trimethoprim/sulfamethoxazole and imipenem) and long-term therapy based on sensitivity testing

Table 12.2 Tests for patients with potential CNS infections[a]

	Primary	Secondary
Radiologic imaging	CT/MRI of the brain	Chest imaging
		Sinus imaging
		PET scans
Cerebrospinal fluid	Opening pressure[b]	Viral PCR
	CBC with differential	Adenovirus
	Glucose	CMV
	Total protein	EBV
	Gram stain	Enteroviral
	Bacterial and fungal cultures	JC virus
	Viral PCR	West Nile virus
	HHV-6	Molecular bacterial DNA analysis
	HSV[c]	AFB cultures/MTB-specific PCR
	VZV[c]	CSF cryptococcal antigen
	Cytology and flow cytometry	Toxoplasma PCR
	Save a tube for later testing	
Antigen testing	–	Serum cryptococcal antigen
		Serum galactomannan
		VDRL
Serologic testing	Toxoplasma serology	Coccidioides immunofixation
		Histoplasma urinary antigen
		Strongyloides antibody
Additional testing	Blood and urine cultures	Electroencephalogram (EEG)
	Neurologic exam	Ophthalmologic exam
	HHV-6 PCR from serum	Brain biopsy[e]
	Drug levels[d]	

Abbreviations: *CNS* central nervous system, *CT* computed tomography, *MRI* magnetic resonance imaging, *PET* positron emission tomography, *CBC* complete blood count, *PCR* polymerase chain reaction, *HHV-6* human herpesvirus-6, *HSV* herpes simplex virus, *VZV* varicella-zoster virus, *CMV* cytomegalovirus, *EBV* Epstein-Barr virus, *AFB* acid-fast bacilli, *MTB* mycobacterium tuberculosis, *VDRL* venereal disease research laboratory test for syphilis
[a]This list is *not* completely inclusive, and decisions should be made based on clinical symptoms and history. Primary and secondary options may be different depending on presentation
[b]Opening pressure should be determined at the time of lumbar puncture whenever possible
[c]May not be necessary in patients taking prophylactic acyclovir
[d]Drug levels will depend on patients' current medications
[e]Brain biopsy may be necessary in some cases to make the diagnosis, but this should be reserved for patients with severe and life-threatening symptoms when possible

once available. Length of therapy is dependent on CT resolution, but most feel that at least a year of therapy is needed [153]. Usual antimicrobial coverage for bacterial meningitis (vancomycin, cephalosporins, and aminoglycosides) will not treat *Listeria monocytogenes*. All immunosuppressed patients with presumed meningitis should have IV ampicillin added to the underlying empiric regimen. Patients with proven listeriosis require prolonged IV ampicillin therapy. *Aspergillus* CNS infections should be guided by sensitivity testing when possible, but usual treatment includes either voriconazole or lipid amphotericin B formulations; treatment guidelines are reviewed by Walsh et al. [154]. Voriconazole, in particular, is known to get excellent CNS penetration [155, 156]. Patients with CNS infection with any of the *Mucorales* species should be treated with either lipid amphotericin B formulations or posaconazole, but overall outcomes are poor [116]. Endemic fungal CNS infections' treatment options are reviewed in references by Wheat et al. [119], Galgiani et al. [120], and Perfect et al. [109]. HSV and VZV CNS infections require high-dose IV acyclovir, and patients with HHV-6 encephalitis should receive either IV foscarnet or IV ganciclovir [157]. Patients with toxoplasmosis should receive intensive therapy with pyrimethamine, sulfadiazine, and folinic acid or high-dose trimethoprim/sulfamethoxazole [158].

Sinopulmonary Infections

Signs and Symptoms

The sinopulmonary system is one of the most frequent sites of infection during leukemia therapy. Symptoms vary depending on the involved site, particularly since both upper and lower tract infections can occur. Classic symptom presentations, however, normally seen in immunocompetent patients are uncommon in this population. Upper tract infection symptoms often involve the sinuses and nasopharynx, including: rhinorrhea, sore throat, facial pain/pressure, headaches, cough, disturbances in taste and smell, among others. Classic symptoms that are consistent with the common cold or sinusitis are not infrequent in mild cases, but the development of bloody/ black nasal discharge, lesions on the palate, facial weakness, periorbital erythema, or proptosis are signs of severe invasive disease.

With lower tract parenchymal involvement, symptoms may include cough, sputum production, shortness of breath, and wheezing. Focal chest pain or hemoptysis are more ominous signs of an invasive fungal infection, and hypoxia can be a harbinger of the development of acute respiratory distress. Still, specific symptoms in transplant are not always pathognomonic for a specific infectious etiology, and patients receiving corticosteroids may have less prominent symptoms. Occasional patients may be asymptomatic with lesions found only on imaging. Noninfectious etiologies such as diffuse alveolar hemorrhage, idiopathic pneumonia syndrome, cryptogenic organizing pneumonia, and drug toxicity can cause symptoms and even radiographic changes that mimic infections, making a prompt diagnosis even more challenging [159, 160].

Differential Diagnosis

Bacterial

Numerous bacterial pathogens can lead to sinusitis. In immunocompetent hosts, sinusitis is caused by predominantly respiratory pathogens such as *S. pneumoniae*, *Haemophilus influenzae*, and *Moraxella catarrhalis*, but in transplantation, other

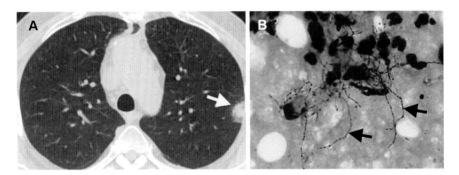

Fig. 12.3 (**a**) A patient found to have a 2-cm pulmonary nodule on a routine CT of the chest (*white arrow*). Standard infectious work-up, including bronchoalveolar lavage, was negative. (**b**) Video-assisted thoracic surgical (*VATS*) biopsy of nodule demonstrated weakly staining gram-positive branching filaments that were partially acid-fast on Kinyoun staining (*black arrows*) consistent with *Nocardia* species, and cultures from lesion grew *Nocardia nova*

GNR, resistant organisms, and polymicrobial infections are more frequent etiologies [75, 161]. Patients with preexisting disease or those with a history of chronic sinus infections prior to transplant are likely at higher risk [162]. Specific pathogens cannot always be identified, and most patients are treated empirically with broad-spectrum antibiotics.

Pneumonia can be caused by a variety of bacterial organisms in leukemic patients, although after transplant, bacterial pneumonias are less frequent [163]. Patients with prolonged neutropenia or undergoing salvage chemotherapy are not surprisingly at higher risk for developing this complication. There are a wide variety of gram-positive and GNR species that can lead to pneumonia in this immunocompromised population, but providers should be aware of specific bacterial pathogens that are more specific to these patients. The gram-positive filamentous bacteria *Nocardia* is an opportunistic infection that after inhalation can develop into pulmonary disease. *Nocardia* are usually resistant to standard antimicrobial prophylaxis regimens, are more frequent in patients not on trimethoprim/sulfamethoxazole prophylaxis [164] and those receiving steroids [165]. *Nocardia* species can have varied presentations in transplantation, but most frequently appear as nodular pulmonary disease; some patients may have asymptomatic nodules found only on imaging (Fig. 12.3) [165]. *Legionella* species can also occur in posttransplant recipients, though nonpneumophila species, particularly *L. micdadei*, are more frequent [166–168]. *Legionella* species can present with lung nodules, mimicking fungal infections, or as pulmonary infiltrates. *Mycoplasma* and other atypical organisms are rare [169, 170]. *Mycobacterium avium-intracellulare* (MAI) is the most frequently isolated mycobacteria from pulmonary specimens in HCT patients, but since many have colonization, not all warrant treatment [55].

Fungal

Fungal infections are one of the most common and vexing problems in patients with leukemia and HCT, and most lead to sinopulmonary infections. Fungal sinusitis can particularly be troubling due to the proximity of the infection and risk for invasion into the CNS and can present initially with similar features to bacterial cases. A high index of suspicion is needed to prevent life-threatening complications particularly in patients who worsen after treatment for bacterial sinusitis or in patients on steroids. *Aspergillus* species are the most common cause of fungal sinusitis [171, 172], but less frequent fungal organisms, such as *Scopulariopsis* [173] and *Paecilomyces* [174], among others, can also lead to sinus disease. The Mucorales are notorious for leading to life-threatening sinus disease [115, 116, 118, 175].

Pulmonary fungal infections are even more common in this patient population, where invasive Aspergillus remains the most common etiology [176–178]. Patients with known GVHD, high-dose steroids, iron overload, CMV infection, and prolonged neutropenia are at increased risk for fungal infections [179–184]. Iron overload is particularly associated with the Mucorales, which may also be more prevalent in patients who are treated or undergo prophylaxis with voriconazole [185, 186]. Because of the severity of immunosuppression, multiple other fungal species manifest as pulmonary disease in hematopoietic transplant recipients [187, 188]. Yeast less commonly causes pulmonary disease, with the exception of *Cryptococcus* species, which can lead to pulmonary nodules [189]. Although resistant *Candida* species can be isolated from bronchoalveolar lavage (BAL) cultures, Candida pneumonia is a rare complication, even more so with the addition of standardized antifungal prophylaxis [190].

The other unique pulmonary fungal pathogen in these patients is PCP. PCP is more common in patients on high-dose steroids and in those who do not receive or discontinue trimethoprim/sulfamethoxazole prophylaxis [191, 192]. Disease usually occurs as a late complication due to current prevention strategies [191]. Even with appropriate treatment and diagnostics, patients who develop PCP can develop major complications [193].

Viral

Multiple viral pathogens lead to sinopulmonary complications during therapy for leukemia. These break down into two main categories: reactivation from latency and community acquisition. Latent herpesviruses, particularly CMV, can lead to invasive pulmonary disease in transplant recipients. Patients typically present with shortness of breath and hypoxia, and most have evidence of CMV reactivation from other sites. Risk factors for the development of CMV pneumonia include: lymphopenia, GVHD, and high-dose steroids, among others [194]. Patients who undergo umbilical cord blood transplant or T-cell depletion are at significantly higher risk [195, 196]. Early CMV pneumonia/pneumonitis is seen within the first 3 months posttransplantation during the period of greatest immunosuppression. Late CMV disease occurs more than 3 months after HSCT, and likely as a result of residual deficits in cell-mediated immunity [194,

197, 198]. HSV, VZV, and other herpesviruses can also rarely lead to pulmonary complications in patients [199]. EBV-associated posttransplant related lymphoproliferative disease (PTLD) can manifest in the lungs as pulmonary nodules [200]. Adenovirus can be latent in the lung and reactivate during the posttransplant period [201], leading to severe pulmonary complications and dissemination [202, 203].

Respiratory viral pathogens are the most frequent sinopulmonary infection in these patients, with up to 30% of patients developing at least one infection (mostly upper respiratory events) during follow-up [204, 205]. These viruses can cause a spectrum of disease, including upper respiratory infection, pneumonia, and/or even late airflow obstruction [206], and are a cause of significant morbidity and mortality [205]. Influenza A and B, parainfluenza virus, metapneumovirus, and RSV can all be associated with both upper and severe lower tract disease. Influenza viruses and RSV are seasonal, while parainfluenza can occur year round. Community-acquired adenovirus can also be associated with high rates of mortality when associated with lower tract disease [207]. Rhinovirus and coronavirus are the most common respiratory viral infections, often limited to only upper respiratory disease [204]. They have been rarely associated with pulmonary complications in transplant recipients [208]. Other novel and emerging respiratory pathogens' (e.g., human bocavirus, WU and KI polyomaviruses) epidemiology in this population has not been well described to date [209].

Diagnostics

Radiologic imaging of the sinopulmonary system has become an important part of any diagnostic evaluation in this population. Bacterial, viral, and fungal infections can opacify sinus spaces on plain film or CT, but more invasive findings, such as bony erosion, suggest fungal sinusitis. Bacterial infections typically present as lobar consolidations or infiltrates. Fungal infections typically present on CT as solitary or multiple pulmonary nodules, and a classic "halo sign" on CT is very suggestive of an underlying fungal nodule (Fig. 12.4) [210, 211]. Lobar consolidation and cavitary disease are less frequent CT presentations [210]. International criteria for the diagnosis of fungal infections, which include radiologic findings, can help providers determine which patients should receive antifungal therapy [212]. Lower tract viral infections primarily present with diffuse interstitial disease or ground-glass infiltrates; other infections such as PCP can have a similar appearance. Pulmonary consolidation [213] and nodular disease [214] have also been described for viral infections (e.g., CMV, HMPV). Since multiple pathogens can occur in a single patient, radiologic findings are only suggestive and need confirmatory testing.

Noninvasive modalities are available for viral and fungal infections. Serum galactomannan (GM) testing has improved diagnostics specifically for *Aspergillus* species and has become an important tool for screening [215–217]. The serum $(1 \rightarrow 3)$-beta-D-glucan assay has also been used for detecting fungal infections in transplant patients [218]. Similar to GM, this assay does not identify *Mucorales* species but may be useful in diagnosing PCP [219]. Serum cryptococcal antigen testing can be useful in patients where *Cryptococcus* is a diagnostic possibility.

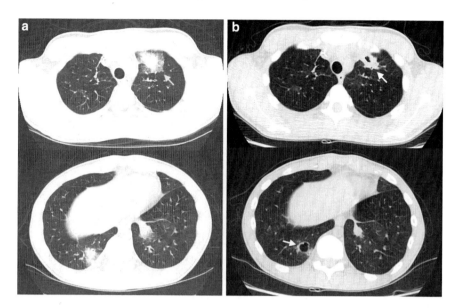

Fig. 12.4 Patient with acute myelogenous leukemia found to have pulmonary nodules during a work-up for neutropenic fever. (**a**) *Upper panel* demonstrates large nodule surrounded by white zone of ground glass which is reflective of a "halo sign" (*yellow arrow*). The patient was diagnosed with *Aspergillus fumigatus* pneumonia after bronchoalveolar lavage. (**b**) The same patient after 2 months of voriconazole therapy with the formation of posttherapy cavitation (*white arrows*)

CMV and adenovirus pneumonia are typically associated with dissemination, so viremia is often found during and before pulmonary infection. Upper respiratory viral infections can be detected by a number of laboratory modalities, including culture, direct fluorescent antigen (DFA) testing, and other rapid commercial antigen detection kits. Comprehensive or multiplex PCR panels are becoming increasingly utilized at many centers, including ours, since these techniques offer greater sensitivity than standard modalities and can detect coinfection [220, 221]. The fact that many of these patients develop prolonged shedding, particularly those on steroids [222], also suggest that PCR-based methods may enhance infection control practices.

Invasive diagnostic modalities are also needed to diagnose patients, and BAL should be considered in all patients with pulmonary findings [216]. Cultures, cytology, and antigen testing (e.g., GM from BAL) [215] can all provide additional microbiologic evidence to avoid the institution of empiric therapies (see Table 12.2). Additionally, this modality may help to evaluate other nonfungal infections, separate specific pathogens from each other, detect coinfections, and provide samples for antimicrobial resistance testing. While PCR-based strategies for specific fungal pathogens are still under development, PCR-based respiratory testing for viral pathogens from BAL samples is becoming standard at many centers [209, 220]. PCP is classically diagnosed from induced sputum samples in other immunocompromised populations (e.g., HIV); however, bronchoscopy may enhance diagnosis in transplant recipients due to the low burden of disease [223, 224]. CMV shell vial assays and cultures from BAL are also necessary criteria for the diagnosis of CMV pneumonia [225].

Table 12.3 Bronchoalveolar lavage infectious work-up[a]

Bacterial	Gram stain
	Quantitative culture
	Special media for specific pathogens (*Legionella/Nocardia*)
	AFB stain and culture
Fungal	KOH preparation with calcofluor[b]
	Cytologic review
	Fungal specific cultures
	Galactomannan antigen by EIA
	PCR for *Aspergillus* or other fungal species[c]
Viral	CMV shell vial
	RSV shell vial
	Viral cultures
	Respiratory DFAs (*rapid*)
	– Adenovirus, influenza A and B, metapneumovirus, parainfluenza, and RSV
	Respiratory PCR testing
	– Adenovirus, bocavirus, coronavirus[d], influenza A and B, metapneumovirus, parainfluenza[e], RSV, and rhinovirus

Abbreviations: *AFB* acid-fast bacillus, *KOH* potassium hydroxide, *EIA* enzyme immunoassay, *PCR* polymerase chain reaction, *CMV* cytomegalovirus, *RSV* respiratory syncytial virus, *DFA* direct fluorescent antibody
[a]These are current strategies used at our center but may not be appropriate at all centers
[b]The KOH preparation dissolves keratin and other cellular in the specimen; calcofluor is a flores-cent dye that binds to polysaccharides in chitin of fungi
[c]PCR for fungal pathogens are not standardized and not currently considered part of standard diag-nostic testing for fungal diagnoses
[d]Specific coronavirus species associated with clinical disease
[e]Includes parainfluenza (1,2,3, and 4)

A microbiologic diagnosis is important to allow targeted treatment and can help determine the duration of therapy. When a diagnosis of a pulmonary process is not made by BAL, video-assisted thoracoscopic biopsy (VATS) or CT-guided biopsy may be necessary to determine the cause of the pulmonary symptoms. For sinus infections, Otolaryngology evaluation should be obtained in all high-risk patients with sinus symptoms, as early nasal/sinus endoscopy with visual inspection, and biopsy can allow for more prompt diagnosis.

Treatment

Bacterial pneumonias should be treated when possible as directed by cultures and sensitivities (Table 12.1). Treatment guidelines for community-acquired pneumonia are reviewed by Mandell [226], and recommendations for treatment of nosocomial or ventilator-associated pneumonia are reviewed by the American Thoracic Society and the Infectious Diseases Society of America [227]. In particular, *Pseudomonas* pneumonia may require prolonged treatment due to the high risk of fatal relapse [71]. Similar to CNS disease, *Nocardia* pulmonary disease should be treated with trimethoprim/sulfamethoxazole or based on microbiologic sensitivities for at least

6 months [108]. Patients with *Legionella* pneumonia should receive 3 weeks of a respiratory fluoroquinolone or azithromycin.

Aspergillus pulmonary infections are most frequently treated with voriconazole or lipid amphotericin B formulations; treatment guidelines are reviewed by Walsh [154]. There is a lack of randomized clinical trials comparing different agents, and the role of combination therapy is controversial; results from a future trial addressing combination therapy are forthcoming. Patients should typically undergo therapy until pulmonary nodules have completely resolved or stabilized for 2–3 months of immunosuppressive therapy. Patients with *Mucorales* pulmonary infections should be treated with either lipid amphotericin B formulations or posaconazole; when possible, sensitivity testing can help tailor therapy. Cardiothoracic surgery consultation should be considered in patients failing therapy and can be considered as adjunctive treatment for patients with solitary fungal nodules. Treatment of less frequent fungal infections (e.g., *Scedosporium* species) should be based on sensitivity testing. Endemic fungal CNS infections' treatment options are reviewed in references by Wheat et al. [119], Galgiani et al. [120], and Perfect et al. [109].

Patients who develop pulmonary CMV should receive IV ganciclovir or foscarnet, with the addition of intravenous immunoglobulin (IVIG) for at least 5 weeks; treatment options are reviewed by Boeckh [19]. Adenovirus pneumonia has no approved therapy, but many centers will attempt IV cidofovir and IVIG, although neither have been studied prospectively [228, 229]. Treatment options for patients with influenza are reviewed by Casper [230] but usually include oseltamivir or inhaled zanamivir as primary therapy. Alternate combination therapy can be considered in patients with life-threatening infections [230], particularly since the development of resistance can occur during therapy [29]. RSV is responsive to aerosolized ribavirin, which has been shown to reduce mortality from lower tract disease [231]. Survival may be improved when aerosolized ribavirin is used in combination therapy with intravenous immunoglobulin or palivizumab [29, 205]. Few options exist for treatment of other viral respiratory pathogens, so although no randomized data exist, oral or inhaled ribavirin can be considered in patients with parainfluenza [232] or metapneumovirus [233].

Cardiovascular

Signs and Symptoms

Cardiac infections are relatively infrequent in patients who undergo therapy for leukemia. A diagnostic clue for a cardiovascular infection is the development of persistently positive blood cultures. Patients who receive appropriate antimicrobial therapy and have continued positive cultures after removal of all hardware (e.g., central catheters) should be evaluated for a cardiac or vascular source of infection (e.g., endocarditis, aortitis, or infected thrombophlebitis). Additionally, patients with cardiovascular infections can present with tachycardia, arrhythmias, acute heart block, heart failure or myocardial infarction, painful phlebitis or limb swelling.

Bacterial and Fungal

The two most common infections associated with cardiopulmonary system are septic thrombophlebitis and endocarditis. Septic thrombophlebitis typically involves the development of bacteremia or fungemia that infects a preexisting thrombus, typically at sites of line placement. *Candida* species are commonly associated with this phenomenon, but any bacteria can lead to this complication [234]. Endocarditis in this population is an uncommon outcome following transplantation. These cases are often due to *Streptococcus*, *Staphylococcus*, or *Enterococcal* species, but other rare GNRs and atypical organisms have occasionally been reported [235, 236]; nearly all cases involve the right side of the heart unless patients have known underlying valvular pathology [235]. Candida or other fungal endocarditis is rare but associated with high rates of morbidity and mortality [237–239]. Interestingly, non-infectious etiologies of endocardial masses (thrombi or marantic changes) can lead to similar symptoms in this population [236, 240]. Invasive fungal infections of the myocardium can also occur, but most are associated with primary pulmonary involvement or dissemination [241, 242]. Rare bacterial and fungal processes can lead to purulent pericarditis [243, 244].

Viral

Viral cardiac complications are uncommon in patients being treated for leukemia. Rare cases of herpesviruses and sporadic community-acquired viral infections and pericarditis or myocarditis have been reported [128, 245–248]. Noninfectious etiologies and adverse drug side effects are significantly more likely as causes of inflammatory heart disease [249, 250].

Diagnosis

Blood cultures remain a staple for the diagnosis of cardiovascular infections. Patients with recurrent bacteremia either during or immediately after completing their antibiotic therapy should be considered for imaging to rule out septic thrombophlebitis. Ultrasound evaluation of veins near either the site of a line placement or involving an edematous limb can help identify suspicious thrombi. Patients who have clinical symptoms concerning for endocarditis should undergo an electrocardiogram and echocardiography. Transthoracic echocardiography can be helpful in diagnosing right-sided endocarditis, but transesophageal echocardiography has higher sensitivity for left-sided lesions and should be pursued in those who are considered high risk [251]. Guidelines for the diagnosis, treatment, and management of infective endocarditis can be found in Baddour [251]. Cardiac MRI may be useful in diagnosing invasive fungal infections [252], but biopsy is the gold standard for diagnosis. Many patients with invasive cardiac mould infections are only diagnosed at autopsy.

Treatment

Patients with infected thrombophlebitis should receive extended antibiotic therapy that is based on antimicrobial sensitivity testing of the organism. In addition to prolonged antibiotic therapy, anticoagulation or surgical thrombus removal may be necessary for cure. Patients with endocarditis need appropriate antibiotics for 4–6 weeks following bacterial clearance. Patients who develop additional complications such as heart failure, or who fail antibiotic therapy may need valve replacement. Patients with Candida or other fungal endocarditis need cardiothoracic surgical consultation as few, if any, recover without surgical valve replacement. Treatment and follow-up of patients with endocarditis are reviewed in detail by Baddour [251]. Patients with invasive cardiac fungal infections have a poor prognosis, but antifungal therapy should be attempted.

Gastrointestinal/Hepatobiliary

Signs and Symptoms

Gastrointestinal (GI) symptoms are frequent during the treatment for leukemia as a consequence of chemotherapy, adverse reactions, GVHD, and infections. Diarrhea, for example, occurs in nearly 80% of patients at some during the posttransplant period [253]. Not surprisingly, it can be difficult to separate infectious from noninfectious etiologies. Typical GI symptoms associated with infections are abdominal or perirectal pain, diarrhea, nausea vomiting, dysphagia, or GI bleeding. Signs of an infectious GI process can also include elevated temperature, tachycardia, jaundice, and liver enzyme abnormalities, but many of these are also seen in noninfectious etiologies such as GVHD or sinusoidal obstruction syndrome [254].

Bacterial

Bacterial GI complications can occur during treatment of leukemia and during the transplant process. Most community-acquired bacterial causes for diarrhea, such as *Salmonella* and *Shigella*, occur only sporadically due to limited oral intake, less frequent exposure, and to standard prophylactic antibiotic therapy [255]. A more frequent infectious etiology for diarrhea is *Clostridium difficile* infection.

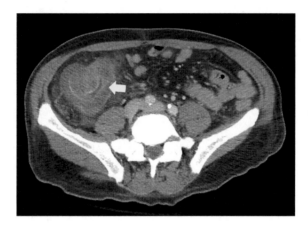

Fig. 12.5 Patient approximately 10 days following induction chemotherapy for acute myeloge-nous leukemia developed increasing right-sided abdominal pain, fever, and shortness of breath. Underwent CT scan of the abdomen which demonstrated bowel wall thickening and edema throughout the cecum and ascending colon with surrounding fat stranding (*yellow arrow*), consistent with neutropenic enterocolitis (typhlitis). Blood cultures from the day of admission were positive for *C. septicum*. The patient improved with broad-spectrum antibiotic therapy and did not need surgical intervention

The use of broad-spectrum antibiotic therapy and prolonged exposure to inpatient care increase the risk for *C. difficile*. Usually *C. difficile*–associated diarrhea occurs within the first 30–40 days posttransplant [253, 256], but patients are at risk through the transplant process. Episodes of *C. difficile* that occur during neutropenia can develop into life-threatening disease [257].

Neutropenic enterocolitis (typhlitis) presents with the triad of right lower quadrant pain, diarrhea, and fever; patients with severe disease may have rebound tenderness and signs of peritonitis (Fig. 12.5) [258]. This condition involves the cecum and is related to loss of integrity of the bowel wall and subsequent bacterial invasion [258]. Classically, this condition is associated with *Clostridium septicum* but likely involves other anaerobic organisms as well [259]. Perirectal abscesses can occur during early conditioning and mucositis, as neutropenic patients may present with minimal swelling or erythema, a high index of suspicion is needed in patients with rectal pain. Necrotizing fasciitis should be ruled out in patients with perineal involvement (see Skin and Soft Tissue section). Intra-abdominal and hepatic abscesses are infrequent.

Fungal

Oral candidiasis (thrush) was a frequent complication following transplantation, but is much less common with the addition of fluconazole to prevention strategies. Thrush can occur as a result of azole-resistant species. Candida esophagitis is less frequent as it is primarily due to *C. albicans* [260] which is reliably sensitive to fluconazole [261]. *Candida* species, primarily *C. albicans*, can also present as involvement in the liver as hepatosplenic candidiasis. Patients with hepatosplenic candidiasis acquire the disease during periods of neutropenia but may develop fever, right upper quadrant pain, and increasing liver function tests only after neutrophil recovery [262]. Patients with hepatosplenic candidiasis do not normally have detectable candidemia, and nearly all cases are thought to be due to *C. albicans* [262]. Similar to other invasive Candida complications, hepatosplenic candidiasis has become less common since the addition of standardized fluconazole prophylaxis.

Mould involvement of the gut can be a devastating complication. Most mould infections in the GI tract are thought to be acquired from ingestion during periods of high risk. Unfortunately, these invasive infections are difficult to diagnosis premortem, due to nonspecific symptoms and imaging (Fig. 12.6). Patients typically present with abdominal pain, but others can have only fever or nonspecific findings; GI bleeding or perforation can be late signs of invasive involvement. The most frequent GI moulds are *Aspergillus* species and the Mucorales which can both lead to disease throughout the GI tract [263, 264] including the liver [265]. Clinical diagnosis can be very challenging, and such a delay leads to high rates of mortality; many are diagnosed only at autopsy [263].

Viral

Herpesviruses, particularly CMV, can lead to invasive disease throughout the GI tract. CMV GI disease in transplant recipients resembles gut GVHD and, not infrequently, is found on biopsy in conjunction with a gut GVHD diagnosis. Patients typically present with abdominal pain, diarrhea (lower tract), nausea, and early satiety (upper tract); most patients are either on high-dose steroids or are T-cell-depleted transplant recipients [194]. The majority of patients have CMV detected in the blood at the time of diagnosis, but since a significant proportion have no blood dissemination, a negative plasma PCR does not preclude invasive CMV disease. GI disease is the most common site of late CMV disease [266]. CMV rarely leads to severe hepatitis [267]. HSV can cause erosive esophagitis [268] and hepatitis [269], but the routine use of acyclovir prophylaxis limits these complications.

VZV reactivation can lead to GI disease. Visceral varicella-zoster is unique to this population and is a life-threatening condition that necessitates treatment with high-dose IV acyclovir. This complication must be considered in any leukemic or transplant patient who presents with the triad of abdominal pain, increasing liver function tests, and hyponatremia [270, 271]. Patients with visceral involvement can also present with hepatitis and pancreatitis as a component of the diagnosis [271]. Importantly, unlike most episodes of VZV reactivation, this presentation is not always associated with the rash or skin lesions usually associated with herpes zoster [272]. Empiric therapy should be started immediately if this diagnosis is suspected.

EBV in posttransplant recipients can cause PTLD in high-risk patients and occurs in about 1% of all HCT patients [273]. PTLD can present anywhere but has a predilection for the gut and liver. Symptoms vary by location, but GI disease can be challenging to diagnose. Risk factors for the development of EBV-associated complications include T-cell depletion, EBV serologic mismatch, splenectomy [274], mismatched or unrelated transplantation, and the development of chronic GVHD. 200 PTLD peaks around 2–3 months posttransplant, and most are polymorphic disease [200]. Umbilical cord blood transplant recipients may be more likely to develop early malignant monomorphic disease [275]. Interestingly, patients over the age of 50 have an increased rate of PTLD [200].

Adenovirus most frequently leads to the development of diarrhea, and in more severe cases lower tract GI bleeding and dissemination [229, 276]. There is a strong correlation between the detection of viremia and the development of invasive disease [277]. Adenovirus reactivation occurs most frequently in patients with mismatched grafts and in those who have received T-cell-depleted transplants [278]. In children, adenovirus occurs more frequently, and earlier posttransplant; invasive disease is more prevalent [279]. Adenovirus can lead to hepatitis and fulminant hepatic failure [280, 281].

Norovirus (Norwalk agent) has been increasingly recognized as a major cause of morbidity and mortality in cancer patients [282, 283]. These patients are more likely to develop chronic diarrhea which has been associated with significant weight loss and need for parenteral nutrition [282, 284]. Patients who develop norovirus from the community are likely to shed the virus for extended periods of time [284], making infection control practices critical for prevention [285]. Rotavirus is also recognized as a potential pathogen [286, 287].

Finally, hepatitis B (HBV) can be a major problem in patients with prior exposure. During treatment for leukemia, patients with quiescent HBV (HBsAg positive or those with occult HBV) can develop reactivation with the development of hepatitis and even fulminant liver failure [288]. Prophylaxis and treatment for patients with a prior history of HBV have led to fewer complications related to the disease [289–291]. While, hepatitis C (HCV) is also known to cause long-term complications in transplant recipients [292], it may also be associated with the development of sinusoidal obstruction syndrome [293].

Diagnosis

Patients who develop GI symptoms, particularly diarrhea and abdominal pain, should be evaluated for infectious etiologies. Routine bacterial cultures and parasite examinations are rarely useful as these pathogens are uncommon [286]. Samples however should routinely be sent for *C. difficile* testing regardless of prior antibiotic exposure. Elevated liver transaminases and alkaline phosphatase, and rising bilirubin, can also suggest potential etiologies [294]. Viral testing including adenovirus PCR, norovirus PCR, and rotavirus EIA from stool can be considered for patients. All patients with known HBV exposure should have a HBV PCR at baseline, and if they develop severe transaminitis, have it repeated. Additionally, although CMV, EBV, and adenovirus PCRs from serum can suggest an underlying diagnosis, VZV and HSV PCRs from serum/plasma in the face of symptoms consistent with visceral zoster or acute hepatitis are of critical importance for diagnosis. Serum GM can be sent in patients who are felt to be at risk for gut-related *Aspergillus* but may be falsely positive in patients with severe mucosal breakdown or in those receiving piperacillin-tazobactam therapy [295, 296]. All patients receiving intensive chemotherapy should have baseline serologic testing for viral hepatitis.

In patients with abdominal pain, CT scans of the abdomen and pelvis can help evaluate potential etiologies, assess for perforation or abscess, and may help to identify diseases with classic appearance on CT. Hepatosplenic candidiasis, for example, presents with multiple hypodense "bull's eye" lesions in the liver and spleen which are indicative of Candida abscesses within the liver [294]. Neutropenic enterocolitis typically demonstrates inflammation and stranding around the cecum (Fig. 12.5). Unfortunately, GI mould infections may be difficult to diagnose from imaging [264], with many diagnosed following death (Fig. 12.6). Intervention may also be important in the work-up of patient's symptoms. In patients at risk for GVHD, gastroenterology consultation is suggested to evaluate by endoscopy. Endoscopic visualization and biopsies can help differentiate between viral infections (CMV and adenovirus) and GVHD and may detect other infectious lesions [297]. It is important to stress that more than one diagnostic method for CMV detection is needed in the GI tract [298] and that CMV PCR still needs to be validated as a diagnostic entity for the diagnosis. Surgical intervention or liver biopsy may be necessary particularly in patients without a clear diagnosis or if CT findings are suspicious for a fungal process. Patients with severe neutropenic enterocolitis or those with severe abdominal pain may need emergent surgical consultation [258].

Treatment

Patients who develop *C. difficile* infections should be treated with either oral metronidazole or oral vancomycin (Table 12.1). Patients with severe infections may have better outcomes with oral vancomycin [299]. Patients with neutropenic enterocolitis and perirectal infections should receive broad-spectrum antibiotics covering anaerobic species (e.g., metronidazole) and GNRs. Surgical consultation should be pursued in all patients with these conditions, as some patients may need early surgical intervention [258]. Patients with invasive Candida infections should receive prolonged fluconazole or echinocandin therapy, and patients diagnosed with invasive moulds should receive mould-active therapy depending on the pathogen identified. Voriconazole, lipid amphotericin B formulations, or posaconazole are the most commonly used agents. All patients should also have a surgical consultation.

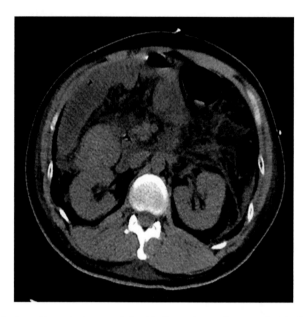

Fig. 12.6 Patient posttransplant presented with *Enterobacter* bacteremia. On broad-spectrum antibiotics, continued to be febrile with increasing abdominal distention and increasing bilirubin despite aggressive antibiotics. Underwent CT scan of the abdomen which demonstrated moderate ascites, but no pneumoperitoneum or obstruction was identified (*above*). The patient developed respiratory distress, anasarca, and dense pulmonary infiltrates. At autopsy found to have disseminated intra-abdominal *Rhizopus* species. Mould invaded into celiac axis (with thrombosis) and also involved liver, diaphragm, stomach, pancreas, spleen, and adrenal glands

CMV infections should be treated with ganciclovir or foscarnet and HSV/VZV infections with high-dose IV acyclovir. Patients who develop PTLD after HCT are often treated with rituximab but may need additional chemotherapy [300, 301]. Few options exist for norovirus therapy, but nitazoxanide may be an option [302]. Treatment of HBV is reviewed in detail by Lok [303] but typically entails lamivudine, entecavir, or adefovir.

Genitourinary

Signs and Symptoms

Patients with genitourinary (GU) infections during treatment for leukemia often present with symptoms that are similar to immunocompetent patients: urinary frequency, dysuria, flank pain, hematuria, and fevers. These patients are at risk for additional complications and are more likely to develop renal dysfunction and invasive infections. Additionally, side effects of numerous medications and chemotherapy agents (e.g., cyclophosphamide and calcineurin inhibitors) can lead to additional GU toxicity. The need for urinary catheters in highly compromised patients may also increase risk. The combination of adverse drug toxicity, GVHD, sepsis, and subsequent multiorgan failure can lead to renal failure and the need for acute renal replacement therapy [304, 305].

Differential Diagnosis

Bacterial

Patients receiving standard therapy for leukemia and patients undergoing transplantation are at risk for developing urinary tract infections (UTI). The use of standard prophylactic antibiotics has limited UTIs, somewhat, but has led to the development of more resistant nosocomial infections particularly in patients who have prolonged hospitalizations and are catheterized [306, 307]. Patients undergoing leukemia therapy have *Escherichia coli* and *Klebsiella pneumonia* as the predominant species detected from urinary samples [307]. In patients with urinary catheters, it is important to separate colonization from symptomatic infection [308]. Patients can also develop complications in the kidney from septic emboli, and more invasive infections of the kidneys and bladder can occur but are infrequent.

Fungal

Fungal infections of pelvic organs are a relatively infrequent phenomenon. Candida is the most frequent organism to infect the GU tract, with urinary tract infections being the typical presentation, but invasive candidal abscesses can occur during episodes of candidemia [309]. Patients who develop candiduria typically have anatomic abnormalities of the GU tract, have been treated with broad-spectrum antibiotics, or have a urinary catheter [310]. Candidal organisms can also lead to asymptomatic colonization of urinary catheters and, in some cases, invasive disease.

GU tract infections are an uncommon manifestation of mould infections. Patients with Aspergillus infection will not infrequently develop parenchymal involvement with disseminated infections [242], but occasionally they can be seen as isolated infections in the bladder [311] or kidney [312, 313]. The Mucorales and other less common fungal species have also been rarely reported to cause invasive disease in the genitourinary tract [314, 315].

Viral

BK virus frequently reactivates in the genitourinary system during immunosuppression and can lead to the development of hemorrhagic cystitis (HC) [316].

Many patients who have detectable BK virus in the urine may be asymptomatic, but those that develop BK-associated HC present with frequent urination, flank pain, frank hematuria, and, in severe cases, the development of severe inflammation and clotting in the bladder that can lead to urinary obstruction [317, 318]. Rarely, BK can lead to nephritis in HCT recipients [319]. Interestingly, the immune response to BK may play an important role in the development of BK-associated symptoms [320]. Adenovirus also leads to HC [320, 321] but is a more common cause of nephritis than BK [322]. Unlike BK virus, risk factors for the development of invasive adenovirus include major changes in immune function, including T-cell depletion [202, 320]. Adenovirus genitourinary infections are also known to be more common in children and in patients with mismatched grafts [202, 229].

Diagnosis

Standard urinalysis and urine and blood cultures are important components of the work-up for patients with urinary symptoms. Urine culture results must be interpreted with caution in patients with urinary catheters, as separating colonization versus invasive disease can be challenging (reviewed by Nicolle) [308]. Viral PCRs for adenovirus and BK, from both blood and urine, can be helpful in evaluating patients with either HC and/or renal failure. A BK viral load in serum $\geq 10,000$ copies/mL may predict patients with BK-associated HC [323]. Ultrasound and CT imaging may also help in determining invasive fungal infections. If there is concern for possible nephritis or fungal infection, kidney biopsy or bladder cystoscopy may be necessary to make a definitive diagnosis.

Treatment

Bacterial infections typically require focused therapy based on sensitivity testing, but length of therapy depends on the severity of infection (Table 12.1). Patients with catheters should have them replaced prior to starting therapy if possible. Candida infections should be treated with fluconazole, echinocandin therapy, or lipid amphotericin B formulations, depending on sensitivity testing. Amphotericin bladder washes are used by some centers as adjunctive therapy or for patients with known colonization [324]. Patients with invasive mould infections should receive voriconazole, lipid amphotericin B formulations, or posaconazole, depending on the pathogen identified; all patients should also have a urology consultation.

BK-virus-related disease is difficult to treat, particularly since reductions in immunosuppression are not possible. In patients with severe disease, cidofovir, leflunomide, IVIG, and fluoroquinolones have all been suggested as possible therapeutic options, but no randomized trials exist [325–327]. Adenovirus HC and nephritis are difficult to treat, but IV cidofovir can be attempted [328].

Skin and Soft Tissue

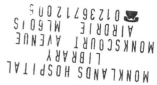

Signs and Symptoms

Leukemia patients can present with a myriad of skin and soft tissue manifestations that can be clues to an underlying infectious etiology. When examining transplant patients and those receiving therapy for leukemia, it is important to do a good skin exam. Cutaneous infections can present in a wide variety of visual appearances as nodules, ulceration, eschars, petechiae, rash/erythema, and/or pustules. Most patients present with fever, but pain suggests a more invasive process. Depending on the appearance and distribution, cutaneous findings can be helpful in making a diagnosis (e.g., dermatomal herpes zoster). Many important noninfectious etiologies such as drug side effects, GVHD, leukemia cutis [329], and neutrophilic dermatosis (Sweet's syndrome) [330] can mimic infectious etiologies. Regardless, any notable lesions or rashes should be promptly evaluated.

Bacterial

Cellulitis is a common manifestation of bacterial infections. The majority of cellulitis cases are due to *Streptococcus* and *Staphylococcus* species, but more frequently, no bacterial etiology is identified. Certain bacterial species present with specific skin manifestations. *Pseudomonas* and other GNRs can present with ecthyma gangrenosum, which in the early stage appears as bullae and later slough to classically form a gangrenous ulcer with a black eschar [331]. *C. jeikeium* often presents with an erythematous papular eruption during episodes of bacteremia [332]. Nocardia and other uncommon organisms have also led to cutaneous manifestations in this population [333, 334]. Gangrenous or necrotizing fasciitis is a life-threatening skin infection and is characterized by necrosis of the deeper subcutaneous fat and fascia. Patients typically present with signs of overwhelming infection, and rates of mortality are very high [335]. In leukemia, necrotizing fasciitis can be either a polymicrobial process or caused by singular primarily GNR species [335]. Patients may present with bacteremia and minimal skin findings which may progress rapidly to a more fulminant course [336]. Clues to this diagnosis include a rapidly expanding cellulitis, black/dusky areas of involvement, pain out of proportion to the cutaneous findings, and laboratory alterations such as an elevated creatinine and lactic acidosis. Surgical consultation and immediate debridement of the affected area are mandatory. A specific form of necrotizing fasciitis that involves the perineum, Fournier's gangrene, can be particularly morbid [337].

Fungal

Fungal skin lesions in transplantation can be similar to their bacterial counterparts. *Candida* species are one of the most common fungal infections to have dermatologic manifestations, and during candidemia, can present with <1 cm scattered erythematous papular nodules with pale centers [338]. *Cryptococcus* also can lead to skin nodules in those with disseminated disease [339]. Solitary nodules are more likely to be caused by moulds, typically *Aspergillus* and the Mucorales, and initially can be subtle in presentation. Mould infections can occur at sites of trauma, such as sites for bone marrow biopsy or IV placement [340]. Typically, lesions will progress rapidly without appropriate treatment. Fusarium is the one mould that presents frequently with dermatologic manifestations, usually appearing in greater than 60% of patients with disseminated fusariosis [341]. Typical lesions are erythematous macules and papules with gray necrotic or ulcerated centers [242]. Any patient with a cutaneous fungal infection should undergo further evaluation to identify others sites of infection.

Viral

HSV is commonly associated with vesicular lesions either around the oropharynx (typically HSV-1) or around anogenital region (HSV-2). Lesions during periods of severe immunosuppression can be much more severe but typically present as erythematous vesicles ("dew drop on a rose petal"). With the standard use of acyclovir, prophylaxis episodes of HSV during transplant and leukemia therapy are less frequent, although acyclovir-resistant cases can occasionally occur, especially in low-dose regimens [38]. Similar to HSV, VZV can present as herpes zoster or disseminated disease. Typical dermatomal reactivations occur late after transplant, but during active chemotherapy and postconditioning, patients are at risk for dissemination which can have an appearance not unlike primary Varicella (chickenpox) [343]. Erythematous rashes can be seen in other viral infections [344].

Diagnosis

As with all infections blood cultures can be helpful in identifying an underlying etiology to skin infections. Dermatology consultation and biopsies can also help in making a diagnosis and may be necessary in some cases that have a large differential diagnosis. Any patient with lesions suspicious for an invasive fungal infection should undergo routine biopsy. In patients with increased concern for necrotizing fasciitis, a high lactate and abnormal chemistry panel (low CO_2 and elevated creatinine) can also be suggestive. Diagnosis must be confirmed by visual inspection of the fascia and on pathologic review, so an urgent surgical consultation is required. Patients with lesions consistent with HSV or VZV should have lesions unroofed and samples from the base of the lesion sent for DFA, shell vial, and PCR. HSV and VZV PCR levels from serum should also be sent in patients who appear to have disseminated disease.

Treatment

Bacterial cellulitis is often treated with empiric regimens, as patients rarely have a known causative organism. Vancomycin is often added gram-positive coverage, but GNR treatment should be added in cases of severe of infection. Patients with identified pathogens should have therapy focused on the sensitivity patterns of that organism (Table 12.1). Patients with evidence of necrotizing fasciitis must undergo immediate surgical consultation and debridement; broad coverage is recommended for empiric therapy while awaiting the operating room. Fungal infections should be treated with fluconazole, echinocandin, voriconazole, lipid amphotericin B formulations, or posaconazole, depending on the species, sensitivities, and severity of disease. Patients with invasive *Aspergillus*, *Mucorales* species, or other mould need more extensive surgical debridement to cure the infection. Patients with localized HSV or VZV reactivation should be treated with high-dose acyclovir or valacyclovir.

Prevention Strategies

Bacterial Prophylaxis

(Guidelines reviewed in Freifeld [39], Tomblyn [31], and Baden [32])

Neutropenic fever is one of the most common complications following therapy for patients with leukemia occurring in greater than 80% of patients undergoing treatment [345]. Fever can be caused by numerous etiologies, and only about 20–30% of patients have documented infections during a neutropenic evaluation [39]. However, due to the high risk for morbidity and mortality associated with infections, most providers give standard prophylaxis during this period of risk. There are numerous risk categories that are reviewed in detail by Freifeld et al. and prevention strategies differ slightly between groups [39]. Patients receiving therapy for leukemia and transplant recipients are expected to have prolonged periods of neutropenia (>7–10 days) so are considered to be higher risk. Most centers and guidelines recommend the use of fluoroquinolone prophylaxis in this population, and this appears to be as effective as IV ceftazidime [31, 57]. Due to the emergence of fluoroquinolone-resistant *S. viridans* (particularly ciprofloxacin) [346], some centers add additional penicillin VK or amoxicillin to fluoroquinolones [347, 348] and others early vancomycin in patients at high risk for this organism [349]. Trimethoprim/sulfamethoxazole can be considered in patients who have an allergy to fluoroquinolones but is often not possible in patients with neutropenia [32]. Prophylaxis should be stopped after neutrophil recovery. Late strategies to prevent posttransplant *S. pneumoniae* and encapsulated bacteria in patients with chronic GVHD should be based on local resistance patterns [31].

Since VRE and MRSA can be major problems in the treatment phase of leuke-mia therapy, standard screening for VRE (rectal) and MRSA (nasal) are recom-mended prior to starting chemotherapy.

Fungal Prevention

Due to the increased risk and significant morbidity associated with fungal infec-tions, most centers use standard antifungal prophylaxis [350]. Fluconazole prophy-laxis has been shown to decrease the rates of major fungal infections [351, 352], but its major effect is on prevention of invasive Candida [22]. Breakthrough candidemia on prophylactic fluconazole can occur typically in the form of *C. glabrata* and *C. krusei* [353]. The echinocandins, particularly micafungin, have been shown to be useful alternative agents [354, 355].

Voriconazole prophylaxis has been shown to be equivalent to fluconazole in patients undergoing myeloablative HCT, but it did not significantly reduce the num-ber of Aspergillus infections during follow-up in a randomized trial [355]; an increase in *Mucorales* species was not seen. Posaconazole prophylaxis has been shown to decrease the risk of invasive mould infections in high-risk patients with GVHD [356] and in patients with neutropenia [357]. Limitation of proton-pump inhibitor use, coadministration with food or acidic beverages, and increases in dos-ing may prevent the development of insufficient drug levels and subsequent break-through infections [358]. Drug levels should be considered in patients receiving voriconazole or posaconazole prophylaxis.

PCP prevention is also an important component of posttransplant prevention. The preferred agent for prevention is postengraftment trimethoprim/sulfamethox-azole [31]. Trimethoprim/sulfamethoxazole is preferred because of superiority to other preventative agents [359] and cross-protection for toxoplasmosis and Nocardia. If patients have a known allergy to sulfa drugs, an attempt at desensitization should be attempted. Second-line agents include dapsone, atovaquone, and aerosolized pentamidine, but pentamidine is clearly inferior [360], and atovaquone has not been studied prospectively.

Viral Prevention

Cytomegalovirus (CMV)

Two major prevention strategies are currently used in practice to prevent the development of CMV disease: primary antiviral prophylaxis and preemptive ther-apy (Fig. 12.7). Clinical trials of ganciclovir prophylaxis have been performed and shown to decrease CMV disease [361, 362], but prophylactic approaches with ganciclovir can cause neutropenia, and increase susceptibility to bacterial or fungal infections [363, 364]. Prolonged exposure to CMV-specific antiviral agents, particularly with minimal immune pressure and subclinical reactivation, can lead to the selection of drug-resistant CMV [365].

At many transplant centers, preemptive therapy is used for CMV prevention in HCT [350]. Although preemptive strategies are similar at most centers, specific cutoffs for starting therapy vary between centers. At our institution, transplant recipients are monitored weekly for CMV viremia by quantitative real-time serum PCR for the first 100 days posttransplant [23]; other centers use the pp65 CMV antigenemia of whole blood PCR assay. Not all patients with detectable CMV will progress to disease, so centers need to develop viral load thresholds for PCR and antigenemia that will maximize effect and minimize toxicity. Alternatively, some centers use a combined strategy with primary prophylaxis with high-dose acyclovir in addition to preemptive therapy [366].

After 100 days posttransplant, PCR surveillance may be discontinued in low-risk patients [19]. High-risk patient, particularly those with ongoing GVHD therapy, should continue weekly surveillance for late CMV disease until they reach minimal immunosuppressant levels and have at least three consecutive negative weekly tests [19]. During late surveillance, our threshold for initiation of therapy is 1,000 copies/mL or greater than fivefold increase in viral load above the patient's established baseline [19].

Epstein-Barr Virus (EBV)

Some centers screen high-risk posttransplant patients (e.g., T-cell-depleted transplants) by weekly EBV PCR. Numerous testing strategies have been advocated, including whole blood, PBMCs, or cell-free plasma. In general, all of these specimens provide good sensitivity, although comparisons suggest that cell-free plasma may provide superior specificity for PTLD [367]. Most authors favor a preemptive therapy similar to what is seen in CMV, in which detection of EBV DNA levels above a certain threshold triggers a reduction in immunosuppression or rituximab therapy [368, 369]. There are no current guidelines for a threshold for EBV viremia due to variances in testing and in transplant populations [31]. Other groups use "prompt" therapy in which treatment is triggered only when detection of EBV DNA is accompanied by overt signs of EBV disease. Prompt therapy has shown similar efficacy to preemptive therapy [370]. Based on the concern that the delay in treatment may lead to increased complications, many groups still favor preemptive approaches [31, 301]. T-cell immunotherapeutic regimens are still experimental and not widely available.

HSV and VZV

Studies using both moderate- and low-dose acyclovir during the posttransplant period have demonstrated a marked decrease in both VZV and HSV complications [6, 371]. The use of acyclovir or valacyclovir is recommended for at least one year posttransplant and through 6 months after cessation of all immunosuppressive

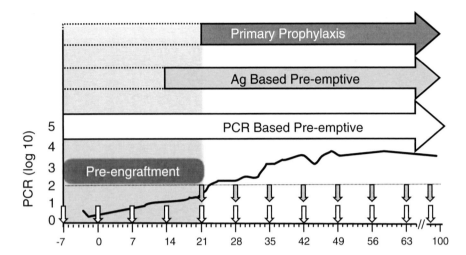

Fig. 12.7 CMV prevention strategies in the posthematopoietic cell transplant period. The *X* axis indicates the approximate CMV PCR level in serum (log10 copies per mL), which is indicated by the *thick solid line*. The *thin solid line* indicates the typical level of PCR detection. The *Y* axis represents days pre- or posttransplant. Primary prophylaxis (*large dark-gray arrow*), with drugs such as ganciclovir (IV or oral), is usually given after the point at which patients engraft. Many centers use an antigenemia-based preemptive testing (pp65) strategy (*large medium-gray arrow*). This can be started earlier and has been shown to prevent CMV disease. PCR-based preemptive therapy (*large white arrow*) is the standard at many other centers, including our own, and allows for testing to begin immediately after conditioning. *Small white arrows* indicate weekly testing by PCR that we do at our center through at least day 100. *Small gray arrows* indicated weekly antigenemia testing that typically starts near engraftment

therapies [31]. Long-term prophylaxis also appears to prevent the emergence of acyclovir-resistant HSV [38]. Low-dose acyclovir has also shown the ability to prevent both HSV and VZV reactivation in smaller studies [371, 372].

Adenovirus

Generally, surveillance is not recommended in low-risk patients. Preemptive monitoring has been advocated for adenovirus [277, 373, 374], particularly in children undergoing transplantation and in other high-risk adults (e.g., T-cell-depleted transplant recipients). Most often, cidofovir is used as the agent of choice for preemptive therapy [374].

Respiratory Viruses

Several nonrandomized studies support the use of prophylactic palivizumab for children ≤2 years throughout RSV season [375, 376], but adults should not receive palivizumab as prophylaxis.

Acknowledgments The authors wish to thank Kyoko Kurosawa for the excellent illustrations.

References

1. Ohno R, Tomonaga M, Kobayashi T, et al. Effect of granulocyte colony-stimulating factor after intensive induction therapy in relapsed or refractory acute leukemia. N Engl J Med. 1990;323(13):871–7.
2. Hersh EM, Bodey GP, Nies BA, Freireich EJ. Causes of death in acute leukemia: a ten-year study of 414 patients from 1954–1963. JAMA. 1965;193:105–9.
3. Chang HY, Rodriguez V, Narboni G, Bodey GP, Luna MA, Freireich EJ. Causes of death in adults with acute leukemia. Medicine (Baltimore). 1976;55(3):259–68.
4. Bucaneve G, Micozzi A, Menichetti F, et al. Levofloxacin to prevent bacterial infection in patients with cancer and neutropenia. N Engl J Med. 2005;353(10):977–87.
5. Gooley TA, Chien JW, Pergam SA, et al. Reduced mortality after allogeneic hematopoietic-cell transplantation. N Engl J Med. Nov 25 2010;363(22):2091–101.
6. Erard V, Guthrie KA, Varley C, et al. One-year acyclovir prophylaxis for preventing varicella-zoster virus disease after hematopoietic cell transplantation: no evidence of rebound varicella-zoster virus disease after drug discontinuation. Blood. 2007;110(8):3071–7.
7. Hofmann WK, Stauch M, Hoffken K. Impaired granulocytic function in patients with acute leukaemia: only partial normalisation after successful remission-inducing treatment. J Cancer Res Clin Oncol. 1998;124(2):113–6.
8. Bassoe CF. Flow cytometric quantification of phagocytosis in acute myeloid leukemia. Acta Haematol. 1999;102(4):163–71.
9. Hamblin AD, Hamblin TJ. The immunodeficiency of chronic lymphocytic leukaemia. Br Med Bull. 2008;87:49–62.
10. Dearden C. Disease-specific complications of chronic lymphocytic leukemia. Hematology Am Soc Hematol Educ Program. 2008:450–6.
11. Beebe JL, Koneman EW. Recovery of uncommon bacteria from blood: association with neoplastic disease. Clin Microbiol Rev. 1995;8(3):336–56.
12. Hakki M, Riddell SR, Storek J, et al. Immune reconstitution to cytomegalovirus after allogeneic hematopoietic stem cell transplantation: impact of host factors, drug therapy, and subclinical reactivation. Blood. 2003;102(8):3060–7.
13. Roux E, Helg C, Chapuis B, Jeannet M, Roosnek E. T-cell repertoire complexity after allogeneic bone marrow transplantation. Hum Immunol. 1996;48(1–2):135–8.
14. Elter T, Vehreschild JJ, Gribben J, Cornely OA, Engert A, Hallek M. Management of infections in patients with chronic lymphocytic leukemia treated with alemtuzumab. Ann Hematol. 2009;88(2):121–32.
15. Hargadon MT, Young VM, Schimpff SC, Wade JC, Minah GE. Selective suppression of alimentary tract microbial flora as prophylaxis during granulocytopenia. Antimicrob Agents Chemother. 1981;20(5):620–4.
16. Murphy BA. Clinical and economic consequences of mucositis induced by chemotherapy and/or radiation therapy. J Support Oncol. 2007;5(9 Suppl 4):13–21.
17. Sallah S, Wan JY, Nguyen NP, Vos P, Sigounas G. Analysis of factors related to the occurrence of chronic disseminated candidiasis in patients with acute leukemia in a non-bone marrow transplant setting: a follow-up study. Cancer. 2001;92(6):1349–53.
18. Armand P, Kim HT, Cutler CS, et al. Prognostic impact of elevated pretransplantation serum ferritin in patients undergoing myeloablative stem cell transplantation. Blood. 2007;109(10):4586–8.
19. Boeckh M, Ljungman P. How we treat cytomegalovirus in hematopoietic cell transplant recipients. Blood. 2009;113(23):5711–9.

20. Bergmann OJ, Mogensen SC, Ellermann-Eriksen S, Ellegaard J. Acyclovir prophylaxis and fever during remission-induction therapy of patients with acute myeloid leukemia: a randomized, double-blind, placebo-controlled trial. J Clin Oncol. 1997;15(6):2269–74.

21. Herbrecht R, Denning DW, Patterson TF, et al. Voriconazole versus amphotericin B for primary therapy of invasive aspergillosis. N Engl J Med. 2002;347(6):408–15.

22. Marr KA, Seidel K, Slavin MA, et al. Prolonged fluconazole prophylaxis is associated with persistent protection against candidiasis-related death in allogeneic marrow transplant recipients: long-term follow-up of a randomized, placebo-controlled trial. Blood. 2000;96(6): 2055–61.

23. Boeckh M, Huang M, Ferrenberg J, et al. Optimization of quantitative detection of cytomegalovirus DNA in plasma by real-time PCR. J Clin Microbiol. 2004;42(3):1142–8.

24. Cortez KJ, Fischer SH, Fahle GA, et al. Clinical trial of quantitative real-time polymerase chain reaction for detection of cytomegalovirus in peripheral blood of allogeneic hematopoietic stem-cell transplant recipients. J Infect Dis. 2003;188(7):967–72.

25. Kuderer NM, Dale DC, Crawford J, Lyman GH. Impact of primary prophylaxis with granulocyte colony-stimulating factor on febrile neutropenia and mortality in adult cancer patients receiving chemotherapy: a systematic review. J Clin Oncol. 2007;25(21):3158–67.

26. Panackal AA, Gribskov JL, Staab JF, Kirby KA, Rinaldi M, Marr KA. Clinical significance of azole antifungal drug cross-resistance in *Candida glabrata*. J Clin Microbiol. 2006;44(5): 1740–3.

27. Alexander BD, Schell WA, Miller JL, Long GD, Perfect JR. Candida glabrata fungemia in transplant patients receiving voriconazole after fluconazole. Transplantation. 2005;80(6): 868–71.

28. Zirakzadeh A, Gastineau DA, Mandrekar JN, Burke JP, Johnston PB, Patel R. Vancomycin-resistant enterococcal colonization appears associated with increased mortality among allogeneic hematopoietic stem cell transplant recipients. Bone Marrow Transplant. 2008;41(4): 385–92.

29. Oseltamivir-resistant novel influenza A (H1N1) virus infection in two immunosuppressed patients – Seattle, Washington, 2009. MMWR Morb Mortal Wkly Rep. 2009;58(32):893–6.

30. Marfori JE, Exner MM, Marousek GI, Chou S, Drew WL. Development of new cytomegalovirus UL97 and DNA polymerase mutations conferring drug resistance after valganciclovir therapy in allogeneic stem cell recipients. J Clin Virol. 2007;38(2):120–5.

31. Tomblyn M, Chiller T, Einsele H, et al. Guidelines for preventing infectious complications among hematopoietic cell transplantation recipients: a global perspective. Biol Blood Marrow Transplant. 2009;15(10):1143–238.

32. Baden LR, Casper C, Dubberke ER, Freifeld AG, Gelfand M, Greene JN, et al. Prevention and treatment of cancer-related infections. 2010. Downloaded from www.nccn.org on April 2011.

33. Scott BL, Park JY, Deeg HJ, et al. Pretransplant neutropenia is associated with poor-risk cytogenetic features and increased infection-related mortality in patients with myelodysplastic syndromes. Biol Blood Marrow Transplant. 2008;14(7):799–806.

34. Peck AJ, Corey L, Boeckh M. Pretransplantation respiratory syncytial virus infection: impact of a strategy to delay transplantation. Clin Infect Dis. 2004;39(5):673–80.

35. Hoover M, Morgan ER, Kletzel M. Prior fungal infection is not a contraindication to bone marrow transplant in patients with acute leukemia. Med Pediatr Oncol. 1997;28(4):268–73.

36. Martino R, Lopez R, Sureda A, Brunet S, Domingo-Albos A. Risk of reactivation of a recent invasive fungal infection in patients with hematological malignancies undergoing further intensive chemo-radiotherapy. A single-center experience and review of the literature. Haematologica. 1997;82(3):297–304.

37. Kinch A, Oberg G, Arvidson J, Falk KI, Linde A, Pauksens K. Post-transplant lymphoproliferative disease and other Epstein-Barr virus diseases in allogeneic haematopoietic stem cell transplantation after introduction of monitoring of viral load by polymerase chain reaction. Scand J Infect Dis. 2007;39(3):235–44.

38. Erard V, Wald A, Corey L, Leisenring WM, Boeckh M. Use of long-term suppressive acyclovir after hematopoietic stem-cell transplantation: impact on herpes simplex virus (HSV) disease and drug-resistant HSV disease. J Infect Dis. 2007;196(2):266–70.

39. Freifeld AG, Bow EJ, Sepkowitz KA, et al. Clinical practice guideline for the use of antimicrobial agents in neutropenic patients with cancer: 2010 update by the infectious diseases society of America. Clin Infect Dis. 2011;52(4):e56–93.

40. Kanathezhath B, Shah A, Secola R, Hudes M, Feusner JH. The utility of routine surveillance blood cultures in asymptomatic hematopoietic stem cell transplant patients. J Pediatr Hematol Oncol. 2010;32(4):327–31.

41. Son YM, Na SY, Lee HY, Baek JO, Lee JR, Roh JY. Ecthyma gangrenosum: a rare cutaneous manifestation caused by *Stenotrophomonas maltophilia* in a leukemic patient. Ann Dermatol. 2009;21(4):389–92.

42. Morgan EA, Henrich TJ, Jarell AD, et al. Infectious granulomatous dermatitis associated with *Rothia mucilaginosa* bacteremia: a case report. Am J Dermatopathol. 2010;32(2):175–9.

43. Gutierrez PEM, Gamez PL, Gonzalez RAJ, Ramon QD, Monteagudo CC, Jorda CE. Disseminated fusariosis in immunocompromised patients. Eur J Dermatol. 2011;21(5):753–6.

44. Ribeiro P, Sousa AB, Nunes O, Aveiro F, Fernandes JP, Gouveia J. Candidemia in acute leukemia patients. Support Care Cancer. 1997;5(3):249–51.

45. Thurlow LR, Hanke ML, Fritz T, et al. *Staphylococcus aureus* biofilms prevent macrophage phagocytosis and attenuate inflammation in vivo. J Immunol. 2011;186(11):6585–96.

46. Kristian SA, Golda T, Ferracin F, et al. The ability of biofilm formation does not influence virulence of *Staphylococcus aureus* and host response in a mouse tissue cage infection model. Microb Pathog. 2004;36(5):237–45.

47. Gunther F, Wabnitz GH, Stroh P, et al. Host defence against *Staphylococcus aureus* biofilms infection: phagocytosis of biofilms by polymorphonuclear neutrophils (PMN). Mol Immunol. 2009;46(8–9):1805–13.

48. Stroh P, Gunther F, Meyle E, Prior B, Wagner C, Hansch GM. Host defence against *Staphylococcus aureus* biofilms by polymorphonuclear neutrophils: oxygen radical production but not phagocytosis depends on opsonisation with immunoglobulin G. Immunobiology. 2011;216(3):351–7.

49. Meyle E, Stroh P, Gunther F, Hoppy-Tichy T, Wagner C, Hansch GM. Destruction of bacterial biofilms by polymorphonuclear neutrophils: relative contribution of phagocytosis, DNA release, and degranulation. Int J Artif Organs. 2010;33(9):608–20.

50. Johansson JE, Ekman T. Gastro-intestinal toxicity related to bone marrow transplantation: disruption of the intestinal barrier precedes clinical findings. Bone Marrow Transplant. 1997; 19(9):921–5.

51. Mermel LA, Allon M, Bouza E, et al. Clinical practice guidelines for the diagnosis and management of intravascular catheter-related infection: 2009 Update by the Infectious Diseases Society of America. Clin Infect Dis. 2009;49(1):1–45.

52. Yamasaki S, Heike Y, Mori S, et al. Infectious complications in chronic graft-versus-host disease: a retrospective study of 145 recipients of allogeneic hematopoietic stem cell transplantation with reduced- and conventional-intensity conditioning regimens. Transpl Infect Dis. 2008; 10(4):252–9.

53. Mikulska M, Del Bono V, Raiola AM, et al. Blood stream infections in allogeneic hematopoietic stem cell transplant recipients: reemergence of Gram-negative rods and increasing antibiotic resistance. Biol Blood Marrow Transplant. 2009;15(1):47–53.

54. Ortega M, Rovira M, Almela M, et al. Bacterial and fungal bloodstream isolates from 796 hematopoietic stem cell transplant recipients between 1991 and 2000. Ann Hematol. 2005;84(1):40–6.

55. Gaviria JM, Garcia PJ, Garrido SM, Corey L, Boeckh M. Nontuberculous mycobacterial infections in hematopoietic stem cell transplant recipients: characteristics of respiratory and catheter-related infections. Biol Blood Marrow Transplant. 2000;6(4):361–9.

56. Frere P, Hermanne JP, Debouge MH, de Mol P, Fillet G, Beguin Y. Bacteremia after hematopoietic stem cell transplantation: incidence and predictive value of surveillance cultures. Bone Marrow Transplant. 2004;33(7):745–9.

57. Guthrie KA, Yong M, Frieze D, Corey L, Fredricks DN. The impact of a change in antibacterial prophylaxis from ceftazidime to levofloxacin in allogeneic hematopoietic cell transplantation. Bone Marrow Transplant. 2010;45(4):675–81.

58. Syrjala H, Ohtonen P, Kinnunen U, et al. Blood stream infections during chemotherapy-induced neutropenia in adult patients with acute myeloid leukemia: treatment cycle matters. Eur J Clin Microbiol Infect Dis. 2010;29(10):1211–8.
59. Cherif H, Kronvall G, Bjorkholm M, Kalin M. Bacteraemia in hospitalised patients with malignant blood disorders: a retrospective study of causative agents and their resistance profiles during a 14-year period without antibacterial prophylaxis. Hematol J. 2003;4(6):420–6.
60. Mihu CN, Schaub J, Kesh S, et al. Risk factors for late *Staphylococcus aureus* bacteremia after allogeneic hematopoietic stem cell transplantation: a single-institution, nested case-controlled study. Biol Blood Marrow Transplant. 2008;14(12):1429–33.
61. Jaffe D, Jakubowski A, Sepkowitz K, et al. Prevention of peritransplantation viridans streptococcal bacteremia with early vancomycin administration: a single-center observational cohort study. Clin Infect Dis. 2004;39(11):1625–32.
62. Spanik S, Trupl J, Kunova A, et al. *Viridans streptococcal* bacteraemia due to penicillin-resistant and penicillin-sensitive streptococci: analysis of risk factors and outcome in 60 patients from a single cancer centre before and after penicillin is used for prophylaxis. Scand J Infect Dis. 1997;29(3):245–9.
63. Huang WT, Chang LY, Hsueh PR, et al. Clinical features and complications of viridans streptococci bloodstream infection in pediatric hemato-oncology patients. J Microbiol Immunol Infect. 2007;40(4):349–54.
64. Meisel R, Toschke AM, Heiligensetzer C, Dilloo D, Laws HJ, von Kries R. Increased risk for invasive pneumococcal diseases in children with acute lymphoblastic leukaemia. Br J Haematol. 2007;137(5):457–60.
65. Sinisalo M, Vilpo J, Itala M, Vakevainen M, Taurio J, Aittoniemi J. Antibody response to 7-valent conjugated pneumococcal vaccine in patients with chronic lymphocytic leukaemia. Vaccine. 2007;26(1):82–7.
66. Lehrnbecher T, Schubert R, Behl M, et al. Impaired pneumococcal immunity in children after treatment for acute lymphoblastic leukaemia. Br J Haematol. 2009;147(5):700–5.
67. Kamboj M, Chung D, Seo SK, et al. The changing epidemiology of vancomycin-resistant Enterococcus (VRE) bacteremia in allogeneic hematopoietic stem cell transplant (HSCT) recipients. Biol Blood Marrow Transplant. 2010;16(11):1576–81.
68. Mikulska M, Del Bono V, Prinapori R, et al. Risk factors for enterococcal bacteremia in allogeneic hematopoietic stem cell transplant recipients. Transpl Infect Dis. 2010;12(6):505–12.
69. Bossaer JB, Hall PD, Garrett-Mayer E. Incidence of vancomycin-resistant enterococci (VRE) infection in high-risk febrile neutropenic patients colonized with VRE. Support Care Cancer. 2010;19(2):231–7.
70. Wang CC, Mattson D, Wald A. Corynebacterium jeikeium bacteremia in bone marrow transplant patients with Hickman catheters. Bone Marrow Transplant. 2001;27(4):445–9.
71. Hakki M, Limaye AP, Kim HW, Kirby KA, Corey L, Boeckh M. Invasive *Pseudomonas aeruginosa* infections: high rate of recurrence and mortality after hematopoietic cell transplantation. Bone Marrow Transplant. 2007;39(11):687–93.
72. Caselli D, Cesaro S, Ziino O, et al. Multidrug resistant *Pseudomonas aeruginosa* infection in children undergoing chemotherapy and hematopoietic stem cell transplantation. Haematologica. 2010;95(9):1612–5.
73. Sefcick A, Tait RC, Wood B. *Stenotrophomonas maltophilia*: an increasing problem in patients with acute leukaemia. Leuk Lymphoma. 1999;35(1–2):207–11.
74. Safdar A, Rolston KV. *Stenotrophomonas maltophilia*: changing spectrum of a serious bacterial pathogen in patients with cancer. Clin Infect Dis. 2007;45(12):1602–9.
75. Yeshurun M, Gafter-Gvili A, Thaler M, Keller N, Nagler A, Shimoni A. Clinical characteristics of *Stenotrophomonas maltophilia* infection in hematopoietic stem cell transplantation recipients: a single center experience. Infection. 2010;38(3):211–5.
76. El-Mahallawy HA, El-Wakil M, Moneer MM, Shalaby L. Antibiotic resistance is associated with longer bacteremic episodes and worse outcome in febrile neutropenic children with cancer. Pediatr Blood Cancer. 2011;57(2):283–8.

77. Pirrotta MT, Bucalossi A, Forconi F, et al. Massive intravascular hemolysis: a fatal complication of *Clostridium perfringens* septicemia in a patient with acute lymphoblastic leukemia. Leuk Lymphoma. 2005;46(5):793.
78. Johnson S, Driks MR, Tweten RK, et al. Clinical courses of seven survivors of *Clostridium septicum* infection and their immunologic responses to alpha toxin. Clin Infect Dis. 1994;19(4):761–4.
79. Pasqualotto AC, Nedel WL, Machado TS, Severo LC. Risk factors and outcome for nosocomial breakthrough candidaemia. J Infect. 2006;52(3):216–22.
80. Fukuda T, Boeckh M, Carter RA, et al. Risks and outcomes of invasive fungal infections in recipients of allogeneic hematopoietic stem cell transplants after nonmyeloablative conditioning. Blood. 2003;102(3):827–33.
81. Mori T, Nakamura Y, Kato J, et al. Fungemia due to *Rhodotorula mucilaginosa* after allogeneic hematopoietic stem cell transplantation. Transpl Infect Dis. 2011. doi:10.1111/j.1399-3062.2011.00647.x.
82. Chan-Tack KM, Nemoy LL, Perencevich EN. Central venous catheter-associated fungemia secondary to mucormycosis. Scand J Infect Dis. 2005;37(11–12):925–7.
83. Passos XS, Sales WS, Maciel PJ, Costa CR, Ferreira DM, do Silva MR. Nosocomial invasive infection caused by *Cunninghamella bertholletiae*: case report. Mycopathologia. 2006;161(1): 33–5.
84. Campo M, Lewis RE, Kontoyiannis DP. Invasive fusariosis in patients with hematologic malignancies at a cancer center: 1998–2009. J Infect. 2010;60(5):331–7.
85. Kerl K, Koch B, Fegeler W, Rossig C, Ehlert K, Groll AH. Catheter-associated aspergillosis of the chest wall following allogeneic hematopoietic stem cell transplantation. Transpl Infect Dis. 2011;13(2):182–5.
86. Leong KW, Crowley B, White B, et al. Cutaneous mucormycosis due to *Absidia corymbifera* occurring after bone marrow transplantation. Bone Marrow Transplant. 1997;19(5): 513–5.
87. Falagas ME, Kazantzi MS, Bliziotis IA. Comparison of utility of blood cultures from intravascular catheters and peripheral veins: a systematic review and decision analysis. J Med Microbiol. 2008;57(Pt 1):1–8.
88. Guembe M, Rodriguez-Creixems M, Sanchez-Carrillo C, Perez-Parra A, Martin-Rabadan P, Bouza E. How many lumens should be cultured in the conservative diagnosis of catheter-related bloodstream infections? Clin Infect Dis. 2010;50(12):1575–9.
89. Abdelkefi A, Achour W, Ben OT, et al. Difference in time to positivity is useful for the diagnosis of catheter-related bloodstream infection in hematopoietic stem cell transplant recipients. Bone Marrow Transplant. 2005;35(4):397–401.
90. Bouza E, Burillo A, Guembe M. Managing intravascular catheter-related infections in heart transplant patients: how far can we apply IDSA guidelines for immunocompromised patients? Curr Opin Infect Dis. 2011;24(4):302–8.
91. Fraser TG, Gordon SM. CLABSI rates in immunocompromised patients: a valuable patient centered outcome? Clin Infect Dis. 2011;52(12):1446–50.
92. Pappas PG, Kauffman CA, Andes D, et al. Clinical practice guidelines for the management of candidiasis: 2009 update by the Infectious Diseases Society of America. Clin Infect Dis. 2009;48(5):503–35.
93. Saiz A, Graus F. Neurologic complications of hematopoietic cell transplantation. Semin Neurol. 2010;30(3):287–95.
94. Zerr DM, Fann JR, Breiger D, et al. HHV-6 reactivation and its effect on delirium and cognitive functioning in hematopoietic cell transplantation recipients. Blood. 2011;117(19):5243–9.
95. Torres HA, Reddy BT, Raad II, et al. Nocardiosis in cancer patients. Medicine (Baltimore). 2002;81(5):388–97.
96. Seeley WW, Marty FM, Holmes TM, et al. Post-transplant acute limbic encephalitis: clinical features and relationship to HHV6. Neurology. 2007;69(2):156–65.
97. Steiner I. Herpes simplex virus encephalitis: new infection or reactivation? Curr Opin Neurol. 2011;24(3):268–74.

98. Fukuno K, Tomonari A, Takahashi S, et al. Varicella-zoster virus encephalitis in a patient undergoing unrelated cord blood transplantation for myelodysplastic syndrome-overt leukemia. Int J Hematol. 2006;84(1):79–82.
99. Baddley JW, Salzman D, Pappas PG. Fungal brain abscess in transplant recipients: epidemiologic, microbiologic, and clinical features. Clin Transplant. 2002;16(6):419–24.
100. Haddad PA, Repka TL, Weisdorf DJ. Penicillin-resistant Streptococcus pneumoniae septic shock and meningitis complicating chronic graft versus host disease: a case report and review of the literature. Am J Med. 2002;113(2):152–5.
101. Engelhard D, Cordonnier C, Shaw PJ, et al. Early and late invasive pneumococcal infection following stem cell transplantation: a European bone marrow transplantation survey. Br J Haematol. 2002;117(2):444–50.
102. Lee AB, Harker-Murray P, Ferrieri P, Schleiss MR, Tolar J. Bacterial meningitis from *Rothia mucilaginosa* in patients with malignancy or undergoing hematopoietic stem cell transplantation. Pediatr Blood Cancer. 2008;50(3):673–6.
103. Gaur AH, Patrick CC, McCullers JA, et al. Bacillus cereus bacteremia and meningitis in immunocompromised children. Clin Infect Dis. 2001;32(10):1456–62.
104. Robin F, Paillard C, Marchandin H, Demeocq F, Bonnet R, Hennequin C. Lactobacillus rhamnosus meningitis following recurrent episodes of bacteremia in a child undergoing allogeneic hematopoietic stem cell transplantation. J Clin Microbiol. 2010;48(11):4317–9.
105. Hakim A, Rossi C, Kabanda A, Deplano A, De Gheldre Y, Struelens MJ. Ommaya-catheter-related Staphylococcus epidermidis cerebritis and recurrent bacteremia documented by molecular typing. Eur J Clin Microbiol Infect Dis. 2000;19(11):875–7.
106. Bartt R. Listeria and atypical presentations of *Listeria* in the central nervous system. Semin Neurol. 2000;20(3):361–73.
107. McLauchlin J. Human listeriosis in Britain, 1967–85, a summary of 722 cases. 2. Listeriosis in non-pregnant individuals, a changing pattern of infection and seasonal incidence. Epidemiol Infect. 1990;104(2):191–201.
108. Yildiz O, Doganay M. Actinomycoses and Nocardia pulmonary infections. Curr Opin Pulm Med. 2006;12(3):228–34.
109. Perfect JR, Dismukes WE, Dromer F, et al. Clinical practice guidelines for the management of cryptococcal disease: 2010 update by the Infectious Diseases Society of America. Clin Infect Dis. 2010;50(3):291–322.
110. Lockhart SR, Wagner D, Iqbal N, et al. Comparison of in vitro susceptibility characteristics of *Candida* species from cases of invasive candidiasis in solid organ and stem cell transplant recipients: Transplant-Associated Infections Surveillance Network (TRANSNET), 2001 to 2006. J Clin Microbiol. 2011;49(7):2404–10.
111. Bacigalupo A, Mordini N, Pitto A, et al. Transplantation of HLA-mismatched CD34+ selected cells in patients with advanced malignancies: severe immunodeficiency and related complications. Br J Haematol. 1997;98(3):760–6.
112. Gabelmann A, Klein S, Kern W, et al. Relevant imaging findings of cerebral aspergillosis on MRI: a retrospective case-based study in immunocompromised patients. Eur J Neurol. 2007;14(5):548–55.
113. Hagensee ME, Bauwens JE, Kjos B, Bowden RA. Brain abscess following marrow transplantation: experience at the Fred Hutchinson Cancer Research Center, 1984–1992. Clin Infect Dis. 1994;19(3):402–8.
114. de Medeiros BC, de Medeiros CR, Werner B, et al. Central nervous system infections following bone marrow transplantation: an autopsy report of 27 cases. J Hematother Stem Cell Res. 2000;9(4):535–40.
115. Skiada A, Pagano L, Groll A, et al. Zygomycosis in Europe: analysis of 230 cases accrued by the registry of the European Confederation of Medical Mycology (ECMM) Working Group on Zygomycosis between 2005 and 2007. Clin Microbiol Infect. 2011. doi:10.1111/j.1469-0691.2010.03456.x.
116. Roden MM, Zaoutis TE, Buchanan WL, et al. Epidemiology and outcome of zygomycosis: a review of 929 reported cases. Clin Infect Dis. 2005;41(5):634–53.

117. Husain S, Munoz P, Forrest G, et al. Infections due to *Scedosporium apiospermum* and *Scedosporium prolificans* in transplant recipients: clinical characteristics and impact of antifungal agent therapy on outcome. Clin Infect Dis. 2005;40(1):89–99.
118. Pagano L, Valentini CG, Caira M, Fianchi L. ZYGOMYCOSIS: current approaches to management of patients with haematological malignancies. Br J Haematol. 2009;146(6):597–606.
119. Wheat LJ, Freifeld AG, Kleiman MB, et al. Clinical practice guidelines for the management of patients with histoplasmosis: 2007 update by the Infectious Diseases Society of America. Clin Infect Dis. 2007;45(7):807–25.
120. Galgiani JN, Ampel NM, Blair JE, et al. Coccidioidomycosis. Clin Infect Dis. 2005; 41(9):1217–23.
121. Glenn TJ, Blair JE, Adams RH. Coccidioidomycosis in hematopoietic stem cell transplant recipients. Med Mycol. 2005;43(8):705–10.
122. Pereira GH, Padua SS, Park MV, Muller RP, Passos RM, Menezes Y. Chronic meningitis by histoplasmosis: report of a child with acute myeloid leukemia. Braz J Infect Dis. 2008; 12(6):555–7.
123. Kauffman CA. Diagnosis of histoplasmosis in immunosuppressed patients. Curr Opin Infect Dis. 2008;21(4):421–5.
124. Schmidt-Hieber M, Schwender J, Heinz WJ, et al. Viral encephalitis after allogeneic stem cell transplantation: a rare complication with distinct characteristics of different causative agents. Haematologica. 2011;96(1):142–9.
125. Zerr DM. Human herpesvirus 6 and central nervous system disease in hematopoietic cell transplantation. J Clin Virol. 2006;37 Suppl 1:S52–6.
126. Nagel MA, Traktinskiy I, Azarkh Y, et al. Varicella zoster virus vasculopathy: analysis of virus-infected arteries. Neurology. 2011;77(4):364–70.
127. Koskiniemi M, Piiparinen H, Rantalaiho T, et al. Acute central nervous system complications in varicella zoster virus infections. J Clin Virol. 2002;25(3):293–301.
128. Hentrich M, Oruzio D, Jager G, et al. Impact of human herpesvirus-6 after haematopoietic stem cell transplantation. Br J Haematol. 2005;128(1):66–72.
129. Romee R, Brunstein CG, Weisdorf DJ, Majhail NS. Herpes simplex virus encephalitis after allogeneic transplantation: an instructive case. Bone Marrow Transplant. 2010;45(4): 776–8.
130. Adour KK. Otological complications of herpes zoster. Ann Neurol. 1994;35(Suppl):S62–4.
131. Diaz GA, Rakita RM, Koelle DM. A case of Ramsay Hunt-like syndrome caused by herpes simplex virus type 2. Clin Infect Dis. 2005;40(10):1545–7.
132. Kremer S, Matern JF, Bilger K, et al. EBV limbic encephalitis after allogeneic hematopoietic stem cell transplantation. J Neuroradiol. 2010;37(3):189–91.
133. Reddy SM, Winston DJ, Territo MC, Schiller GJ. CMV central nervous system disease in stem-cell transplant recipients: an increasing complication of drug-resistant CMV infection and protracted immunodeficiency. Bone Marrow Transplant. 2010;45(6):979–84.
134. Lee S, Kim SH, Choi SM, et al. Cytomegalovirus ventriculoencephalitis after unrelated double cord blood stem cell transplantation with an alemtuzumab-containing preparative regimen for Philadelphia-positive acute lymphoblastic leukemia. J Korean Med Sci. 2010;25(4):630–3.
135. Kittan NA, Beier F, Kurz K, et al. Isolated cerebral manifestation of Epstein-Barr virus-associated post-transplant lymphoproliferative disorder after allogeneic hematopoietic stem cell transplantation: a case of clinical and diagnostic challenges. Transpl Infect Dis. 2011; 13(5):524–30.
136. D'Souza A, Wilson J, Mukherjee S, Jaiyesimi I. Progressive multifocal leukoencephalopathy in chronic lymphocytic leukemia: a report of three cases and review of the literature. Clin Lymphoma Myeloma Leuk. 2010;10(1):E1–9.
137. Kharfan-Dabaja MA, Ayala E, Greene J, Rojiani A, Murtagh FR, Anasetti C. Two cases of progressive multifocal leukoencephalopathy after allogeneic hematopoietic cell transplantation and a review of the literature. Bone Marrow Transplant. 2007;39(2):101–7.
138. Fernandez-Ruiz M, de la Serna J, Ruiz J, Lopez-Medrano F. Progressive multifocal leukoencephalopathy in a patient with acute myeloid leukaemia after allogeneic hematopoietic-cell transplantation. Enferm Infecc Microbiol Clin. 2011;29(8):636–7.

139. Kotton CN. Zoonoses in solid-organ and hematopoietic stem cell transplant recipients. Clin Infect Dis. 2007;44(6):857–66.
140. Brenner W, Storch G, Buller R, Vij R, Devine S, DiPersio J. West Nile Virus encephalopathy in an allogeneic stem cell transplant recipient: use of quantitative PCR for diagnosis and assessment of viral clearance. Bone Marrow Transplant. 2005;36(4):369–70.
141. Tan PL, Verneris MR, Charnas LR, Reck SJ, van Burik JA, Blazar BR. Outcome of CNS and pulmonary enteroviral infections after hematopoietic cell transplantation. Pediatr Blood Cancer. 2005;45(1):74–5.
142. Mulanovich VE, Ahmed SI, Ozturk T, Khokhar FA, Kontoyiannis DP, de Lima M. Toxoplasmosis in allo-SCT patients: risk factors and outcomes at a transplantation center with a low incidence. Bone Marrow Transplant. 2011;46(2):273–7.
143. Martino R, Maertens J, Bretagne S, et al. Toxoplasmosis after hematopoietic stem cell transplantation. Clin Infect Dis. 2000;31(5):1188–95.
144. Small TN, Leung L, Stiles J, et al. Disseminated toxoplasmosis following T cell-depleted related and unrelated bone marrow transplantation. Bone Marrow Transplant. 2000;25(9): 969–73.
145. Roemer E, Blau IW, Basara N, et al. Toxoplasmosis, a severe complication in allogeneic hematopoietic stem cell transplantation: successful treatment strategies during a 5-year single-center experience. Clin Infect Dis. 2001;32(1):E1–8.
146. Walker M, Zunt JR. Parasitic central nervous system infections in immunocompromised hosts. Clin Infect Dis. 2005;40(7):1005–15.
147. Smallman LA, Young JA, Shortland-Webb WR, Carey MP, Michael J. Strongyloides stercoralis hyperinfestation syndrome with *Escherichia coli* meningitis: report of two cases. J Clin Pathol. 1986;39(4):366–70.
148. Sauter A, Ernemann U, Beck R, et al. Spectrum of imaging findings in immunocompromised patients with HHV-6 infection. AJR Am J Roentgenol. 2009;193(5):W373–80.
149. Shah R, Bag AK, Chapman PR, Cure JK. Imaging manifestations of progressive multifocal leukoencephalopathy. Clin Radiol. 2010;65(6):431–9.
150. Ionita C, Wasay M, Balos L, Bakshi R. MR imaging in toxoplasmosis encephalitis after bone marrow transplantation: paucity of enhancement despite fulminant disease. AJNR Am J Neuroradiol. 2004;25(2):270–3.
151. Nishiguchi T, Mochizuki K, Shakudo M, Takeshita T, Hino M, Inoue Y. CNS complications of hematopoietic stem cell transplantation. AJR Am J Roentgenol. 2009;192(4):1003–11.
152. Fricker-Hidalgo H, Bulabois CE, Brenier-Pinchart MP, et al. Diagnosis of toxoplasmosis after allogeneic stem cell transplantation: results of DNA detection and serological techniques. Clin Infect Dis. 2009;48(2):e9–15.
153. Martinez R, Reyes S, Menendez R. Pulmonary nocardiosis: risk factors, clinical features, diagnosis and prognosis. Curr Opin Pulm Med. 2008;14(3):219–27.
154. Walsh TJ, Anaissie EJ, Denning DW, et al. Treatment of aspergillosis: clinical practice guidelines of the Infectious Diseases Society of America. Clin Infect Dis. 2008;46(3):327–60.
155. Schwartz S, Ruhnke M, Ribaud P, et al. Improved outcome in central nervous system aspergillosis, using voriconazole treatment. Blood. 2005;106(8):2641–5.
156. Lutsar I, Roffey S, Troke P. Voriconazole concentrations in the cerebrospinal fluid and brain tissue of guinea pigs and immunocompromised patients. Clin Infect Dis. 2003;37(5): 728–32.
157. de Pagter PJ, Schuurman R, Meijer E, van Baarle D, Sanders EA, Boelens JJ. Human herpesvirus type 6 reactivation after haematopoietic stem cell transplantation. J Clin Virol. 2008;43(4):361–6.
158. Torre D, Casari S, Speranza F, et al. Randomized trial of trimethoprim-sulfamethoxazole versus pyrimethamine-sulfadiazine for therapy of toxoplasmic encephalitis in patients with AIDS. Italian Collaborative Study Group. Antimicrob Agents Chemother. 1998;42(6):1346–9.
159. Afessa B, Abdulai RM, Kremers WK, Hogan WJ, Litzow MR, Peters SG. Risk factors and outcome of pulmonary complications after autologous hematopoietic stem cell transplant (HSCT). Chest. 2011. doi:10.1378/chest.10-2889.

160. Panoskaltsis-Mortari A, Griese M, Madtes DK, et al. An official American Thoracic Society research statement: noninfectious lung injury after hematopoietic stem cell transplantation: idiopathic pneumonia syndrome. Am J Respir Crit Care Med. 2011;183(9): 1262–79.
161. Imamura R, Voegels R, Sperandio F, et al. Microbiology of sinusitis in patients undergoing bone marrow transplantation. Otolaryngol Head Neck Surg. 1999;120(2):279–82.
162. Shibuya TY, Momin F, Abella E, et al. Sinus disease in the bone marrow transplant population: incidence, risk factors, and complications. Otolaryngol Head Neck Surg. 1995;113(6):705–11.
163. Chen CS, Boeckh M, Seidel K, et al. Incidence, risk factors, and mortality from pneumonia developing late after hematopoietic stem cell transplantation. Bone Marrow Transplant. 2003;32(5):515–22.
164. van Burik JA, Hackman RC, Nadeem SQ, et al. Nocardiosis after bone marrow transplantation: a retrospective study. Clin Infect Dis. 1997;24(6):1154–60.
165. Martinez TR, Menendez VR, Reyes CS, et al. Pulmonary nocardiosis: risk factors and outcomes. Respirology. 2007;12(3):394–400.
166. Schwebke JR, Hackman R, Bowden R. Pneumonia due to Legionella micdadei in bone marrow transplant recipients. Rev Infect Dis. 1990;12(5):824–8.
167. Meyer R, Rappo U, Glickman M, et al. Legionella jordanis in hematopoietic SCT patients radiographically mimicking invasive mold infection. Bone Marrow Transplant. 2011;46(8): 1099–103.
168. Harrington RD, Woolfrey AE, Bowden R, McDowell MG, Hackman RC. Legionellosis in a bone marrow transplant center. Bone Marrow Transplant. 1996;18(2):361–8.
169. Banov L, Garanata C, Dufour C, et al. Pneumonia due to Mycoplasma pneumoniae in granulocytopenic children with cancer. Pediatr Blood Cancer. 2009;53(2):240–2.
170. Geisler WM, Corey L. Chlamydia pneumoniae respiratory infection after allogeneic stem cell transplantation. Transplantation. 2002;73(6):1002–5.
171. Drakos PE, Nagler A, Or R, et al. Invasive fungal sinusitis in patients undergoing bone marrow transplantation. Bone Marrow Transplant. 1993;12(3):203–8.
172. Choi SS, Milmoe GJ, Dinndorf PA, Quinones RR. Invasive Aspergillus sinusitis in pediatric bone marrow transplant patients. Evaluation and management. Arch Otolaryngol Head Neck Surg. 1995;121(10):1188–92.
173. Beltrame A, Sarmati L, Cudillo L, et al. A fatal case of invasive fungal sinusitis by Scopulariopsis acremonium in a bone marrow transplant recipient. Int J Infect Dis. 2009; 13(6):e488–92.
174. Gucalp R, Carlisle P, Gialanella P, Mitsudo S, McKitrick J, Dutcher J. Paecilomyces sinusitis in an immunocompromised adult patient: case report and review. Clin Infect Dis. 1996;23(2):391–3.
175. Bethge WA, Schmalzing M, Stuhler G, et al. Mucormycoses in patients with hematologic malignancies: an emerging fungal infection. Haematologica. 2005;90(Suppl:ECR22): e62–4.
176. Kontoyiannis DP, Marr KA, Park BJ, et al. Prospective surveillance for invasive fungal infections in hematopoietic stem cell transplant recipients, 2001–2006: overview of the Transplant-Associated Infection Surveillance Network (TRANSNET) Database. Clin Infect Dis. 2010;50(8):1091–100.
177. Wingard JR, Carter SL, Walsh TJ, et al. Randomized, double-blind trial of fluconazole versus voriconazole for prevention of invasive fungal infection after allogeneic hematopoietic cell transplantation. Blood. 2010;116(24):5111–8.
178. Neofytos D, Horn D, Anaissie E, et al. Epidemiology and outcome of invasive fungal infection in adult hematopoietic stem cell transplant recipients: analysis of Multicenter Prospective Antifungal Therapy (PATH) Alliance registry. Clin Infect Dis. 2009;48(3):265–73.
179. Garcia-Vidal C, Upton A, Kirby KA, Marr KA. Epidemiology of invasive mold infections in allogeneic stem cell transplant recipients: biological risk factors for infection according to time after transplantation. Clin Infect Dis. 2008;47(8):1041–50.
180. Marr KA, Carter RA, Boeckh M, Martin P, Corey L. Invasive aspergillosis in allogeneic stem cell transplant recipients: changes in epidemiology and risk factors. Blood. 2002;100(13): 4358–66.

181. Thursky K, Byrnes G, Grigg A, Szer J, Slavin M. Risk factors for post-engraftment invasive aspergillosis in allogeneic stem cell transplantation. Bone Marrow Transplant. 2004;34(2): 115–21.
182. Maertens J, Demuynck H, Verbeken EK, et al. Mucormycosis in allogeneic bone marrow transplant recipients: report of five cases and review of the role of iron overload in the pathogenesis. Bone Marrow Transplant. 1999;24(3):307–12.
183. Villarroel M, Aviles CL, Silva P, et al. Risk factors associated with invasive fungal disease in children with cancer and febrile neutropenia: a prospective multicenter evaluation. Pediatr Infect Dis J. 2010;29(9):816–21.
184. Bow EJ, Loewen R, Cheang MS, Schacter B. Invasive fungal disease in adults undergoing remission-induction therapy for acute myeloid leukemia: the pathogenetic role of the antileukemic regimen. Clin Infect Dis. 1995;21(2):361–9.
185. Marty FM, Cosimi LA, Baden LR. Breakthrough zygomycosis after voriconazole treatment in recipients of hematopoietic stem-cell transplants. N Engl J Med. 2004;350(9):950–2.
186. Trifilio S, Singhal S, Williams S, et al. Breakthrough fungal infections after allogeneic hematopoietic stem cell transplantation in patients on prophylactic voriconazole. Bone Marrow Transplant. 2007;40(5):451–6.
187. Rivier A, Perny J, Debourgogne A, et al. Fatal disseminated infection due to *Scedosporium prolificans* in a patient with acute myeloid leukemia and posaconazole prophylaxis. Leuk Lymphoma. 2011;52(8):1607–10.
188. Mullane K, Toor AA, Kalnicky C, Rodriguez T, Klein J, Stiff P. Posaconazole salvage therapy allows successful allogeneic hematopoietic stem cell transplantation in patients with refractory invasive mold infections. Transpl Infect Dis. 2007;9(2):89–96.
189. Sun HY, Wagener MM, Singh N. Cryptococcosis in solid-organ, hematopoietic stem cell, and tissue transplant recipients: evidence-based evolving trends. Clin Infect Dis. 2009;48(11): 1566–76.
190. van Burik JH, Leisenring W, Myerson D, et al. The effect of prophylactic fluconazole on the clinical spectrum of fungal diseases in bone marrow transplant recipients with special attention to hepatic candidiasis. An autopsy study of 355 patients. Medicine (Baltimore). 1998; 77(4):246–54.
191. De Castro N, Neuville S, Sarfati C, et al. Occurrence of Pneumocystis jiroveci pneumonia after allogeneic stem cell transplantation: a 6-year retrospective study. Bone Marrow Transplant. 2005;36(10):879–83.
192. Souza JP, Boeckh M, Gooley TA, Flowers ME, Crawford SW. High rates of Pneumocystis carinii pneumonia in allogeneic blood and marrow transplant recipients receiving dapsone prophylaxis. Clin Infect Dis. 1999;29(6):1467–71.
193. Festic E, Gajic O, Limper AH, Aksamit TR. Acute respiratory failure due to pneumocystis pneumonia in patients without human immunodeficiency virus infection: outcome and associated features. Chest. 2005;128(2):573–9.
194. Boeckh M, Nichols WG, Papanicolaou G, Rubin R, Wingard JR, Zaia J. Cytomegalovirus in hematopoietic stem cell transplant recipients: current status, known challenges, and future strategies. Biol Blood Marrow Transplant. 2003;9(9):543–58.
195. Yoo KH, Lee SH, Sung KW, et al. Current status of pediatric umbilical cord blood transplantation in Korea: a multicenter retrospective analysis of 236 cases. Am J Hematol. 2011;86(1): 12–7.
196. van Burik JA, Carter SL, Freifeld AG, et al. Higher risk of cytomegalovirus and aspergillus infections in recipients of T cell-depleted unrelated bone marrow: analysis of infectious complications in patients treated with T cell depletion versus immunosuppressive therapy to prevent graft-versus-host disease. Biol Blood Marrow Transplant. 2007;13(12): 1487–98.
197. Zaia JA, Gallez-Hawkins GM, Tegtmeier BR, et al. Late cytomegalovirus disease in marrow transplantation is predicted by virus load in plasma. J Infect Dis. 1997;176(3):782–5.
198. Krause H, Hebart H, Jahn G, Muller CA, Einsele H. Screening for CMV-specific T cell proliferation to identify patients at risk of developing late onset CMV disease. Bone Marrow Transplant. 1997;19(11):1111–6.

199. Taplitz RA, Jordan MC. Pneumonia caused by herpesviruses in recipients of hematopoietic cell transplants. Semin Respir Infect. 2002;17(2):121–9.
200. Landgren O, Gilbert ES, Rizzo JD, et al. Risk factors for lymphoproliferative disorders after allogeneic hematopoietic cell transplantation. Blood. 2009;113(20):4992–5001.
201. Kojaoghlanian T, Flomenberg P, Horwitz MS. The impact of adenovirus infection on the immunocompromised host. Rev Med Virol. 2003;13(3):155–71.
202. Symeonidis N, Jakubowski A, Pierre-Louis S, et al. Invasive adenoviral infections in T-cell-depleted allogeneic hematopoietic stem cell transplantation: high mortality in the era of cidofovir. Transpl Infect Dis. 2007;9(2):108–13.
203. Feuchtinger T, Lang P, Handgretinger R. Adenovirus infection after allogeneic stem cell transplantation. Leuk Lymphoma. 2007;48(2):244–55.
204. Milano F, Campbell AP, Guthrie KA, et al. Human rhinovirus and coronavirus detection among allogeneic hematopoietic stem cell transplantation recipients. Blood. 2010;115(10):2088–94.
205. Boeckh M. The challenge of respiratory virus infections in hematopoietic cell transplant recipients. Br J Haematol. 2008;143(4):455–67.
206. Erard V, Chien JW, Kim HW, et al. Airflow decline after myeloablative allogeneic hematopoietic cell transplantation: the role of community respiratory viruses. J Infect Dis. 2006;193(12): 1619–25.
207. Whimbey E, Englund JA, Couch RB. Community respiratory virus infections in immunocompromised patients with cancer. Am J Med. 1997;102(3A):10–8.
208. Gutman JA, Peck AJ, Kuypers J, Boeckh M. Rhinovirus as a cause of fatal lower respiratory tract infection in adult stem cell transplantation patients: a report of two cases. Bone Marrow Transplant. 2007;40(8):809–11.
209. Renaud C, Campbell AP. Changing epidemiology of respiratory viral infections in hematopoietic cell transplant recipients and solid organ transplant recipients. Curr Opin Infect Dis. 2011;24(4):333–43.
210. Greene RE, Schlamm HT, Oestmann JW, et al. Imaging findings in acute invasive pulmonary aspergillosis: clinical significance of the halo sign. Clin Infect Dis. 2007;44(3):373–9.
211. Georgiadou SP, Sipsas NV, Marom EM, Kontoyiannis DP. The diagnostic value of halo and reversed halo signs for invasive mold infections in compromised hosts. Clin Infect Dis. 2011;52(9):1144–55.
212. De Pauw B, Walsh TJ, Donnelly JP, et al. Revised definitions of invasive fungal disease from the European Organization for Research and Treatment of Cancer/Invasive Fungal Infections Cooperative Group and the National Institute of Allergy and Infectious Diseases Mycoses Study Group (EORTC/MSG) Consensus Group. Clin Infect Dis. 2008;46(12):1813–21.
213. Shiley KT, Van Deerlin VM, Miller Jr WT. Chest CT features of community-acquired respiratory viral infections in adult inpatients with lower respiratory tract infections. J Thorac Imaging. 2010;25(1):68–75.
214. Shimada A, Koga T, Shimada M, et al. Cytomegalovirus pneumonitis presenting small nodular opacities. Intern Med. 2004;43(12):1198–200.
215. Luong ML, Filion C, Labbe AC, et al. Clinical utility and prognostic value of bronchoalveolar lavage galactomannan in patients with hematologic malignancies. Diagn Microbiol Infect Dis. 2010;68(2):132–9.
216. Forslow U, Remberger M, Nordlander A, Mattsson J. The clinical importance of bronchoalveolar lavage in allogeneic SCT patients with pneumonia. Bone Marrow Transplant. 2010; 45(5):945–50.
217. Park SH, Choi SM, Lee DG, et al. Serum galactomannan strongly correlates with outcome of invasive aspergillosis in acute leukaemia patients. Mycoses. 2011;54:523–30.
218. Koo S, Bryar JM, Page JH, Baden LR, Marty FM. Diagnostic performance of the (1−>3)-beta-D-glucan assay for invasive fungal disease. Clin Infect Dis. 2009;49(11):1650–9.
219. Marty FM, Koo S, Bryar J, Baden LR. (1−>3)beta-D-glucan assay positivity in patients with Pneumocystis (carinii) jiroveci pneumonia. Ann Intern Med. 2007;147(1):70–2.
220. Kuypers J, Campbell AP, Cent A, Corey L, Boeckh M. Comparison of conventional and molecular detection of respiratory viruses in hematopoietic cell transplant recipients. Transpl Infect Dis. 2009;11(4):298–303.

221. Kuypers J, Wright N, Ferrenberg J, et al. Comparison of real-time PCR assays with fluorescent-antibody assays for diagnosis of respiratory virus infections in children. J Clin Microbiol. 2006;44(7):2382–8.
222. Choi SM, Boudreault AA, Xie H, Englund JA, Corey L, Boeckh M. Differences in clinical outcomes after 2009 influenza A/H1N1 and seasonal influenza among hematopoietic cell transplant recipients. Blood. 2011;117(19):5050–6.
223. Thomas Jr CF, Limper AH. Pneumocystis pneumonia: clinical presentation and diagnosis in patients with and without acquired immune deficiency syndrome. Semin Respir Infect. 1998;13(4):289–95.
224. Thomas Jr CF, Limper AH. Pneumocystis pneumonia. N Engl J Med. 2004;350(24): 2487–98.
225. Ljungman P, Griffiths P, Paya C. Definitions of cytomegalovirus infection and disease in transplant recipients. Clin Infect Dis. 2002;34(8):1094–7.
226. Mandell LA, Wunderink RG, Anzueto A, et al. Infectious Diseases Society of America/American Thoracic Society consensus guidelines on the management of community-acquired pneumonia in adults. Clin Infect Dis. 2007;44 Suppl 2:S27–72.
227. American Thoracic Society; Infectious Diseases Society of America. Guidelines for the management of adults with hospital-acquired, ventilator-associated, and healthcare-associated pneumonia. Am J Respir Crit Care Med. 2005;171(4):388–416.
228. Bordigoni P, Carret AS, Venard V, Witz F, Le Faou A. Treatment of adenovirus infections in patients undergoing allogeneic hematopoietic stem cell transplantation. Clin Infect Dis. 2001;32(9):1290–7.
229. Echavarria M. Adenoviruses in immunocompromised hosts. Clin Microbiol Rev. 2008; 21(4):704–15.
230. Casper C, Englund J, Boeckh M. How I treat influenza in patients with hematologic malignancies. Blood. 2010;115(7):1331–42.
231. Boeckh M, Englund J, Li Y, et al. Randomized controlled multicenter trial of aerosolized ribavirin for respiratory syncytial virus upper respiratory tract infection in hematopoietic cell transplant recipients. Clin Infect Dis. 2007;44(2):245–9.
232. Shima T, Yoshimoto G, Nonami A, et al. Successful treatment of parainfluenza virus 3 pneumonia with oral ribavirin and methylprednisolone in a bone marrow transplant recipient. Int J Hematol. 2008;88(3):336–40.
233. Bonney D, Razali H, Turner A, Will A. Successful treatment of human metapneumovirus pneumonia using combination therapy with intravenous ribavirin and immune globulin. Br J Haematol. 2009;145(5):667–9.
234. Bodey GP, Mardani M, Hanna HA, et al. The epidemiology of Candida glabrata and Candida albicans fungemia in immunocompromised patients with cancer. Am J Med. 2002;112(5): 380–5.
235. Martino P, Micozzi A, Venditti M, et al. Catheter-related right-sided endocarditis in bone marrow transplant recipients. Rev Infect Dis. 1990;12(2):250–7.
236. Kuruvilla J, Forrest DL, Lavoie JC, et al. Characteristics and outcome of patients developing endocarditis following hematopoietic stem cell transplantation. Bone Marrow Transplant. 2004;34(11):969–73.
237. Otaki M, Omiya H, Matsumoto T, et al. Candida endocarditis in association with myelodysplastic syndromes: review of the literature and report of a case. J Med. 1999;30(3–4): 176–84.
238. Kalokhe AS, Rouphael N, El Chami MF, Workowski KA, Ganesh G, Jacob JT. Aspergillus endocarditis: a review of the literature. Int J Infect Dis. 2010;14(12):e1040–7.
239. Chim CS, Ho PL, Yuen ST, Yuen KY. Fungal endocarditis in bone marrow transplantation: case report and review of literature. J Infect. 1998;37(3):287–91.
240. Kupari M, Volin L, Suokas A, Timonen T, Hekali P, Ruutu T. Cardiac involvement in bone marrow transplantation: electrocardiographic changes, arrhythmias, heart failure and autopsy findings. Bone Marrow Transplant. 1990;5(2):91–8.

241. Uckay I, Chalandon Y, Sartoretti P, et al. Invasive zygomycosis in transplant recipients. Clin Transplant. 2007;21(4):577–82.
242. Hori A, Kami M, Kishi Y, Machida U, Matsumura T, Kashima T. Clinical significance of extra-pulmonary involvement of invasive aspergillosis: a retrospective autopsy-based study of 107 patients. J Hosp Infect. 2002;50(3):175–82.
243. Schaumann R, Ponisch W, Helbig JH, et al. Pericarditis after allogeneic peripheral blood stem cell transplantation caused by *Legionella pneumophila* (non-serogroup 1). Infection. 2001;29(1):51–3.
244. Kraus WE, Valenstein PN, Corey GR. Purulent pericarditis caused by *Candida*: report of three cases and identification of high-risk populations as an aid to early diagnosis. Rev Infect Dis. 1988;10(1):34–41.
245. Broliden K. Parvovirus B19 infection in pediatric solid-organ and bone marrow transplantation. Pediatr Transplant. 2001;5(5):320–30.
246. Adachi N, Kiwaki K, Tsuchiya H, Migita M, Yoshimoto T, Matsuda I. Fatal cytomegalovirus myocarditis in a seronegative ALL patient. Acta Paediatr Jpn. 1995;37(2):211–6.
247. Midulla M, Marzetti G, Borra G, Sabatino G. Myocarditis associated with Echo type 7 infection in a leukemic child. Acta Paediatr Scand. 1976;65(5):649–51.
248. Galama JM, de Leeuw N, Wittebol S, Peters H, Melchers WJ. Prolonged enteroviral infection in a patient who developed pericarditis and heart failure after bone marrow transplantation. Clin Infect Dis. 1996;22(6):1004–8.
249. Silberstein L, Davies A, Kelsey S, et al. Myositis, polyserositis with a large pericardial effusion and constrictive pericarditis as manifestations of chronic graft-versus-host disease after non-myeloablative peripheral stem cell transplantation and subsequent donor lymphocyte infusion. Bone Marrow Transplant. 2001;27(2):231–3.
250. Yamamoto R, Kanda Y, Matsuyama T, et al. Myopericarditis caused by cyclophosphamide used to mobilize peripheral blood stem cells in a myeloma patient with renal failure. Bone Marrow Transplant. 2000;26(6):685–8.
251. Baddour LM, Wilson WR, Bayer AS, et al. Infective endocarditis: diagnosis, antimicrobial therapy, and management of complications: a statement for healthcare professionals from the Committee on Rheumatic Fever, Endocarditis, and Kawasaki Disease, Council on Cardiovascular Disease in the Young, and the Councils on Clinical Cardiology, Stroke, and Cardiovascular Surgery and Anesthesia, American Heart Association: endorsed by the Infectious Diseases Society of America. Circulation. 2005;111(23):e394–434.
252. Salanitri GC, Huo E, Miller FH, Gupta A, Pereles FS. MRI of mycotic sinus of valsalva pseudoaneurysm secondary to Aspergillus pericarditis. AJR Am J Roentgenol. 2005;184(3 Suppl):S25–7.
253. Leung S, Metzger BS, Currie BP. Incidence of Clostridium difficile infection in patients with acute leukemia and lymphoma after allogeneic hematopoietic stem cell transplantation. Infect Control Hosp Epidemiol. 2010;31(3):313–5.
254. DeLeve LD, Shulman HM, McDonald GB. Toxic injury to hepatic sinusoids: sinusoidal obstruction syndrome (veno-occlusive disease). Semin Liver Dis. 2002;22(1):27–42.
255. Dadwal SS, Tegtmeier B, Nakamura R, et al. Nontyphoidal Salmonella infection among recipients of hematopoietic SCT. Bone Marrow Transplant. 2011;46(6):880–3.
256. Chopra T, Chandrasekar P, Salimnia H, Heilbrun LK, Smith D, Alangaden GJ. Recent epidemiology of Clostridium difficile infection during hematopoietic stem cell transplantation. Clin Transplant. 2011;25(1):E82–7.
257. Gorschluter M, Glasmacher A, Hahn C, et al. Clostridium difficile infection in patients with neutropenia. Clin Infect Dis. 2001;33(6):786–91.
258. Cunningham SC, Fakhry K, Bass BL, Napolitano LM. Neutropenic enterocolitis in adults: case series and review of the literature. Dig Dis Sci. 2005;50(2):215–20.
259. Pouwels MJ, Donnelly JP, Raemaekers JM, Verweij PE, de Pauw BE. Clostridium septicum sepsis and neutropenic enterocolitis in a patient treated with intensive chemotherapy for acute myeloid leukemia. Ann Hematol. 1997;74(3):143–7.

260. Calderone RA, Fonzi WA. Virulence factors of *Candida albicans*. Trends Microbiol. 2001;9(7):327–35.
261. Chen YC, Chang SC, Luh KT, Hsieh WC. Stable susceptibility of Candida blood isolates to fluconazole despite increasing use during the past 10 years. J Antimicrob Chemother. 2003;52(1):71–7.
262. Kontoyiannis DP, Luna MA, Samuels BI, Bodey GP. Hepatosplenic candidiasis. A manifestation of chronic disseminated candidiasis. Infect Dis Clin North Am. 2000;14(3):721–39.
263. Kazan E, Maertens J, Herbrecht R, et al. A retrospective series of gut aspergillosis in haematology patients. Clin Microbiol Infect. 2011;17(4):588–94.
264. Mantadakis E, Samonis G. Clinical presentation of zygomycosis. Clin Microbiol Infect. 2009;15 Suppl 5:15–20.
265. Padmanabhan S, Battiwalla M, Hahn T, et al. Two cases of hepatic zygomycosis in allogeneic stem cell transplant recipients and review of literature. Transpl Infect Dis. 2007;9(2):148–52.
266. Boeckh M, Leisenring W, Riddell SR, et al. Late cytomegalovirus disease and mortality in recipients of allogeneic hematopoietic stem cell transplants: importance of viral load and T-cell immunity. Blood. 2003;101(2):407–14.
267. Beschorner WE, Pino J, Boitnott JK, Tutschka PJ, Santos GW. Pathology of the liver with bone marrow transplantation. Effects of busulfan, carmustine, acute graft-versus-host disease, and cytomegalovirus infection. Am J Pathol. 1980;99(2):369–86.
268. Spencer GD, Hackman RC, McDonald GB, et al. A prospective study of unexplained nausea and vomiting after marrow transplantation. Transplantation. 1986;42(6):602–7.
269. Johnson JR, Egaas S, Gleaves CA, Hackman R, Bowden RA. Hepatitis due to herpes simplex virus in marrow-transplant recipients. Clin Infect Dis. 1992;14(1):38–45.
270. Szabo F, Horvath N, Seimon S, Hughes T. Inappropriate antidiuretic hormone secretion, abdominal pain and disseminated varicella-zoster virus infection: an unusual triad in a patient 6 months post mini-allogeneic peripheral stem cell transplant for chronic myeloid leukemia. Bone Marrow Transplant. 2000;26(2):231–3.
271. Rau R, Fitzhugh CD, Baird K, et al. Triad of severe abdominal pain, inappropriate antidiuretic hormone secretion, and disseminated varicella-zoster virus infection preceding cutaneous manifestations after hematopoietic stem cell transplantation: utility of PCR for early recognition and therapy. Pediatr Infect Dis J. 2008;27(3):265–8.
272. Yagi T, Karasuno T, Hasegawa T, et al. Acute abdomen without cutaneous signs of varicella zoster virus infection as a late complication of allogeneic bone marrow transplantation: importance of empiric therapy with acyclovir. Bone Marrow Transplant. 2000;25(9):1003–5.
273. Weinstock DM, Ambrossi GG, Brennan C, Kiehn TE, Jakubowski A. Preemptive diagnosis and treatment of Epstein-Barr virus-associated post transplant lymphoproliferative disorder after hematopoietic stem cell transplant: an approach in development. Bone Marrow Transplant. 2006;37(6):539–46.
274. Sundin M, Le Blanc K, Ringden O, et al. The role of HLA mismatch, splenectomy and recipient Epstein-Barr virus seronegativity as risk factors in post-transplant lymphoproliferative disorder following allogeneic hematopoietic stem cell transplantation. Haematologica. 2006;91(8):1059–67.
275. Jeon TY, Kim JH, Eo H, et al. Posttransplantation lymphoproliferative disorder in children: manifestations in hematopoietic cell recipients in comparison with liver recipients. Radiology. 2010;257(2):490–7.
276. Ison MG. Adenovirus infections in transplant recipients. Clin Infect Dis. 2006;43(3):331–9.
277. Chakrabarti S, Milligan DW, Moss PA, Mautner V. Adenovirus infections in stem cell transplant recipients: recent developments in understanding of pathogenesis, diagnosis and management. Leuk Lymphoma. 2004;45(5):873–85.
278. Suparno C, Milligan DW, Moss PA, Mautner V. Adenovirus infections in stem cell transplant recipients: recent developments in understanding of pathogenesis, diagnosis and management. Leuk Lymphoma. 2004;45(5):873–85.
279. Flomenberg P, Babbitt J, Drobyski WR, et al. Increasing incidence of adenovirus disease in bone marrow transplant recipients. J Infect Dis. 1994;169(4):775–81.

280. Wang WH, Wang HL. Fulminant adenovirus hepatitis following bone marrow transplantation. A case report and brief review of the literature. Arch Pathol Lab Med. 2003; 127(5):e246–8.
281. Chakrabarti S, Collingham KE, Fegan CD, Milligan DW. Fulminant adenovirus hepatitis following unrelated bone marrow transplantation: failure of intravenous ribavirin therapy. Bone Marrow Transplant. 1999;23(11):1209–11.
282. Roddie C, Paul JP, Benjamin R, et al. Allogeneic hematopoietic stem cell transplantation and norovirus gastroenteritis: a previously unrecognized cause of morbidity. Clin Infect Dis. 2009;49(7):1061–8.
283. Schwartz S, Vergoulidou M, Schreier E, et al. Norovirus gastroenteritis causes severe and lethal complications after chemotherapy and hematopoietic stem cell transplantation. Blood. 2011;117(22):5850–6.
284. Saif MA, Bonney DK, Bigger B, et al. Chronic norovirus infection in pediatric hematopoietic stem cell transplant recipients: a cause of prolonged intestinal failure requiring intensive nutritional support. Pediatr Transplant. 2011;15(5):505–9.
285. Division of Viral Diseases; National Center for Immunization and Respiratory Diseases; Centers for Disease Control and Prevention. Updated norovirus outbreak management and disease prevention guidelines. MMWR Recomm Rep. 2011;60(RR-3):1–18.
286. Kamboj M, Mihu CN, Sepkowitz K, Kernan NA, Papanicolaou GA. Work-up for infectious diarrhea after allogeneic hematopoietic stem cell transplantation: single specimen testing results in cost savings without compromising diagnostic yield. Transpl Infect Dis. 2007;9(4):265–9.
287. Sugata K, Taniguchi K, Yui A, Nakai H, Asano Y, Hashimoto S, et al. Analysis of rotavirus antigenemia in hematopoietic stem cell transplant recipients. Transpl Infect Dis. 2011. doi:10.1111/j.1399-3062.2011.00668.x.
288. Marinone C, Mestriner M. HBV disease: HBsAg carrier and occult B infection reactivation in haematological setting. Dig Liver Dis. 2011;43 Suppl 1:S49–56.
289. Idilman R, Arat M, Soydan E, et al. Lamivudine prophylaxis for prevention of chemotherapy-induced hepatitis B virus reactivation in hepatitis B virus carriers with malignancies. J Viral Hepat. 2004;11(2):141–7.
290. Moses SE, Lim ZY, Sudhanva M, et al. Lamivudine prophylaxis and treatment of hepatitis B Virus-exposed recipients receiving reduced intensity conditioning hematopoietic stem cell transplants with alemtuzumab. J Med Virol. 2006;78(12):1560–3.
291 Hsiao LT, Chiou TJ, Liu JH, et al. Extended lamivudine therapy against hepatitis B virus infection in hematopoietic stem cell transplant recipients. Biol Blood Marrow Transplant. 2006;12(1):84–94.
292. Peffault Latour R, Levy V, Asselah T, et al. Long-term outcome of hepatitis C infection after bone marrow transplantation. Blood. 2004;10(5):1618–24.
293. Strasser SI, Myerson D, Spurgeon CL, et al. Hepatitis C virus infection and bone marrow transplantation: a cohort study with 10-year follow-up. Hepatology. 1999;29(6):1893–9.
294. Thaler M, Pastakia B, Shawker TH, O'Leary T, Pizzo PA. Hepatic candidiasis in cancer patients: the evolving picture of the syndrome. Ann Intern Med. 1988;108(1):88–100.
295. Asano-Mori Y, Kanda Y, Oshima K, et al. False-positive Aspergillus galactomannan antigenaemia after haematopoietic stem cell transplantation. J Antimicrob Chemother. 2008;61(2): 411–6.
296. Orlopp K, von Lilienfeld-Toal M, Marklein G, et al. False positivity of the Aspergillus galactomannan Platelia ELISA because of piperacillin/tazobactam treatment: does it represent a clinical problem? J Antimicrob Chemother. 2008;62(5):1109–12.
297. Chung CS, Wang WL, Liu KL, Lin JT, Wang HP. Green ulcer in the stomach: unusual mucormycosis infection. Gastrointest Endosc. 2008;68(3):566–7. discussion 567.
298. Hackman RC, Wolford JL, Gleaves CA, et al. Recognition and rapid diagnosis of upper gastrointestinal cytomegalovirus infection in marrow transplant recipients. A comparison of seven virologic methods. Transplantation. 1994;57(2):231–7.
299. Al-Nassir WN, Sethi AK, Nerandzic MM, Bobulsky GS, Jump RL, Donskey CJ. Comparison of clinical and microbiological response to treatment of Clostridium difficile-associated disease with metronidazole and vancomycin. Clin Infect Dis. 2008;47(1):56–62.

300. Everly MJ, Bloom RD, Tsai DE, Trofe J. Posttransplant lymphoproliferative disorder. Ann Pharmacother. 2007;41(11):1850–8.
301. Meijer E, Cornelissen JJ. Epstein-Barr virus-associated lymphoproliferative disease after allogeneic haematopoietic stem cell transplantation: molecular monitoring and early treatment of high-risk patients. Curr Opin Hematol. 2008;15(6):576–85.
302. Rossignol JF, El-Gohary YM. Nitazoxanide in the treatment of viral gastroenteritis: a randomized double-blind placebo-controlled clinical trial. Aliment Pharmacol Ther. 2006; 24(10):1423–30.
303. Lok AS, McMahon BJ. Chronic hepatitis B: update 2009. Hepatology. 2009;50(3):661–2.
304. Kersting S, Koomans HA, Hene RJ, Verdonck LF. Acute renal failure after allogeneic myeloablative stem cell transplantation: retrospective analysis of incidence, risk factors and survival. Bone Marrow Transplant. 2007;39(6):359–65.
305. Parikh CR, Schrier RW, Storer B, et al. Comparison of ARF after myeloablative and nonmyeloablative hematopoietic cell transplantation. Am J Kidney Dis. 2005;45(3):502–9.
306. Matar MJ, Tarrand J, Raad I, Rolston KV. Colonization and infection with vancomycin-resistant Enterococcus among patients with cancer. Am J Infect Control. 2006;34(8):534–6.
307. Ashour HM, El-Sharif A. Species distribution and antimicrobial susceptibility of gram-negative aerobic bacteria in hospitalized cancer patients. J Transl Med. 2009;7:14.
308. Nicolle LE, Bradley S, Colgan R, Rice JC, Schaeffer A, Hooton TM. Infectious Diseases Society of America guidelines for the diagnosis and treatment of asymptomatic bacteriuria in adults. Clin Infect Dis. 2005;40(5):643–54.
309. Li WY, Wu VC, Lin WC, Chen YM. Renal Candida tropicalis abscesses in a patient with acute lymphoblastic leukemia. Kidney Int. 2007;72(3):382.
310. Oravcova E, Lacka J, Drgona L, et al. Funguria in cancer patients: analysis of risk factors, clinical presentation and outcome in 50 patients. Infection. 1996;24(4):319–23.
311. Gonzalez-Vicent M, Lassaletta A, Lopez-Pino MA, Romero-Tejada JC, de la Fuente-Trabado M, Diaz MA. Aspergillus "fungus ball" of the bladder after hematopoietic transplantation in a pediatric patient: successful treatment with intravesical voriconazole and surgery. Pediatr Transplant. 2008;12(2):242–5.
312. Park H, Lee MJ, Kim Y, Min YH, Kim SJ, Kim D. Primary renal aspergillosis and renal stones in both kidneys associated with hematopoietic stem cell transplant. Korean J Hematol. 2010;45(4):275–8.
313. Marchand R, Ahronheim GA, Patriquin H, Benoit P, Laberge I, de Repentigny L. Aspergilloma of the renal pelvis in a leukemic child. Pediatr Infect Dis. 1985;4(1):103–5.
314. Leithauser M, Kahl C, Aepinus C, et al. Invasive zygomycosis in patients with graft-versus-host disease after allogeneic stem cell transplantation. Transpl Infect Dis. 2010;12(3): 251–7.
315. Carrillo-Esper R, Elizondo-Argueta S, Vicuna-Gonzalez RM, Gonzalez-Trueba EF. Isolated renal mucormycosis. Gac Med Mex. 2006;142(6):511–4.
316. Erard V, Storer B, Corey L, et al. BK virus infection in hematopoietic stem cell transplant recipients: frequency, risk factors, and association with postengraftment hemorrhagic cystitis. Clin Infect Dis. 2004;39(12):1861–5.
317. Khan H, Oberoi S, Mahvash A, et al. Reversible ureteral obstruction due to Polyomavirus infection after percutaneous nephrostomy catheter placement. Biol Blood Marrow Transplant. 2011;17:1551–5.
318. Hirsch HH. BK virus: opportunity makes a pathogen. Clin Infect Dis. 2005;41(3):354–60.
319. Lekakis LJ, Macrinici V, Baraboutis IG, Mitchell B, Howard DS. BK virus nephropathy after allogeneic stem cell transplantation: a case report and literature review. Am J Hematol. 2009;84(4):243–6.
320. Mori Y, Miyamoto T, Kato K, et al. Different risk factors related to Adenovirus- or BK virus-associated hemorrhagic cystitis following allogeneic stem cell transplantation. Biol Blood Marrow Transplant. 2011. doi:10.1016/j.bbmt.2011.07.025.
321. Bil-Lula I, Ussowicz M, Rybka B, et al. Hematuria due to adenoviral infection in bone marrow transplant recipients. Transplant Proc. 2010;42(9):3729–34.

322. Bruno B, Zager RA, Boeckh MJ, et al. Adenovirus nephritis in hematopoietic stem-cell transplantation. Transplantation. 2004;77(7):1049–57.
323. Erard V, Kim HW, Corey L, et al. BK DNA viral load in plasma: evidence for an association with hemorrhagic cystitis in allogeneic hematopoietic cell transplant recipients. Blood. 2005;106(3):1130–2.
324. Tuon FF, Amato VS, Penteado Filho SR. Bladder irrigation with amphotericin B and fungal urinary tract infection – systematic review with meta-analysis. Int J Infect Dis. 2009; 13(6):701–6.
325. Savona MR, Newton D, Frame D, Levine JE, Mineishi S, Kaul DR. Low-dose cidofovir treatment of BK virus-associated hemorrhagic cystitis in recipients of hematopoietic stem cell transplant. Bone Marrow Transplant. 2007;39(12):783–7.
326. Ramos E, Drachenberg CB, Wali R, Hirsch HH. The decade of polyomavirus BK-associated nephropathy: state of affairs. Transplantation. 2009;87(5):621–30.
327. Liacini A, Seamone ME, Muruve DA, Tibbles LA. Anti-BK virus mechanisms of sirolimus and leflunomide alone and in combination: toward a new therapy for BK virus infection. Transplantation. 2010;90(12):1450–7.
328. Neofytos D, Ojha A, Mookerjee B, et al. Treatment of adenovirus disease in stem cell transplant recipients with cidofovir. Biol Blood Marrow Transplant. 2007;13(1):74–81.
329. Cronin DM, George TI, Sundram UN. An updated approach to the diagnosis of myeloid leukemia cutis. Am J Clin Pathol. 2009;132(1):101–10.
330. Dabade TS, Davis MD. Diagnosis and treatment of the neutrophilic dermatoses (pyoderma gangrenosum, Sweet's syndrome). Dermatol Ther. 2011;24(2):273–84.
331. Jones SG, Olver WJ, Boswell TC, Russell NH. Ecthyma gangrenosum. Eur J Haematol. 2002;69(5–6):324.
332. Olson JM, Nguyen VQ, Yoo J, Kuechle MK. Cutaneous manifestations of Corynebacterium jeikeium sepsis. Int J Dermatol. 2009;48(8):886–8.
333. Hodohara K, Fujiyama Y, Hiramitu Y, et al. Disseminated subcutaneous Nocardia asteroides abscesses in a patient after bone marrow transplantation. Bone Marrow Transplant. 1993;11(4):341–3.
334. Doucette K, Fishman JA. Nontuberculous mycobacterial infection in hematopoietic stem cell and solid organ transplant recipients. Clin Infect Dis. 2004;38(10):1428–39.
335. Duncan BW, Adzick NS, de Lorimier AA, et al. Necrotizing fasciitis in two children with acute lymphoblastic leukemia. J Pediatr Surg. 1992;27(5):668–71.
336. Kusne S, Eibling DE, Yu VL, et al. Gangrenous cellulitis associated with gram-negative bacilli in pancytopenic patients: dilemma with respect to effective therapy. Am J Med. 1988;85(4):490–4.
337. Mantadakis E, Pontikoglou C, Papadaki HA, Aggelidakis G, Samonis G. Fatal Fournier's gangrene in a young adult with acute lymphoblastic leukemia. Pediatr Blood Cancer. 2007;49(6):862–4.
338. Grossman ME, Silvers DN, Walther RR. Cutaneous manifestations of disseminated candidiasis. J Am Acad Dermatol. 1980;2(2):111–6.
339. Kim JH, Shin DH, Oh MD, Park S, Kim BK, Choe KW. A case of disseminated Cryptococcosis with skin eruption in a patient with acute leukemia. Scand J Infect Dis. 2001;33(3):234–5.
340. Salati SA, Rabah SM. Cutaneous mucormycosis in a leukemic patient. J Coll Physicians Surg Pak. 2011;21(2):109–10.
341. Bushelman SJ, Callen JP, Roth DN, Cohen LM. Disseminated Fusarium solani infection. J Am Acad Dermatol. 1995;32(2 Pt 2):346–51.
342. Boutati EI, Anaissie EJ. Fusarium, a significant emerging pathogen in patients with hematologic malignancy: ten years' experience at a cancer center and implications for management. Blood. 1997;90(3):999–1008.
343. Steer CB, Szer J, Sasadeusz J, Matthews JP, Beresford JA, Grigg A. Varicella-zoster infection after allogeneic bone marrow transplantation: incidence, risk factors and prevention with low-dose aciclovir and ganciclovir. Bone Marrow Transplant. 2000;25(6):657–64.

344. Betts BC, Young JA, Ustun C, Cao Q, Weisdorf DJ. Human herpesvirus 6 infection after hematopoietic cell transplntation: is routine surveillance necessary? Biol Blood Marrow Transplant. 2011;17:1562–8.
345. Klastersky J. Management of fever in neutropenic patients with different risks of complications. Clin Infect Dis. 2004;39 Suppl 1:S32–7.
346. Prabhu RM, Piper KE, Litzow MR, Steckelberg JM, Patel R. Emergence of quinolone resistance among viridans group streptococci isolated from the oropharynx of neutropenic peripheral blood stem cell transplant patients receiving quinolone antimicrobial prophylaxis. Eur J Clin Microbiol Infect Dis. 2005;24(12):832–8.
347. Freifeld A, Marchigiani D, Walsh T, et al. A double-blind comparison of empirical oral and intravenous antibiotic therapy for low-risk febrile patients with neutropenia during cancer chemotherapy. N Engl J Med. 1999;341(5):305–11.
348. Bliziotis IA, Michalopoulos A, Kasiakou SK, et al. Ciprofloxacin vs an aminoglycoside in combination with a beta-lactam for the treatment of febrile neutropenia: a meta-analysis of randomized controlled trials. Mayo Clin Proc. 2005;80(9):1146–56.
349. Cruciani M, Malena M, Bosco O, Nardi S, Serpelloni G, Mengoli C. Reappraisal with meta-analysis of the addition of Gram-positive prophylaxis to fluoroquinolone in neutropenic patients. J Clin Oncol. 2003;21(22):4127–37.
350. Pollack M, Heugel J, Xie H, et al. An international comparison of current strategies to prevent herpesvirus and fungal infections in hematopoietic cell transplant recipients. Biol Blood Marrow Transplant. 2011;17(5):664–73.
351. Winston DJ, Chandrasekar PH, Lazarus HM, et al. Fluconazole prophylaxis of fungal infections in patients with acute leukemia. Results of a randomized placebo-controlled, double-blind, multicenter trial. Ann Intern Med. 1993;118(7):495–503.
352. Rotstein C, Bow EJ, Laverdiere M, Ioannou S, Carr D, Moghaddam N. Randomized placebo-controlled trial of fluconazole prophylaxis for neutropenic cancer patients: benefit based on purpose and intensity of cytotoxic therapy. The Canadian Fluconazole Prophylaxis Study Group. Clin Infect Dis. 1999;28(2):331–40.
353. Marr KA, Seidel K, White TC, Bowden RA. Candidemia in allogeneic blood and marrow transplant recipients: evolution of risk factors after the adoption of prophylactic fluconazole. J Infect Dis. 2000;181(1):309–16.
354. Hirata Y, Yokote T, Kobayashi K, et al. Antifungal prophylaxis with micafungin in neutropenic patients with hematological malignancies. Leuk Lymphoma. 2010;51(5):853–9.
355. van Burik JA, Ratanatharathorn V, Stepan DE, et al. Micafungin versus fluconazole for prophylaxis against invasive fungal infections during neutropenia in patients undergoing hematopoietic stem cell transplantation. Clin Infect Dis. 2004;39(10):1407–16.
356. Ullmann AJ, Lipton JH, Vesole DH, et al. Posaconazole or fluconazole for prophylaxis in severe graft-versus-host disease. N Engl J Med. 2007;356(4):335–47.
357. Cornely OA, Maertens J, Winston DJ, et al. Posaconazole vs. fluconazole or itraconazole prophylaxis in patients with neutropenia. N Engl J Med. 2007;356(4):348–59.
358. Winston DJ, Bartoni K, Territo MC, Schiller GJ. Efficacy, safety, and breakthrough infections associated with standard long-term posaconazole antifungal prophylaxis in allogeneic stem cell transplantation recipients. Biol Blood Marrow Transplant. 2011;17(4):507–15.
359. Green H, Paul M, Vidal L, Leibovici L. Prophylaxis of Pneumocystis pneumonia in immunocompromised non-HIV-infected patients: systematic review and meta-analysis of randomized controlled trials. Mayo Clin Proc. 2007;82(9):1052–9.
360. Vasconcelles MJ, Bernardo MV, King C, Weller EA, Antin JH. Aerosolized pentamidine as pneumocystis prophylaxis after bone marrow transplantation is inferior to other regimens and is associated with decreased survival and an increased risk of other infections. Biol Blood Marrow Transplant. 2000;6(1):35–43.
361. Atkinson K, Downs K, Golenia M, et al. Prophylactic use of ganciclovir in allogeneic bone marrow transplantation: absence of clinical cytomegalovirus infection. Br J Haematol. 1991;79(1):57–62.

362. Winston DJ, Ho WG, Bartoni K, et al. Ganciclovir prophylaxis of cytomegalovirus infection and disease in allogeneic bone marrow transplant recipients. Results of a placebo-controlled, double-blind trial. Ann Intern Med. 1993;118(3):179–84.
363. Salzberger B, Bowden RA, Hackman RC, Davis C, Boeckh M. Neutropenia in allogeneic marrow transplant recipients receiving ganciclovir for prevention of cytomegalovirus disease: risk factors and outcome. Blood. 1997;90(6):2502–8.
364. Burns LJ, Miller W, Kandaswamy C, et al. Randomized clinical trial of ganciclovir vs acyclovir for prevention of cytomegalovirus antigenemia after allogeneic transplantation. Bone Marrow Transplant. 2002;30(12):945–51.
365. Eid AJ, Arthurs SK, Deziel PJ, Wilhelm MP, Razonable RR. Emergence of drug-resistant cytomegalovirus in the era of valganciclovir prophylaxis: therapeutic implications and outcomes. Clin Transplant. 2008;22(2):162–70.
366. Ljungman P, de La Camara R, Milpied N, et al. Randomized study of valacyclovir as prophylaxis against cytomegalovirus reactivation in recipients of allogeneic bone marrow transplants. Blood. 2002;99(8):3050–6.
367. Wagner HJ, Wessel M, Jabs W, et al. Patients at risk for development of posttransplant lymphoproliferative disorder: plasma versus peripheral blood mononuclear cells as material for quantification of Epstein-Barr viral load by using real-time quantitative polymerase chain reaction. Transplantation. 2001;72(6):1012–9.
368. Coppoletta S, Tedone E, Galano B, et al. Rituximab treatment for Epstein-Barr virus DNAemia after alternative-donor hematopoietic stem cell transplantation. Biol Blood Marrow Transplant. 2011;17(6):901–7.
369. Blaes AH, Cao Q, Wagner JE, Young JA, Weisdorf DJ, Brunstein CG. Monitoring and preemptive rituximab therapy for Epstein-Barr virus reactivation after antithymocyte globulin containing nonmyeloablative conditioning for umbilical cord blood transplantation. Biol Blood Marrow Transplant. 2010;16(2):287–91.
370. Wagner HJ, Cheng YC, Huls MH, et al. Prompt versus preemptive intervention for EBV lymphoproliferative disease. Blood. 2004;103(10):3979–81.
371. Asano-Mori Y, Kanda Y, Oshima K, et al. Long-term ultra-low-dose acyclovir against varicella-zoster virus reactivation after allogeneic hematopoietic stem cell transplantation. Am J Hematol. 2008;83(6):472–6.
372. Uchiyama M, Tamai Y, Ikeda T. Low-dose acyclovir against reactivation of varicella zoster virus after unrelated cord blood transplantation. Int J Infect Dis. 2010;14(5):e451–2.
373. Anderson EJ, Guzman-Cottrill JA, Kletzel M, et al. High-risk adenovirus-infected pediatric allogeneic hematopoietic progenitor cell transplant recipients and preemptive cidofovir therapy. Pediatr Transplant. 2008;12(2):219–27.
374. Lindemans CA, Leen AM, Boelens JJ. How I treat adenovirus in hematopoietic stem cell transplant recipients. Blood. 2010;116(25):5476–85.
375. Thomas NJ, Hollenbeak CS, Ceneviva GD, Geskey JM, Young MJ. Palivizumab prophylaxis to prevent respiratory syncytial virus mortality after pediatric bone marrow transplantation: a decision analysis model. J Pediatr Hematol Oncol. 2007;29(4):227–32.
376. Manzoni P, Leonessa M, Farina D, Gomirato G. Respiratory syncytial virus infection and prophylaxis with palivizumab in immunosuppressed children: the experience of a large Italian neonatal care setting. Pediatr Transplant. 2007;11(4):456–7.

Index

E.H. Estey and F.R. Appelbaum (eds.), *Leukemia and Related Disorders:*
Integrated Treatment Approaches, Contemporary Hematology,
DOI 10.1007/978-1-60761-565-1, © Springer Science+Business Media, LLC 2012